MW00810389

# The Breast Thermography Revolution
## Boot Camp for an Estrogen Free® Life

# Wendy Sellens, DACM, LAc

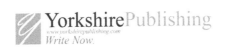

Yorkshire Publishing
www.yorkshirepublishing.com
*Write Now.*

# Contents

To my rebel friend, teacher, surgeon, and giant,
William Bell Hobbins M.D.
I was the answer to your prayers and in return you gave me
my life's purpose.


"If I have seen further it is by standing on the shoulders
of Giants."

Isaac Newton


Rest well, Wild Bill.
In your honor, your groundbreaking research will procced.
I am standing on the shoulders of a medical giant.

With love and respect, your rebel protégée, Wendy.

Dear Readers:

Accredited thermography consists of a thermobiological – or TH – score ranging from 1 to 5 for each breast. To simplify explanations and reduce confusion, the term "abnormal" will be used for any thermogram outside of normal limits. The term "at-risk" will be used for a thermogram that is within normal limits but is concerning due to specific vascular patterns that may be a potential risk factor for the individual's breasts.

Many thanks to the women who consented to have their breast thermograms presented as evidence in this book. Please keep in mind that there are some incredible thermogram examples for which we were not given consent and did not use, though I attempt to exemplify each concept or condition with the appropriate thermogram. We have several thousand examples on which we base our information, but unfortunately we do not have permission to share a majority of these images. Another aspect to keep in mind about thermography is that changes are very subtle most of the time. We have thousands of repeat thermograms, but with such minor changes an untrained eye would not notice. It took years to accumulate the thermograms we are presenting in *The Breast Thermography Revolution*. We hope you learn and incorporate the survival tips provided in this book. Enjoy!

# Introduction

## The Unsung Hero: William Hobbins, MD

D r. Hobbins and I regard each other as "war buddies." The resistance that we have faced from the medical community and even the thermographic community has been tremendous. Throughout our years together, Dr. Hobbins has shared his regrets with me and told me of sacrifices made by him with regard to family, friends, and medical practice. He sees me following in his footsteps, but I have entered this battle with open eyes. I realized that if his lifelong studies were not shared with the world it would most likely be lost. We are comrades for truth and knowledge in this war against women. This book is our mission, our purpose, and our legacy in this long journey which Dr. Hobbins started decades ago.

I knew after Chinese medical school I would continue my study with a Master. Never in my wildest dreams did I think when I began my journey that my path would lead me to a Western medically trained neurosurgeon and thermologist as a mentor. I met my business partner Martin Bales during our first semester at graduate school. He is the son of Maurice Bales, the inventor of the first digital infrared camera in 1979 and first ever infrared camera FDA-approved for breast thermography. After five years I finally convinced Martin to start our breast thermography business, Pink Image. Martin has known Dr. Hobbins most of his life and he naturally was our interpreter. Immediately after we began I had questions which he answered with non-traditional responses. His experience and knowledge fascinated me. I was immediately drawn to him and asked him to teach me. He gruffly responded that he was retired. It took me a few months to convince him, but from then on we were teacher and student. The knowledge I received is immeasurable! This book is written from the notes I accumulated over five years of studying with Dr. Hobbins.

Dr. Hobbins has trained thousands of physicians, but I am proud to say I am his protégée, as he is Dr. Ray Lawson's. He encourages me to stand tall on his shoulders, as he does on Dr. Lawson's, and to carry on all of our work. It is our hope that you review our evidence and explanations with common sense, as logic will lead you to the truth. Set aside the tirelessly repeated myths you hear every day and listen to another side of the story…another chance to save women.

The letter below is in response to my desire for women to understand the immense experience, talents and research Dr. Hobbins has acquired throughout his lifetime. Thermography is only a part of his broad and fascinating career. To view his CV (Curriculum Vitae) please view Hobbins' page at our website: womensacademyofbreastthermography.com.

Dear Wendy,

I wish to congratulate you on your last five years of study with me in the use of thermography in breast diseases and the excellent summary of these diseases that you've written in this book. A job well done and one that will be worthwhile for some time.

You asked how, as a general thoracic surgeon, I became interested in thermography, which has been the major focus of my medical practice of 63 years.

I graduated from Northwestern Medical School in 1944 at age 21, started my internship at Cook County hospital, and a year later, commenced my surgical residency. I became interested in pathology and began my Masters in it. I finished my residency in 1951, and after a short practice, was drafted to run a thoracic center at Fort Carson in Colorado.

After returning to Madison, I continued my medical practice performing general and thoracic surgery. I enjoyed playing bridge and found an excellent partner, a 40-year-old woman. In May, she went for a physical exam and was told that her breasts were okay. In August, she was diagnosed with cancer, which was removed and radiated; but by December, she was dead. As a young surgeon, after losing such a close friend, I prayed that the Lord would allow me to spend half of my surgical career trying to help women with breast cancer.

As seventy-five women a day die in the United States of cancer of the breast and because it is the number one killer between the ages of 35 and 50 of women in the United States, a great deal of attention was placed upon the breast examination in my practice. In 1964, as a private practicing physician of general and thoracic surgery… it became apparent that I was not affording the patient who came for breast examination all that was available with our present knowledge. So I resolved that any female patient over the age of 30 who presented herself for any complaint or examination, would be mammogrammed." [Dr. Hobbins conducted 3,175 mammograms from 1965 to 1971.]

William Hobbins, MD, "Seven Year Mammography in Private Practice"

In 1962, Bob Egan, a radiologist who helped Dr. Gershon-Cohen develop thermography in the United States, took me on as a student, and I began studying thermography under him and others from around the world. I started to concentrate on mammography in my patients 50 and over, and had accumulated 1,000 mammograms by 1968. Of those 1,000, my radiologist, Dr. Arthur Steenen, and I found some 123 shadows that needed further study. That fall at the Wisconsin Surgical Society, I presented as an associate surgical at the University of Wisconsin, the first series to be presented of this work. We found 23 cancers out of the 120 shadows that were nonpalpable by the patient, the nurse, or my resident. I obtained a letter of accommodation from Dr. Robert Hickey, Chief of Surgery at the University of Wisconsin, for this original work.

Earlier detection of breast cancer is necessary to reduce the mortality rate of this disease… mammography will detect breast cancer… earlier than waiting for the female to find the lump. Earlier detection will hopefully change the present cure rate from 45 percent to 90 percent and nationally save 20,000 lives annually". In 1971, he believed every woman over 35 should receive an annual mammogram. At this time in our medical history, "The practical problems of reaching this goal are insurmountable. There are not enough personnel or equipment affordable in the country today to mammograph every female.

William Hobbins, MD, "Seven Year Mammography in Private Practice," 1971

In my study of mammography, I found much advance in Sweden, France and Italy and that they had initiated thermography in their practice. In 1955, Ray Lawson wrote the first use in this continent for thermography in the detection of breast cancer. I contacted Dr. Lawson and asked him if I might be his student and he invited me to come and stay with him in Montreal. As a retired Hudson Bay surgeon at McGill University, he was an amazing teacher and person and became a life-long friend.

As early as 1965, Dr. Gershon-Cohen and associates, including Dr. JoAnn Haberman… established their recommended use of mammography, as well as the great significance of an abnormal thermogram in monitoring of breast health. This work was highly accepted abroad, particularly in France, England, and Italy, and later, in Germany and the Netherlands. Thermography has been utilized effectively and extensively in these countries for the past 20 years."

William Hobbins, MD, "Breast Thermography—A Vital Screening Tool for the 1983 Woman"

In 1972, I formed and incorporated the Wisconsin Breast Cancer Foundation after acquiring my first thermographic equipment, a spectratherm, at its original cost of $50,000. Using a truck and trailer of 28 feet, with its own generator and triple air conditioning system, my wife's staff screened some 37,000 women in five states, sending reports to their physicians with a request of their follow up.

> In 1971, Dr. Hobbins surmised that they could "proceed with programs of mass screening large segments of the population... In the initial step, thermography is used to determine the high risk population and these results are turned over to the private physician for follow up x-ray." He believed that "this brings good screening immediately to all areas at the least expense and helps to expand mammography faculties and education." [Dr. Hobbins' Wisconsin Breast Cancer Foundation imaged over 100,000 women from 1971 to 1975.]
>
> William Hobbins, MD, 1973

In 1974, the board of directors of the Wisconsin Breast Cancer Foundation ignited thermal image analysis, which pioneered instructional training and use of thermography throughout the United States. This was further emphasized by my studies and teaching presentations around the world, and allowed me to meet some of the most outstanding and educated physicians, not only in thermography, but in breast cancer treatment and study. I stopped practicing thermography in 2005, but have remained active in the American Thermographic Society and many other organizations around the world, with writings of more than 40 papers in this regard.

I wish to encourage your continued emphasis on the importance of early detection of breast cancer, as well as the use of thermography to study the female breast. It is the only device to date that can physiologically classify the health and problems in the breast. May you in your future work continue to add to this to realize that the angiogenesis of a breast cancer is not only the earliest sign, but the greatest sign for detection and prognosis in treatment.

With respect, I send you this message so that you may pass on the work of Dr. Lawson that I have continued and make it knowledgeable for others to come.

Sincerely,
William B Hobbins, MD

> In 1956, Dr. Ray Lawson...recorded temperature differences in the circulating fluids of the breast. Breast cancer showed a hotter circulation in most cases. Lawson recorded, in the *Canadian Medical Journal* in 1956, that the skin of the surface of the breast containing a malignant tumor was hotter than that of the normal breast. Thus, as in other medical disciplines, it became apparent that an increased temperature of the breast had great significance. This established the present understanding that any thermal abnormality of the breast has to be studied to rule out the possibility of tumor growth or any other pathology.
>
> William Hobbins, MD, "Breast Thermography—A Vital Screening Tool For The 1983 Woman"
>
> In the United States, as early as 1969, Dr. Dowdy of UCLA reported in a public health grant on the significance of thermography. He established mammography in a free Pap clinic and included thermography. He concluded that had only abnormal thermogram patients been mammogrammed, the early cancer detection per 1,000 mammograms performed would have increased from 12.9 cancers to 129. Such discriminations set forth efforts to use thermography as a prescreening tool.
>
> William Hobbins, MD, "Breast Thermography—A Vital Screening Tool For The 1983 Woman

Dr. Hobbins was a man ahead of his time. He spearheaded the creation of the certified thermography model and was the only original doctor who made thermography a lifelong career. His conviction and determination is why you have heard of mammography and thermography. Dr. Hobbins overcame much adversity, and with perseverance and dedication, saved thousands of lives. He is a brilliant, loving, and generous doctor. He is my mentor.

This book is the result of nearly five years of studying breast thermography, breast health, and breast diseases with Dr. Hobbins. For those unfamiliar with the world of breast thermography, virtually every interpreter attends a weekend course, followed by reading a hundred reviewed reports, and then begin their practice in breast cancer screening. I spent almost two years having Dr. Hobbins approve [over] seven hundred reports, plus an additional two years studying breast cancer with regard to thermography. No other physician has completed this training with Dr. Hobbins. It was and remains my intention to seek the most thorough and highest level of education in order to provide women with the most qualified interpretation possible.

My breast-health education and this book are solely due to Dr. Hobbins' accomplishments and unparalleled knowledge. I hope the fortunate women who come across this book realize the long and difficult journey that Dr. Hobbins has made in efforts to bring the information and technology that saves women's lives to as many as possible. Hold on for an amazing and life-changing experience, as that is what breast thermography and Dr. Hobbins have created for me. Until now, he has truly been an unsung hero.

> I was invited to be the main speaker at the Asian Pacific Congress of Thermology in Seoul Korea. My address was 'Breast Infrared Imaging Paradigm for Eradication of Breast Cancer.'" This was a wonderful honor, as most of the 350 Korean thermographers were introduced and trained by me. Most, if not all, Korean hospitals practice thermography. It was great to see my students and

old friends again. It has been three years. What a terrific time, and I am here to say that they are ahead of the United States.

William Hobbins, MD, *Christian Medical Center Newsletter*, 2002

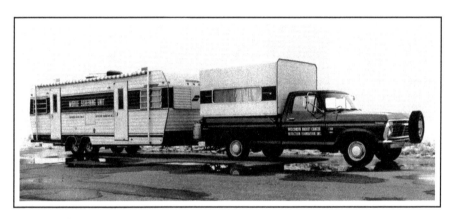

From 1971-1975 Dr. Hobbins screened around 100,000 women, many in his mobile breast thermography clinic which toured the mid-west. The vital information gathered from Dr. Hobbins' mass screenings was used in several breast thermography studies.

"If you know your enemy and know yourself, you need not fear the result of a hundred battles. If you know yourself but not the enemy, for every victory gained, you will also suffer a defeat. If you know neither your enemy nor yourself, you will succumb in every battle."

Sun Tzu, *The Art of War*

This book is dedicated to a small group of brave women
who listened to my evidence and found health in my advice.
Your accomplishments and encouragement kept me marching
strongly forward through the opposition and obstacles
in order to educate more courageous women.
I am also grateful to all the women who consented to having
their breast thermograms included in this book so that
their experiences and thermograms may be a powerful
learning tool to other women.

# 1. The Battle

W omen today are caught in a battle for our breasts and our lives. Every year, more women fall victim to breast cancer, and the United States leads the way with one of the highest occurrences of this horrific disease, as well as other cancers. It is time to take up arms and expose the deceptions surrounding breast health.

Unfortunately, we are inundated with propaganda that tells us we can "stay young" with bioidentical estrogen, flax, and soy-based products, when in fact, these recommendations are literally killing women. Excessive estrogen is the main culprit of breast cancer, yet estrogen therapies have become the mantra of breast health. When a statement is repeated enough times, people believe it to be fact, even without evidence to support it. If these types of estrogen are truly "healthy," why are breast cancer numbers rising, even amongst men? Do not let our fallen comrades become more statistics to fill headlines and further the "cause" for more walks.

This information may be overwhelming, but it is vital to understand the causes and conditions of breast cancer so that they can be treated and defeated. The first signs of overexposure to estrogen include the onset of menstruation before age fourteen, premenstrual syndrome (PMS), weight gain or inability to lose weight despite diet and exercise, abnormal hair loss, fibroids, menstrual disorders, infertility, irritability, insomnia, and hot flashes among many others.

This book will evoke powerful emotions. The images and facts stated within will show women the opposite of what they have been told by trusted professionals. It will anger many, while some may not want to believe the evidence. We have been touted the benefits of estrogen for so long that we actually believe it. Some of us even question and flinch when a specialized physician, like Dr. Hobbins and myself, tells us that estrogen isn't helpful but harmful.

It is socially challenging to argue that excess estrogen is harmful, but we all know that discovering the truth can be scary. In order to defeat an enemy, we must know who or what they are. To shun the truth only promotes failure to take control of our health and future.

Let's return to the basics when estrogen wasn't prescribed and we were actually healthy. This book is meant to serve as a reminder of how in the past, we didn't turn to a pill to solve our issues, but instead employed common sense.

Breast cancer causes fear. This fear is the chain that keeps us locked in the cold manipulation of propaganda's promise of a cure. Prepare—be strong for the battle. Join the revolution. Arm yourself with knowledge—with knowledge comes power, and with power, victory is attainable. This book will change your breast health and your life.

Don't focus on a cure to an illness; focus on strengthening your health to prevent it! The only sure cure is prevention.

# Welcome to the
# Breast Thermography Revolution

# Breast thermography 101

Breast thermography is a superficial breast screening that monitors the blood vessels in your breasts. It is an incredible screening device because it has the possibility of detecting a concern, sometimes years before other imaging modalities. This is due to the blood vessels; cancers and other breast disorders, from benign masses to hormone imbalances, tend to form specific patterns in the blood vessels.

Think of thermography as a thermometer providing a warning signal. It is vital that your thermologist/interpreter discuss your blood vessel patterns during your thermography consult. If a pattern can be identified early, it can possibly be treated. Monitoring begins around the age of 25 to detect changes early.

*"Thermography is the highest marker for the possibility of the immediate presence of breast cancer. Most fevers of the breast are not associated with cancer, but most cancers have a fever of some degree. The more the fever (delta T) and type of pattern of its display relate to the host survival. Simple and inexpensive thermography should be performed on women over 30 years of age."*

*— Willaim Hobbins, M.D., 1982*

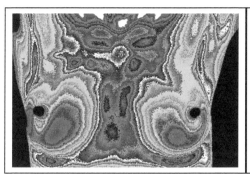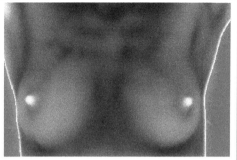

Healthy, normal thermogram.

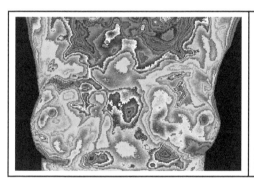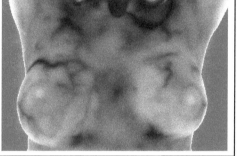

Unhealthy,"at risk" thermogram. Undetectable with mammogram or ultrasound.

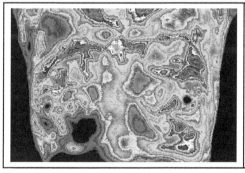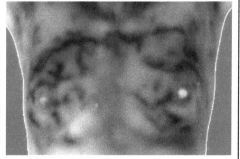

Unhealthy, abnormal thermogram. Undetectable with mammogram or ultrasound.

# How to understand a breast thermogram

Left vs right:

Thermograms are mirror images; left breast is on the right side of the image and right breast is on the left side of the image.

Bilateral (both breasts) vs. unilateral (one breast):

Healthy thermogram patterns should be bilateral symmetrical versus unhealthy thermograms which have unilateral and asymmetrical patterns.

Vascular Patterns, Neoangiogenesis and Nipplar Delta T:

Thermograms analyze vascular patterns in black hot or reverse grey images. Non-vascular, healthy breasts are hormonally balanced. At risk breasts have increased vascularity or neoangiogenesis due to disease or excess estrogen. The strongest indicator of disease is a temperature difference between the nipples, nipplar delta T. Eighty-three percent of all breast cancers have hot nipple.

## Example of Healthy Normal Thermogram

Symmetrical Bilateral Smooth Color Gradient        Symmetrical (Black Hot/ Reverse Grey)

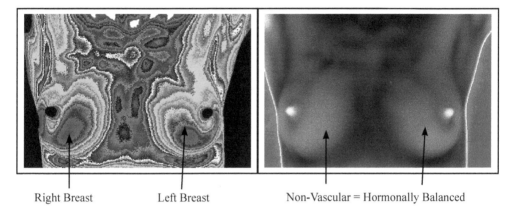

Right Breast        Left Breast        Non-Vascular = Hormonally Balanced

## Example of Unhealthy Abnormal Thermogram

Asymmetrical Unilateral Color Gradient        Asymmetrical Unilateral (Black Hot/Reverse Grey)

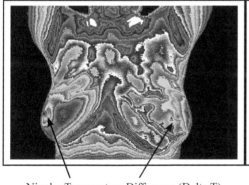
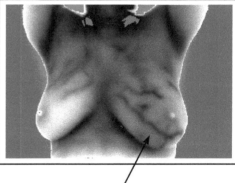

Nipplar Temperature Difference (Delta T)
Note cold color tones in right nipple (blue) and
warm color tones in left nipple (green).

Neoangiogenesis in left breast.

# Thermography interpretation is done in reverse gray or black hot

Thermography monitors blood vessels, which are only visible in the reverse gray or gray images. Color is *only* used as a secondary interpretation. Avoid clinics only using color images because the blood vessels are the "key" to understanding your breast health.

Normal thermograms are non-vascular to mild vascular, meaning you can't see the blood vessels.

At risk (vascular uniform) thermograms, the blood vessels are visible, but within normal limits.

Abnormal thermograms, the blood vessels are visible, but outside of normal limits.

Unilateral vascular patterns, or one-sided, usually means a disease.

Bilateral vascular patterns, both sides, usually means an endocrine imbalance or excess estrogen.

The strongest indicator of disease is a temperature difference between the nipples, nipplar delta T.

What are your blood vessels trying to tell you about your breast health?

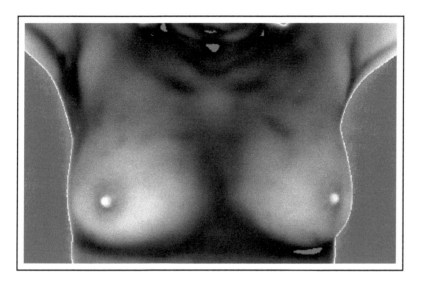

Healthy breasts - normal or non-vascular to mild vascular. Normal thermogram.

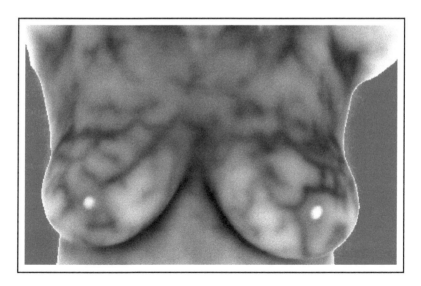

Unhealthy breasts - unusual hypervascular pattern. "At risk."

# Breast thermography is NOT diagnostic and does NOT replace a mammogram

Breast thermography was FDA-approved as an adjunct to mammography in 1982. Thermography can only measure the skin temperature; it is not diagnostic and does not replace a mammogram. Thermography is not "better" than mammography, it is different; comparing thermography to mammography is like comparing cars to airplanes.

Sensitivity – ability to detect. Thermography is 90 percent sensitive at monitoring abnormal vascular structures. Accuracy – the issue detected was what you wanted to find. Accuracy with mammography changes with age due to denseness of the breasts. Mammograms have high false negatives – missing issues, especially at younger ages due to dense breasts. Thermograms have high false positives – finding too many issues, due to high sensitivity; however, this is what makes it beneficial.

In 2009, the age for a mammogram was changed from 40-50 by the U.S. Preventive Services Task Force, and in 2016, from 40 to 45 by the American Cancer Society. In addition, mammograms are only recommended every two years. Estrogen causes the breasts to be dense. This is why mammography is only **48** percent accurate for *women age 40–50, since most women are still menstruating. From the age of 22–50, when the breasts are dense,* thermography could be another option for screening, along with ultrasound annually. At menopause the breasts are no longer stimulated from estrogen and will mature or soften, and this is when a mammogram is more accurate. From age 50–60 a mammogram is **68** percent accurate, and for those aged 60+ it is **88** percent accurate.

Normal healthy breasts should be non-vascular to a mild vascular pattern, especially after menopause when the breasts are mature. There should be *no* stimulation causing vascularity since the body has stopped producing estrogen. Stimulation after the breasts have matured increases breast health risk.

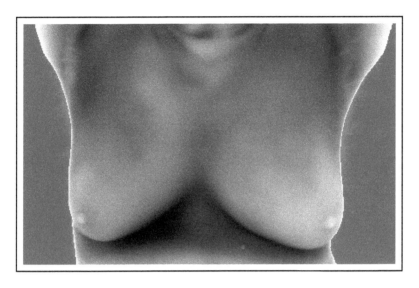

Normal, non-vascular healthy breasts.

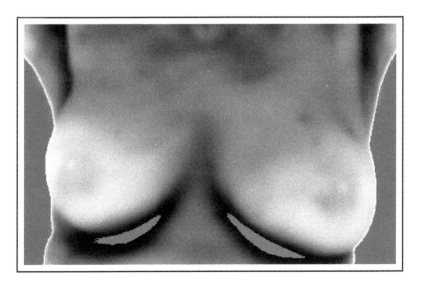

Normal, mild vascular healthy breasts.

# What are your blood vessels trying to tell you about your breast health?

Thermography monitors for vascularity - stimulation of the existing blood vessels, which is considered atypical or abnormal and increases risk. Constant stimulation may lead to neoangiogenesis. Breast thermography also monitors for neoangiogenesis - new blood vessel growth, which may cause a cancer to become invasive.

Avoid thermography clinics using incorrect terms. Vascularity is not inflammation, congestion, stagnation, or toxic build-up.

Mastitis is the only true inflammation of the breast and is very rare in breast thermography; due to the pain with this infection, most women are already being treated. Breast thermography can't monitor past the skin into the tissue. It can only view the blood vessels, not what is inside of the blood vessels including circulation, congestion, stagnation or the tissue, which are all too deep. Toxic build-up is a fad word and not a correct term in breast health.

In this woman's view the progression from vascularity to neoangiogenesis over three years' time. Thermogram reported risk three years before positive mammogram and ultrasound. Continuous stimulation of the breasts increases risk.

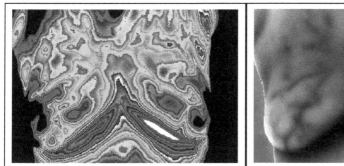
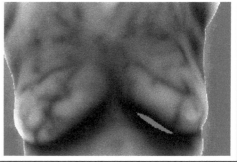

First thermogram is reported as a potential risk due to unusual vascular pattern.

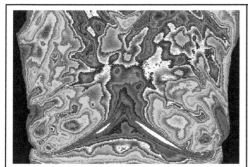
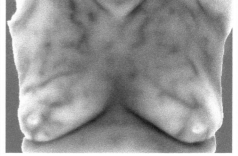

Repeat, 2nd, thermogram is evidence of increased vascularity.

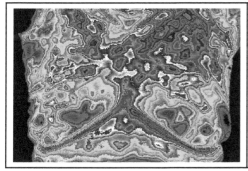
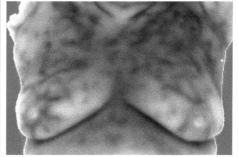

Repeat, 3rd, thermogram is evidence of neoangiogenesis in the upper left breast.

# Breast thermography monitors the blood vessels

Breast cancer tumors cause neoangiogenesis (new blood vessels) which is necessary for neoplasia (abnormal growth of tissue) to move from *in situ* (inside duct) to an invasive cancer. Neoangiogenesis forms specific vascular patterns seen in the black hot or reverse gray images.

Thermography cannot detect if a tumor is malignant or benign. All diseases, including benign or malignant tumors and breast infections (mastitis), may look the same in a thermogram because some benign masses and/or infections may have vascular stimulation. This is why thermography is *only a screening*; it cannot tell the difference, it can only monitor the vascular structures or blood vessels.

What thermography *can* do is alert you to a problem, so you can get further testing done, if necessary and/or start treatment protocols to remove excess estrogen stimulation.

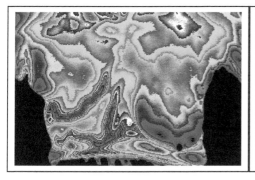

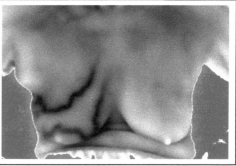

Breast cancer – note unilateral warm colors.       Breast cancer – note neoangiogenesis.

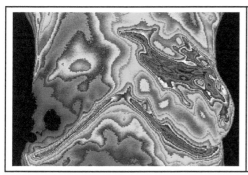

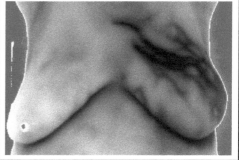

Breast cancer – note unilateral warm colors.       Breast cancer – note neoangiogenesis.

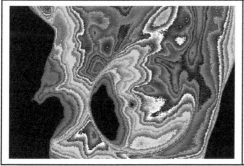

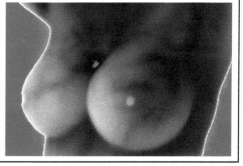

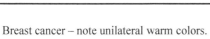

Breast cancer – note unilateral warm colors.       Breast cancer – note neoangiogenesis.

# Breast thermography is safe

Breast thermography is safe, non-contact, non-radiation breast health risk screening. It is safe for pregnant women, nursing mothers, women with implants and dense breasts.

Breast thermography is ideal for dense breasts and implants. Breast thermography is a completely non-contact procedure, which makes it ideal for women with implants, no risk of rupture. Fibroids, scars and implants are "cold" and cannot been "seen" or interfere with a thermogram.

Thermography is safe, non-radiation, ideal for pregnant women. Unlike many other imaging modalities, the infrared camera used in thermography does not emit any radiation, require any injections, and is non-contact and pain-free, and is biologically safe. Since no radiation is involved with this screening procedure, pregnant women or nursing mothers may use this imaging without any harm to fetus or infant.

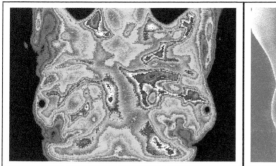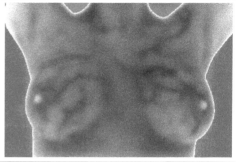

Thermogram of pregnant woman. Normal vascular pattern.
Blood vessels are dilated preparing for lactation.

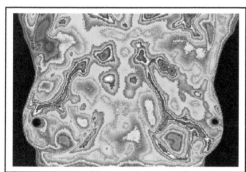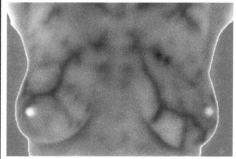

Thermogram of nursing mother. Normal vascular pattern.
Nursing causes dilation of blood vessels.

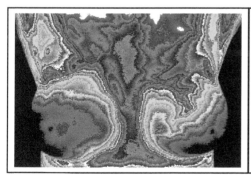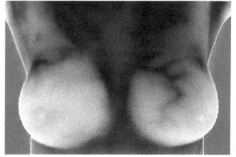

Thermogram of woman with implants.

# Baseline exam and recall

Breast thermography can view the entire breast including the lymph, without contact or compression. Breast thermography reports should include a minimum of four images – front, under, right oblique and left oblique.

A mandatory three-month follow-up is *not* required! Some thermography clinics claim, "a baseline cannot be established with one study because we have no way of knowing if this is your normal pattern...a three-month interval is used because this is the time it takes blood vessels to show change." Incorrect; changes in the blood vessels can been seen quickly, as soon as a month.

They are using the term "baseline" incorrectly; your first thermogram is your baseline. It is used as a reference point to see an increase, decrease or no change in the blood vessel patterns. These clinics have to "double check" in three months because the camera they use is cheap, with an optical line of 120 or 240. Breast thermography requires an optical line of 480 or higher for greater detail. In addition, the majority of interpreters, including M.D.'s, aren't following the minimum standard requirements, are also using this mandatory recall to reduce error.

3 months - for abnormal reports or women monitoring their breast cancer treatments.

6 months - for equivocal reports or women monitoring their hormone treatments.

9 – 12 months - for women who are within normal limits.

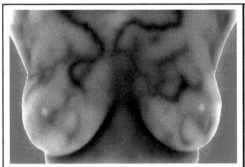

Front view

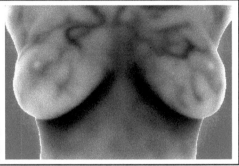

Under view

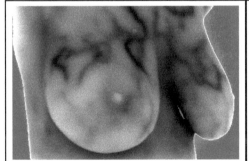

Right side view

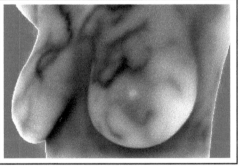

Left side view

# Breast thermography can begin early and monitor women with concerns

The breasts don't finish developing until the age of 22, which makes that a wonderful time to begin breast health screening to establish a baseline, especially since cancers that begin at a younger age are more aggressive. However, breast thermography can begin with the onset of puberty. If you (or your daughter) have a concern, a mass or pain, and you're under the age of 22, then thermography could be a safe tool for monitoring the breasts.

We recommend getting a thermogram in your early 20s, and then if deemed "normal," following up every three years. From the ages of 30 to 40, thermograms should be done every two years, and then annually after the age of 40, in conjunction with an ultrasound, which is another biologically safe test. The risk of breast cancer increases to 1 in 219 women after the age of 40. These two imaging modalities complement each other well and together reduce oversight or risk, especially with women who have a family history. If a qualified breast thermography clinic is not available in your area, it is strongly recommended to choose ultrasound and to pass on the amateur thermogram.

Thermography is the highest risk marker for the possibility of the presence of breast cancer, 10 times more so than family history. This woman has a family history of breast cancer. She monitors her breast health annually with thermograms and MRI.

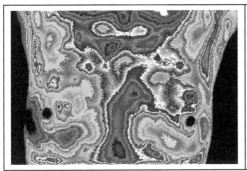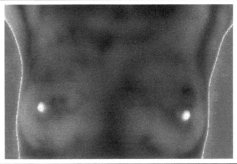

Initial, first thermogram.

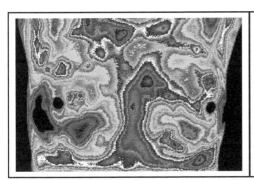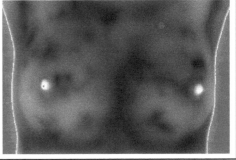

Repeat, 2nd thermogram – Stable.

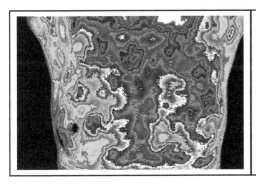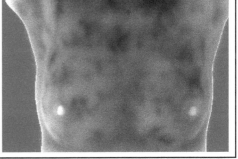

Repeat 3rd, thermogram. Abnormal Thermogram. Negative MRI
(*left*) Note unusual unilateral warm tones in left breast.
(*right*) Evidence of increased vascularity, especially in left breast, seen in black hot.

# Thermography score of each breast is required

Each breast should be graded with a thermographic score (TH). From TH-1 (normal) to TH-5 (severely abnormal). A report of "Normal" and "Abnormal" is not an appropriate score for the breasts.

Thermographic score, TH, of each breast and is determined by asymmetries in the breasts from temperature differences (delta T)

TH-1 Non-Vascular - Normal
TH-2 Vascular Uniform (Potential risk for post-menopausal women)
TH-3 Equivocal
TH-4 Abnormal
TH-5 Severely Abnormal

Many thermography academies and uncertified thermography clinics claim TH score isn't relevant since thermography isn't diagnostic. Then why would you be there? How would you assess the breasts? Good or bad? That is unacceptable. You can't say abnormal or normal because without a baseline, how do you know what "normal" is? What were the factors involved to determine the health of a breast? It would involve assigning a type of score. Medical imaging requires an accepted scoring system to determine health. Mammograms use the accepted BRAID system which is 1-6. A TH score does not make thermography diagnostic, it's a tool to analyze the breast and determine if that breast is abnormal or normal.

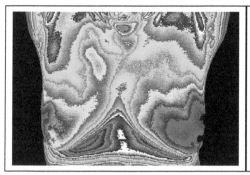

TH Scores
Right Breast: TH-1
Left Breast: TH-1

TH Scores
Right Breast: TH-1
Left Breast: TH-1

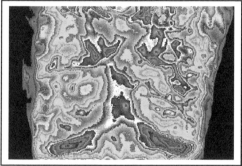

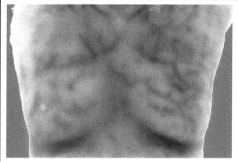

TH Scores
Right Breast: TH-2
Left Breast: TH-3

TH Scores
Right Breast: TH-2
Left Breast: TH-3

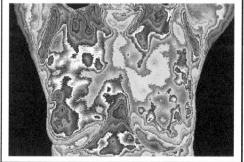

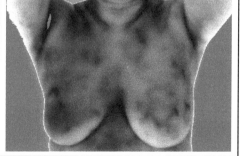

TH Scores
Right Breast: TH-5 – Breast cancer
Left Breast: TH-2

TH Scores
Right Breast: TH-5 – Breast cancer
Left Breast: TH-2

# Major and Minor signs in breast thermography

Cancers tend to form specific patterns that were categorized and classified by several studies and catalogued as Major and Minor Signs. These signs can determine the TH score or risk of each breast, which is why it is vital to be screened in a certified clinic. Black hot or reverse gray is mandatory in thermography in order to view patterns generated by blood vessels in the breasts.

Asymmetries are determined by Major and Minor Signs (blood vessels patterns) or a hyperthermia, which is measured by the Delta T. Delta T is the temperature difference recorded between the breasts. Any hyperthermia noted in breasts must have accompanying Major or Minor sign if applicable. Uncertified clinics do not interpret major and minor signs.

Eighty-three percent of all cancers will have a hot nipple. Nipplar delta T must be reported.

Delta T measurements must be recorded and included in report.

$1.0°$ C or higher at nipple
$1.0°$ C or higher with finding
$1.5°$ C or higher at periareolar
$1.5°$ C or higher global heat
$2.0°$ C or higher in isolated area (Major or Minor sign)
$2.5°$ C or higher with finding in unilateral breast – mastectomy
$3.0°$ C or higher in unilateral breast – mastectomy

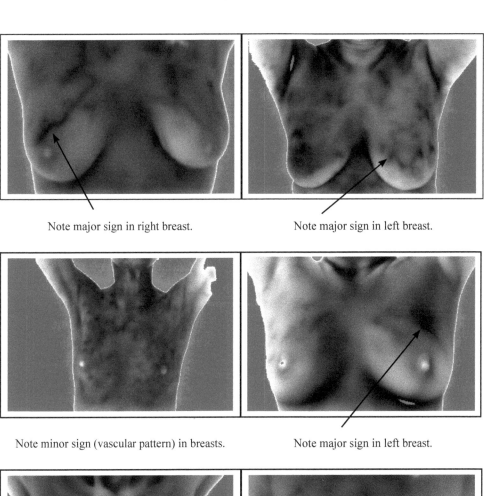

Note major sign in right breast.                    Note major sign in left breast.

Note minor sign (vascular pattern) in breasts.        Note major sign in left breast.

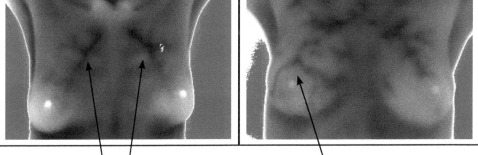

Note minor signs in the breasts.                    Note major sign in right breast.

# Breast thermography's cold stress test

A cold stress challenge or also called a sympathetic stress test is required to constrict the "normal" blood vessels. The camera will capture the blood vessels that are being stimulated, creating thermal activity or heat.

The room temperature must be kept at or below 68-72 degrees Fahrenheit and patient cooled for around 10 minutes. Another option is to apply an ice pack for 2-5 minutes, to the forehead or upper back. A cold stress challenge is not required for a first-time thermogram, but it is always required for a repeat thermographic score of TH-3, TH-4, and TH-5. However, we recommend both modalities just mentioned at every screening to ensure a quality thermogram.

The patient must be undressed from the waist up with no gown; any covering would leave a thermal imprint and corrupt the thermogram.

The hands must be above the head at all times, which lifts the breasts off the abdomen. Heat from the abdomen can reflect onto the breasts and corrupt the thermogram. This is the reason hands placed in cold water isn't effective. Women with large breasts should arch their back to lift breasts off abdomen.

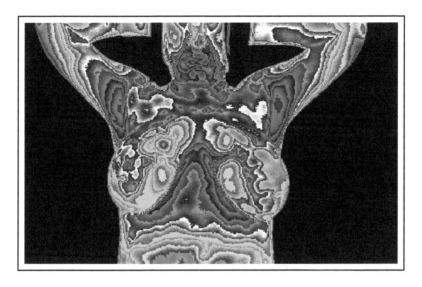

Before cold stress challenge. Note unusual warm color pattern.

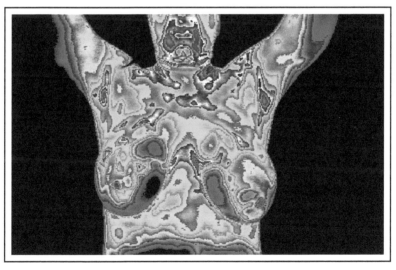

After cold stress challenge. Note breasts have cooled properly showing
a smoother color gradient.

# An infrared camera with an optical line resolution of 480 is required for the breasts

When imaging the breasts, a high-resolution infrared camera is required. The minimum optical line resolution should be no less than 480. This resolution captures small details which are crucial to proper interpretation. Cancer tends to form specific vascular patterns which are seen in black hot (reverse grey) images that are required for interpretation in order to view vascular patterns which are a potential risk. Look for cameras FDA-approved for breast thermography. Most cameras are only FDA-approved for skin temperature variation.

One of the reasons possible breast cancers are being missed in breast thermography reports is cheap cameras. Most thermography clinics are using cameras with an optical line of 120. The higher the optical line resolution, the more detailed the breast image, therefore the greater possibility of earlier detection.

When researching local breast thermography clinics, ask for the infrared camera's make and model to search and confirm the optical line. If they don't give you an answer, don't give them your business. Research make and model. If it reads like this: 480 x 240, then it is only 240 optical line. Or 240 x 120, then it is only 120 optical line. The second number is the optical line. If still unsure call camera company for explanation.

Maurice Bales, is a pioneer in camera technology. All thermography clinics are trained to tell you that their camera is the highest resolution. My business partner's father, Maurice, invented the first digital infrared camera in 1979 and it was the first camera FDA approved for breast thermography in 1982. When you see that fact, that was my partner's father. After getting FDA approval in 1982 with the 600 optical line, his camera dominated the marketplace for 30 years. Most infrared camera companies still consult with him since he is the expert in infrared technology.

Which camera would you choose when screening your breasts?

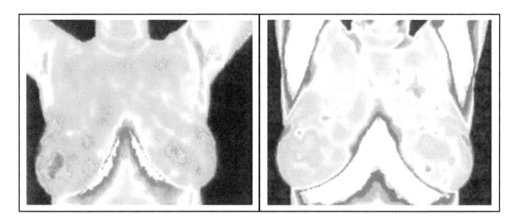

Note lack of detail in inferior camera's color images with optical line of 120. With inferior detail, small changes, which could be potential risks, can be missed. Most clinics do not provide black hot images which display vascular patterns that indicate potential breast health risk.

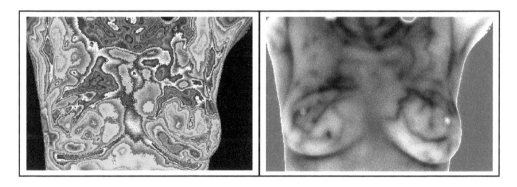

(*left*) Note rich detailed color gradients in color image.
Small changes are easily observed with a 600 optical line camera.
(*right*) Note *specific* vascular patterns, which may be potential risk.

# Avoid full-body thermography

Thermography is a superficial screening procedure that measures skin temperature *only*. Be aware of false claims about thermography. Many clinics recommend full-body scans with breast thermography. This is *not* required. Thermography can only measure the heat emitted from the skin, it cannot analyze heat deep in the body or see into the tissue, lymph, muscles, organs or bones. The blood vessels directly above the organs are not associated with that organ, they are a part of the circulatory system, which is different. The breasts are unique because they are glands, mammary glands, and the blood vessels in the skin are associated with these special glands.

Thermography is a superficial screening – it cannot diagnose lymph, digestive, coronary, uterus, gallbladder disorders, and adrenal or chronic fatigue. It cannot diagnose any organ disorders either– kidney, heart, lung, liver, spleen.

Full-body thermography is a gimmick. Thermography clinics doing full-body thermography are trying to sell you supplements. These false claims are surprisingly made and promoted by M.D.'s, teaching breast thermography and full body-thermography.

Thermography is excellent at pain diagnosis as muscles have referral patterns on the skin, called dermatomes, that thermography can monitor.

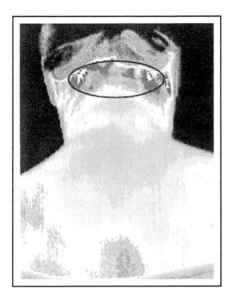

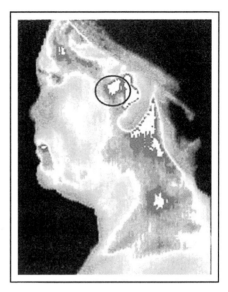

Above—*Cannot* diagnose fibromyalgia, chronic fatigue, and autoimmune disorders.

Above—*Cannot* diagnose pre-stroke conditions.

Right—*Cannot* directly detect heart disease, lung disease, liver disease, gallbladder disease, (kidney disease from back image) uterine or ovarian disease, adrenal exhaustion, all digestive disorders including irritable bowel syndrome, diverticulitis, and Crohns disease.

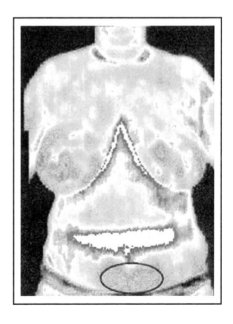

# Avoid computer programs or a point scoring system for breast thermography

Interpretation done by a computer program usually includes a point scoring system. Point scoring programs were popular in the 1970s. A large study found interpretation by a computer program had a 28 percent error rate as compared to interpretation by doctors. A radiologist interprets your mammogram, why would you accept less with thermography?

Many interpreters and some camera software use an *untested* scoring system which has a high error rate. Be sure your interpreter is certified in vascular pattern interpretation as this is what breast thermography studies are based upon. MRI, ultrasound, and mammogram are done by a trained doctor, not software.

A point system score or full rating system. A score is tallied from the thermographic findings. The TH score will have an actual score associated with it from 1-200.

For example -  Right Breast = 50 is TH 2 or normal.
Left Breast = 150 is TH 4 or abnormal.

See conflicting reports, point scoring versus breast thermography interpretation, in same patient.

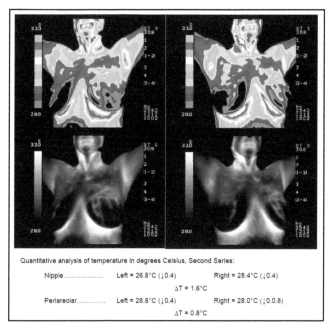

Quantitative analysis of temperature in degrees Celsius, Second Series:

| | | |
|---|---|---|
| Nipple.................. | Left = 26.8°C (↓0.4) | Right = 28.4°C (↓0.4) |
| | ΔT = 1.6°C | |
| Periareolar............. | Left = 28.8°C (↓0.4) | Right = 28.0°C (↓0.0.8) |
| | ΔT = 0.8°C | |

The CTA Scoring System = "Breasts are considered *within normal limits*" (for above images of same woman)

Left Breast TH-2; Score = 70        Right Breast TH-2; Score = 50

1.6 degree C left nipplar delta T (which is outside of normal limits, but score does not recognize this).

Certified Breast Thermography TH Scoring System = Abnormal Thermogram (for below images of same woman)
Left breast is TH-4 (Abnormal), Right Breast TH-2
A 1.6 degree C left nipplar delta T with unilateral vascular pattern with a major sign is an *Abnormal Thermogram*

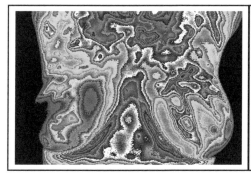

Note unilateral warm tones in left breast and hot nipple (light blue).

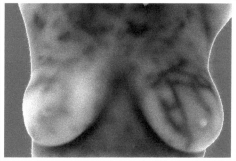

Note unilateral vascular pattern.

33

## Breast thermography may confirm intuition

Many women will perform a self-breast exam or may "feel" something unusual and want to screen with breast thermography even after their mammogram is negative. Most of these concerns are not significant. Many women choose thermography as it may be the *only* screening that detects a concern they are "feeling." Listen to your body and trust your instincts.

All breast imaging complements each other when needed. This is the order breast cancer screening should proceed. Why are these in this particular order? Breast thermography signals, ultrasound confirms, mammography locates, MRI with contrast confirms neoangiogenesis and biopsy establishes diagnosis.

Thermography
Ultrasound
Mammogram
MRI with gadolinium contrast
Biopsy

Mammography uses X-rays to differentiate normal tissue from physical tumors and other breast abnormalities based on their densities. Mammography can see inside or deeper in the breasts. However, it cannot usually detect small changes and is not early detection. In many cases it detects tumors that are already of significant size (>1cm in most cases) or the size of pencil eraser, which usually took about 6 years to grow to that size. Thermography may confirm women who have a "feeling" due to fact that it monitors small changes in the blood vessels, vascularity.

What do you think by looking at these thermograms? Were these women's instincts correct this time?

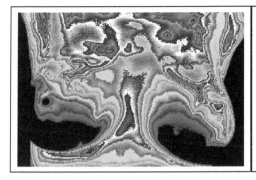

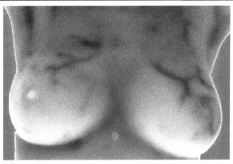

Note unusual color pattern in left breast and warm left nipple (green) versus cool right nipple (blue). Abnormal Thermogram.

Note unusual vascular pattern in black hot. Abnormal Thermogram.

Above two and right images—This woman performed a self breast exam. She reported that her left nipple is hot, itchy, painful, with a lump. Her concerns were confirmed with breast thermography. Notice left breast unilateral vascular pattern, possible neoangiogenesis in black hot. Abnormal Thermogram.

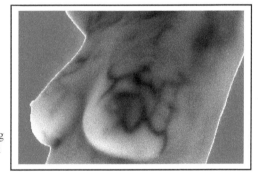

Below—This woman "felt" something was wrong with her breasts. Breast thermography confirmed her intuition. Note unilateral vascular pattern in left breast. Abnormal thermogram.

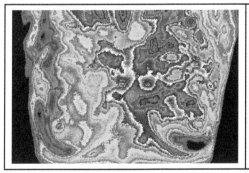

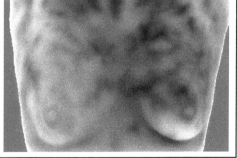

# Thermography for men

Environmental and commercial grade estrogens, found in most food products, household products, skincare products, commercial products, and pollutants are increasing the risk for breast cancer.

The evidence of this increase can be seen in the rise in *male* breast cancer. In 2010 2,000 cases of male breast cancer were reported with 400 deaths. The American Cancer Society predicted 2,470 cases of bresat cancer in men and 460 men were expected to die from breast cancer in 2017.

In the U.S., between the years 1975-2006, the incidence rate for breast cancer in *men* increased 0.9 percent per year! The American Cancer Society reported, "In the U.S., between 1975-2006, the incidence of rate for men increased 0.9 percent per year. The reason for this increase is unknown (not attributed to detection)."

Why are low testosterone rates increasing? Excess estrogen.

Low testosterone? "See" for yourself. With the rising numbers of men experiencing Low T, Man-opause, and infertility issues, more men are turning to breast thermography to monitor their hormones as well.

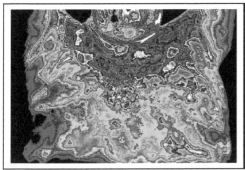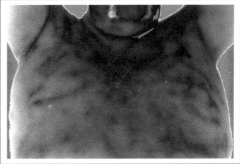

Male patient diagnosed with breast cancer in left breast *twice*, 1994 and 2009.

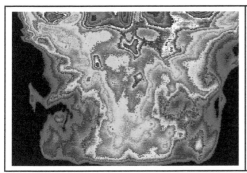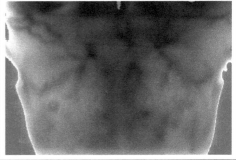

Average thirty-two-year-old male. Excess estrogen or low testosterone.
Note "at risk" unusual vascular pattern in black hot.

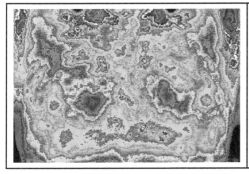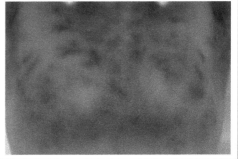

Average thirty-three-year-old male. Excess estrogen or low testosterone.
Note "at risk" unusual vascular pattern in black hot.

# Breast thermography monitors breast health – hormone imbalances

Adding breast thermography to your health regime allows you to "see" your hormone imbalance (not FDA-approved). Hormonally balanced women will have no vascularity because the blood vessels are not being stimulated. Bilateral hypervascular thermograms are usually evidence of a hormone imbalance due to excess estrogen stimulation. Unilateral patterns are abnormal and usually evidence of a disease or benign disorder.

Forty years of breast thermography research is demonstrating that most women are progesterone deficient or have excess estrogen. Eighty percent of breast cancers are stimulated by estrogen, which causes the cancer to grow. We have been told for decades that women are estrogen deficient. If this was true, then breast cancer would be significantly lower and not increasing.

If there is an endocrine imbalance – and not a disease – the use of bio-identical progesterone creams usually decreases bilateral vascularity and breasts return to a non-vascular state or minimal vascular state. Compounded progesterone cream increases breast health by decreasing stimulation and balances hormones. Apply daily and directly to the breasts only; this is where progesterone receptors are located. When applied to arms, legs, and thighs, this won't decrease risk, or vascularity, since there are no receptors in these areas. Progesterone pills, drops, and sublingual are ineffective at reducing vascularity and risk in the breasts as they are not applied locally, not fat soluble, and dissipate in the circulatory or digestive system.

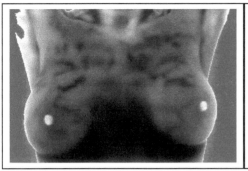
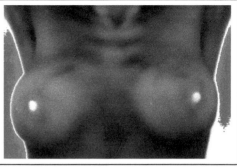

Before progesterone cream.
Note unusual vascular pattern.
"At risk." Progesterone deficiency imbalance.

After progesterone cream. Note reduction in
vascularity. Normal thermogram.

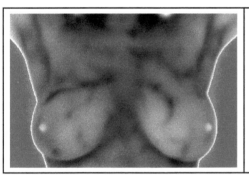
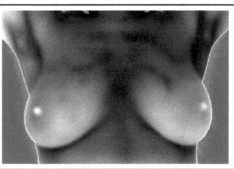

Before progesterone cream.

After progesterone cream.

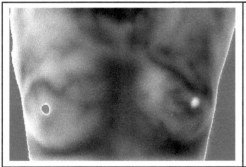
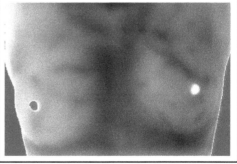

IUD containing hormones
plus progesterone cream usage.

After IUD was removed and continued
progesterone cream usage.

## Estrogen therapies increase risk of breast cancer

Around 80 percent of all breast cancers are estrogen driven, which means estrogen stimulates the cancer. Estrogen does not cause breast cancer but rather "feeds" the cancer. Our body makes the exact same amount of estrogen as is does progesterone. We were never estrogen deficient; it was the biggest lie to sell estrogen therapies. Estrogen therapies increase risk of breast cancer. Decrease your risk for cancer by being estrogen free®.

Thermography clinics that are recommending estrogen supplementation do not understand the basic fundamentals of thermography. Estrogen supplementation includes HRTs, bio-identical estrogen, flax, soy, red clover, black cohosh, primrose, estradiol, estriol, patches, pellets, estrogen essential oils and much more.

Do you think it is possible popular estrogen therapies could have "fed" these estrogen positive breast cancers?

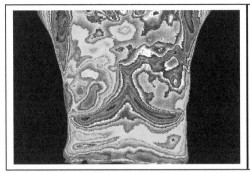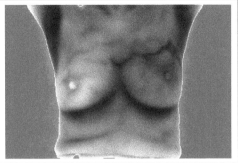

Current diagnosis of DCIS with history of bioidentical estrogen pellet usage for last two years.

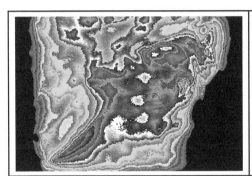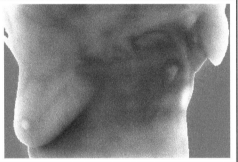

Recurrent breast cancer with history of flax use.

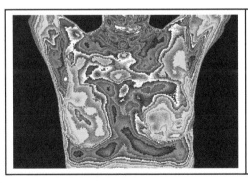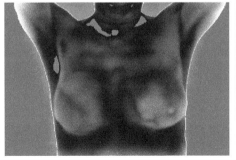

Breast cancer survivor – right breast. Woman has history of eighteen years of HRT usage and is currently using bioidentical estrogen. Note unusual vascular pattern.

## Synthetic estrogen increased breast cancer

Synthetic estrogen including HRTs, hormone replacement therapy, increase breast health risks by stimulating vascularity and possible neo-angiogenesis. The Women's Health Initiative shut down the largest study ever to investigate the effects of estrogen and progestin (synthetic form of progesterone) early due to increased risk in female subjects. They concluded that synthetic estrogen and progestin caused increased risk of breast cancer, heart attack, stroke, blood clots and pulmonary embolism. Thermograms support this conclusion. A few women in this book are currently in class action suits for breast cancer due to their HRTs.

This woman uses HRTs and reports an abnormal mammogram. Do HRTs look healthy?

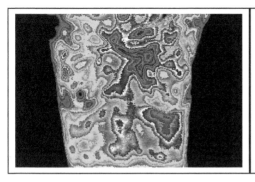 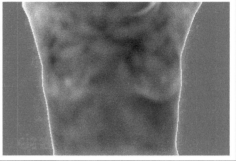

First thermogram with HRT usage. Abnormal thermogram. Severe progesterone deficiency imbalance.
*(left)* Note unusual unilateral color pattern in left breast.
*(right)* Note unusual severe vascular pattern in black hot.

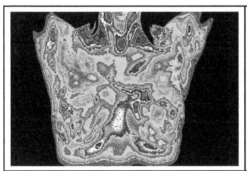 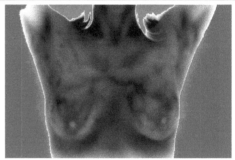

Repeat, 2nd thermogram continued HRT usage.

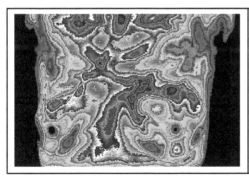 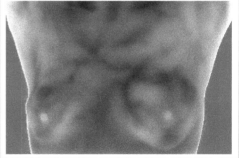

Repeat 3rd thermogram continued HRT usage.

# IUD and risk of breast cancer

Many doctors believe IUDs, vaginal creams and e-rings are *not* systemic and do *not* affect the breasts. This is false. All of these products list breast cancer as a risk by the manufacturer. IUDs containing estrogen, estrogen vaginal creams and e-rings increase breast health risk by stimulating vascularity and possible neoangiogenesis.

Do you think an IUD or vaginal cream can affect the breasts? Do you think IUDs, estrogen vaginal creams and e-rings are healthy?

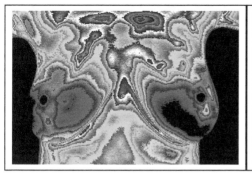
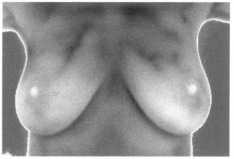

Before use of IUD. Slight bilateral vascular pattern in black hot.

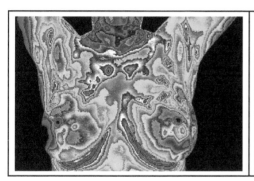
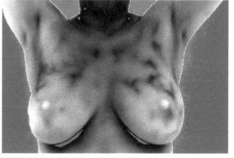

Six months after use of IUD with hormones. (*left*) Note unusual warm color tone changes (right) Note evidence of increased vascularity in black hot. Abnormal thermogram. Progesterone deficiency imbalance.

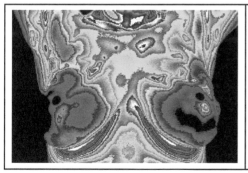
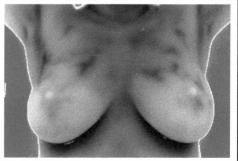

Six months after IUD is removed. Note decrease in vascular pattern in black hot.

## Our breast thermography research is proving phytoestrogens increase risk

Phytoestrogens, plant estrogens, stimulate the estrogen receptors because they are bioidentical. Bioidentical does not mean "safe" or "natural," it means similar chemical structure. Birth control pills and hormone replacement therapy are bioidentical. Dr. Hobbins was one of the first doctors in the 1980s to warn women about the risk of breast cancer due to soy, a phytoestrogen, from abnormal thermograms.

If a plant estrogen can occupy a receptor it is stimulating that receptor, not blocking it from other bioidentical estrogens. In fact, scientists have discovered that synthetic estrogens, which are also bioidentical, can produce more binding sites! You can't pick and choose saying one plant estrogen is harmful, like soy, and then say another is beneficial, like flax. They all stimulate our receptors, but with different strengths.

Looking at this lady's images do you think a bioidentical estrogen patch is healthy? Do you think exposure to bioidentical estrogen may increase risk?

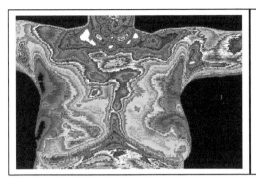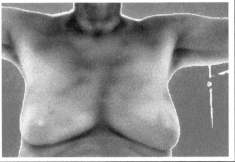

First thermogram. Normal thermogram. Healthy breasts

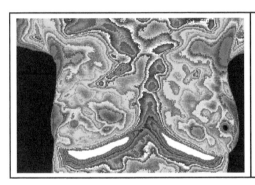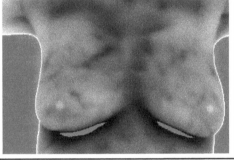

Repeat, second thermogram after bioidentical estrogen patch use for eight months.
Abnormal thermogram. Progesterone deficiency imbalance.
*(right)* Note evidence of vascularity in black hot.

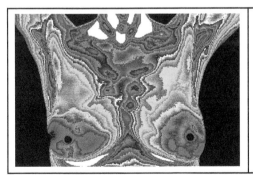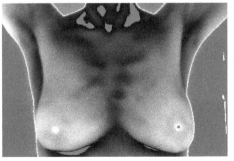

Repeat, third thermogram. After stopping bioidentical estrogen patch use.
Normal thermogram.

# Our breast thermography research is proving bioidentical estrogen increases risk

All these women go to doctors who specializes in bioidentical hormones. Bioidentical means same molecular structure. This definition means HRTs (hormone replacement therapy) and BCPs (birth control pills) are also considered bioidentical. Stop being fooled by the word "natural," it's not! There have been no studies to prove bioidentical estrogen is safe. Once again, just like HRTs, you are the lab rats.

Estrogen accelerates aging. Excess estrogen from estrogen therapies causes a hormone imbalance in the body. Aging occurs when the body is out of balance. The body is overworked by having to fix a hormone imbalance in addition to normal daily functions. Think about having to over-compensate that imbalance every day. Overworking the body is what ages us and leaves the body susceptible to disease. Slow down the aging process by having a functional, balanced body every day. Exposure to excess estrogen causes the body to hold onto excess weight, increases infertility, and creates PMS. Hormonally balanced women don't experience PMS. Estrogen is a stimulator which increases insomnia, anxiety and symptoms of menopause. Symptoms of menopause are *not* normal.

Do these women look healthy to you? Do these images look healthy? Do these images look hormonally balanced? Do you think these women are aging themselves? Or promoting their youth?

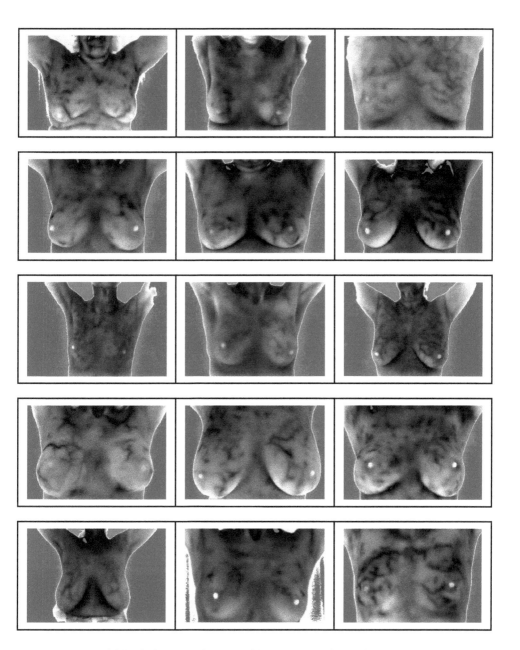

Bioidentical estrogen increases risk. Note unusual vascular patterns.

## Your breast can't lie about your hormone therapy

Breast thermography can determine if your hormone treatment is working correctly. Bio-identical estrogen is a popular hormone fad, but does it work? If it worked at balancing hormones, then the breasts should be non-vascular or normal after treatment.

This woman goes to a "famous" doctor who specializes in bioidentical hormones. Excess estrogen can simulate the blood vessels, which is activity that creates heat which will be captured by the camera.

Let's determine this doctor's ability at balancing hormones. Look at her first thermogram, is she hormonally balanced? Or does she have excess estrogen? Does she look healthy?

This patient wanted to believe her doctor was correct in needing estrogen therapy, but she couldn't deny her images and therefore cut her bioidentical estrogen dose by half after her first thermogram. Her second thermogram confirmed the bioidentical estrogen cream was increasing risk and causing excess estrogen or progesterone deficiency.

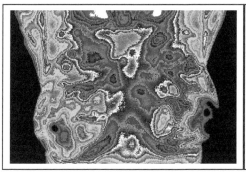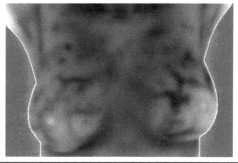

First thermogram. Note severe unusual vascular pattern and suspected neoangiogenesis in left breast.
Severe progesterone deficiency imbalance.

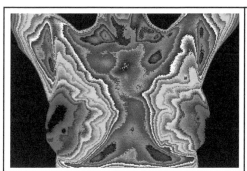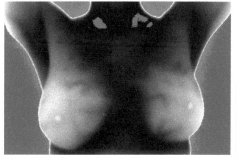

Repeat, second thermogram. Half estrogen dose. Note decrease in vascularity.

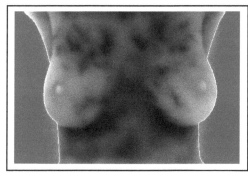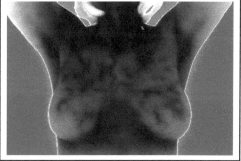

Another woman who goes to a doctor who specializes in bioidenticals. Note "at risk" pattern in first
thermogram. Note increase vascularity with repeat thermogram and continued estrogen use.

# Our breast thermography research is proving bioidentical estrogen and progesterone used together is ineffective

Many doctors believe that progesterone and bioidentical estrogen can be used as a therapy together to balance hormones and prevent aging. Theory sounds reasonable. Let's see if this theory is correct. Thermography will determine if this popular hormone therapy is effective by monitoring the blood vessels.

Do you think progesterone and bioidentical estrogen are effective when used together? Do these women look hormonally balanced? Do they look healthy?

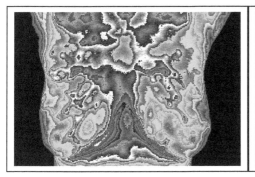 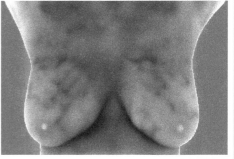

Therapy of bioidentical estrogen with progesterone. Progesterone deficiency imbalance.

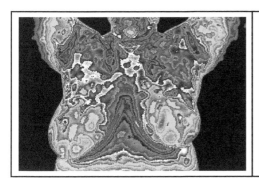 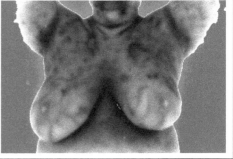

Therapy of bioidentical estrogen with progesterone. Progesterone deficiency imbalance.

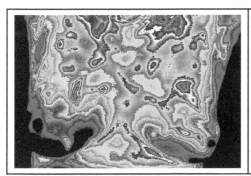 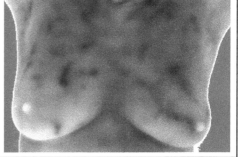

Therapy of bioidentical estrogen with progesterone. Progesterone deficiency imbalance.

*Wendy Sellens, DACM, LAc*

# Our breast thermography research has been proving soy increases risk for over 40 years

The reason breast thermography research is proving what is beneficial or harmful to the breasts before other imaging or tests is due to fact that we can "see" or monitor the blood vessels. The blood vessels are what feed or stimulate disorders and diseases. Thermography can see the stimulation of the blood vessels that are possible feeding a disease or disorder in the early stage.

That is why thermography research discovers medical evidence first because we can "see" changes in the blood vessels – good or bad. We are the first line of defense; that is why our research is so progressive. We then publish and share our research with other doctors, but change takes time.

Remember when everyone thought soy was safe? Dr. Hobbins was telling women in the '80s, from his thermography research, to avoid soy, a plant estrogen, because it increased risk of cancer and progesterone deficiency or excess estrogen seen as PMS and symptoms of menopause.

Due to her cultural tradition, this estrogen receptor positive (ER+) breast cancer patient was raised to believe soy milk was healthy. She followed tradition and enjoyed growing and making her own soy milk. Even after the spread of breast cancer from her left breast to her right, she continued to make her own homemade organic soy milk.

Do you still think organic soy is healthy and "blocks" harmful estrogen? Did homemade organic soy milk stimulate breast cancer?

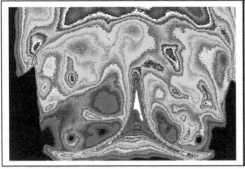 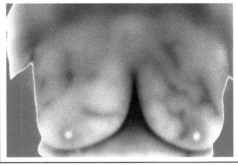

2012 Carcinoma at 9 o'clock left breast.

2012 ER+ invasive ductal carcinoma left breast. Consuming homemade soy milk.

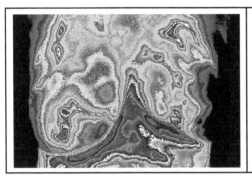 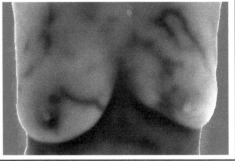

2014 Carcinoma at 5 o'clock right breast.

2014 ER+ invasive ductal carcinoma right breast. Continuing use of soy milk.

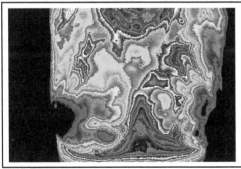 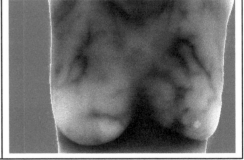

2016 Possible reoccurrence at 8 o'clock left breast.

2012 lumpectomy left breast 2014 lumpectomy right breast. Continuing use of soy milk.

# Our breast thermography research is proving flax increases risk

When our first book was published in 2013 it was the first medical evidence, thermograms, proving flax increased risk of breast cancer and excess estrogen.

Flax is a popular "women's health" supplement. Flax is a plant estrogen, the seed and oils increase vascularity and risk. But what about all those flax studies? A study's theories need to be implemented into a human body's system with success in order to be considered valid and not just a hypothesis. There has been no proof showing flax is beneficial when given to women. It is all based on assumptions or hearsay. In fact, thermographic evidence demonstrates that these hypotheses are incorrect.

Many women are trusting their "alternative" doctors or breast cancer clinics, who are treating their estrogen receptor positive (ER+) breast cancer with flax, which is a phytoestrogen. Estrogen, including phytoestrogens, stimulate or feed ER+ breast cancer causing the tumors to grow. The Budwig Diet does *not* "cure" ER+ breast cancer, in fact it causes it to grow.

After looking at the images do you think flax increases risk? Do you think flax is healthy for women?

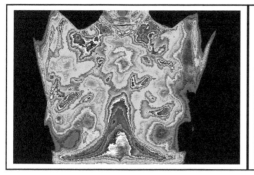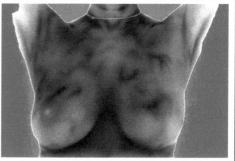

Patient diagnosed with estrogen positive breast cancer in left breast.

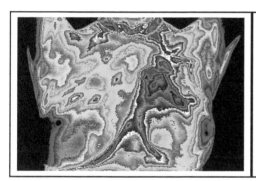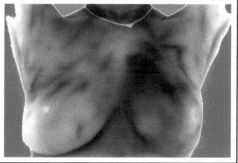

Nine months of treating breast cancer with flax. Note evidence of neoangiogenesis.

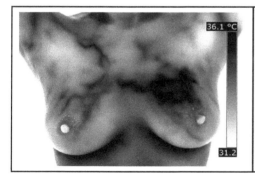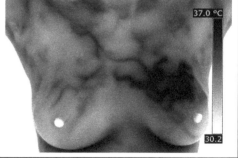

Diagnosed with ER+ breast cancer left breast.

One year treating breast cancer with Budwig Diet, flax. Tumors increased in size. Note neoangiogenesis.

# Our breast thermography research is proving natural estrogen blockers are ineffective

Popular women's supplements, DIM and calcium d-glucarate, broccoli and cauliflower extracts, claim to be "natural" estrogen blockers. Sounds healthy?

Thermograms cannot support these false claims made by most "natural estrogen blockers." Many "alternative" doctors and breast cancer clinics are using these "natural blockers" to treat breast cancer. Most of the women I monitor continue to try this treatment due to the manipulated studies supporting these supplements hoping to "cure" their breast cancer, when in fact it is increasing their risk. Stop being deceived by "women's health" supplements.

Hormone specialist are using "natural estrogen blockers" in their protocols. What is absurd is they will put women on a bioidentical estrogen then also add these blockers. Estrogen is the culprit. These "natural estrogen blockers" aren't effective. Stop using all estrogen therapies to reduce excess estrogen.

These thermograms are from a pilot study challenging claims of natural estrogen blockers. Due to incredible adverse reactions in only 30 days (abnormal thermogram, painful breasts, and six pounds of weight gain), the study had to be discontinued early due to increased health risk. If therapy had worked correctly by blocking harmful estrogen, then vascularity should have decreased.

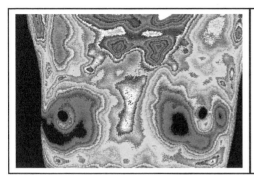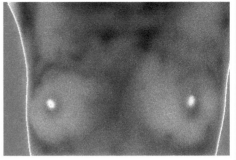

Before supplemental use of calcium d-glucarate.

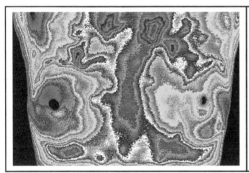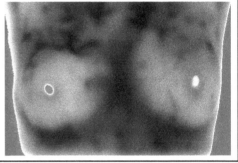

After thirty days of calcium d-glucarate: Left breast-Note warm color tones. Black hot- note nipple temperature difference and increased vascularity.

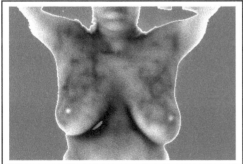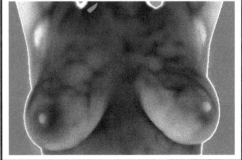

Both of these women are currently using DIM. Note unusual vascular patterns in each woman's breasts. Thermograms cannot support claims that supplements "block estrogen."

# Our breast thermography research is proving supplements may increase risk

Most surprising is supplements increase risk. The American Cancer Society claims there is little evidence proving supplements and vitamins are healthy for the breasts and actually lists them under risk factors. One study showed 19 percent of women increased breast cancer risk from multivitamin use. Thermography supports these studies since most women using numerous supplements rarely have healthy or normal thermograms. Supplements and vitamins can increase risk because they may contain preservatives, cheap product or fillers, contaminates, toxic or antagonist ingredients.

We have been brainwashed to believe a pill is healthy. A pill is not a substitute for fresh foods! Now, some people who have disorders or disease will need to supplement. To be clear we are not anti-supplement, we just want to reduce the amount and ensure that the ones you are using are actually working.

Like many women, this woman uses numerous supplements and vitamins. After two years of abnormal thermograms this woman was finally convinced to stop all her supplements in order observe if they were the cause of her abnormal thermograms. Six months after removing supplements, her breast's health risk was reduced.

Do you think supplements may increase risk?

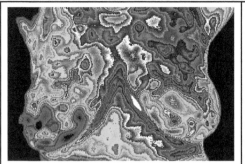
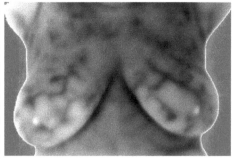

Use of supplements increases risk. First thermogram. (*left*) Note unusual color pattern and warmer tones in left breast. (*right*) Note unusual vascular pattern in black hot. Abnormal thermogram.

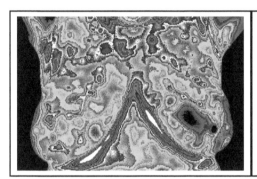
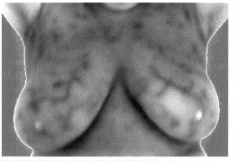

Use of supplements increases risk one year later. Repeat, second thermogram (*left*) Note unusual color pattern and warmer tones in right breast now. (*right*) Note unusual vascular patter in black hot. Abnormal thermogram. Abnormal thermogram. Severely progesterone deficient.

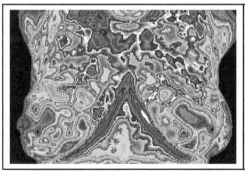
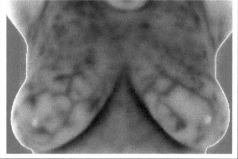

Six months after supplement discontinuation, third thermogram. (*left*) Note unusual color pattern, however, is symmetrical now. (*right*) Note unusual vascular pattern still present in black hot.

# Our breast thermography research is proving environmental estrogens increase risk

The effects of environmental estrogens, commercial grade estrogens, have become more prevalent. This is seen in the majority of thermograms which are rated abnormal or "at risk"

Presently, there are very few non-vascular or normal thermograms. The majority of women are progesterone deficient and "at risk." In fact, the entire family is exposed to environmental estrogens causing early puberty, low testosterone, symptoms of excess estrogen and increase risk of breast cancer.

This may be exposure from estrogens found in foods, household products, skincare, supplements, and pollution. Environmental estrogens are a contributing factor to the rise in breast cancer. Be careful what you eat and place on your skin, you are what you eat...*and* put on your skin.

These women are not currently using any estrogen therapies, notice the unusual vascular patterns.

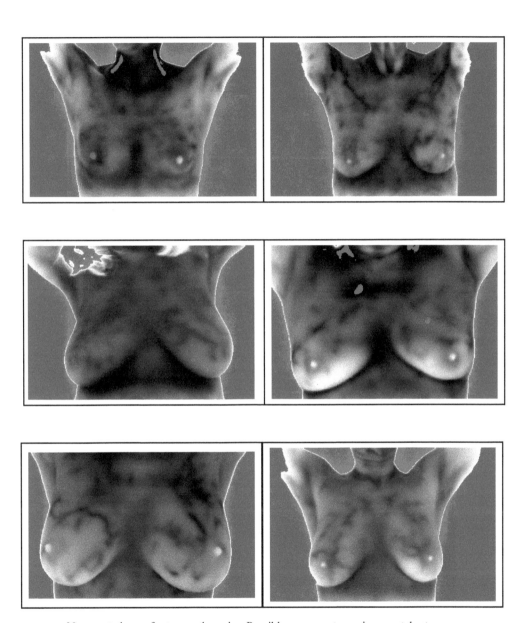

No reported use of estrogen therapies. Possible exposure to environmental estrogens.

# What are your blood vessels telling you about your breast health?

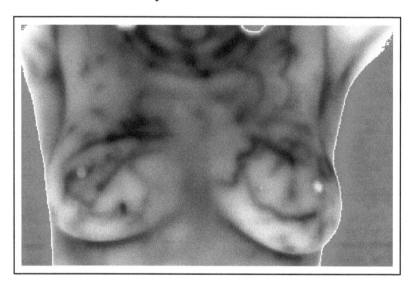

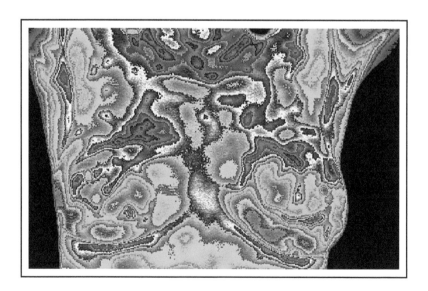

# 2. Intel

If estrogen supplementation is healthy, then why are breast cancer numbers rising? Why do studies on estrogen replacement therapies (ERTs) and hormone replacement therapies (HRTs) show an increase in breast cancer with use? Why are rates in men with breast cancer rising? Why do all synthetic estrogen therapies list breast cancer as a side effect? If flax and soy (plant estrogens) are being consumed more than ever, then why are rates in breast cancer rising? Why are breast cancer numbers increasing in third-world countries? Why do animals given estrogen in studies suffer physical and developmental disorders?

These are important questions to ask, especially as the incidence of breast cancer increases and the age range of those affected grows wider. The 2011-2012 American Cancer Society Breast Cancer Facts & Figures reports that the probability of a thirty year old woman developing invasive breast cancer in the next decade is 1 in 232, while that for a forty year old increases to 1 in 69, and increasing to 1 in 42 for a now fifty year old woman. In addition, they state that the chance of developing breast cancer is one in eight in a woman's lifetime.

The reason for the nearly exponential growth of this ruthless disease is simple— supplemental estrogen is the enemy! The American Cancer Society reported, "Breast-cancer incidence rises from 68,000 to 184,300 between 1970 and 1996. Rise =171 percent... There is no way that the female population increase alone can account for the enormous rise in breast-cancer incidence… During the same period (1970-1996), the number of breast-cancer deaths rose to 44,300 from 30,100. Rise =47 percent." A 171 percent increase in breast cancer incidences! Coincidentally, these numbers reflect breast cancer after the increased popularity and usage of ERTs and HRTs.

Breast cancer is increasing in men as well. Breast cancer in men is considered a rare disease. Less than one percent of all breast cancers occur in men. In 2018, about 2,550 men are expected to be diagnosed and the lifetime risk of being diagnosed with breast cancer is about 1 in 1,000. The American Cancer Society also reported, "In the U.S., between 1975-2006, the incidence rate for men increased 0.9 percent PER year. The reasons for this increase are unknown (not attributed to detection)."

Welcome to the revolution, troops! Women are caught up in a battle for their lives and their breasts. It is time to take up arms and expose the deceptions, misinformation, and propaganda regarding breast health. The battle started in the 1940s, when ERTs were first introduced to women to reduce the signs of aging. Since then, women have unflinchingly swallowed this deceitful directive with the belief they could prolong their youth. Instead, they have actually accelerated the aging process with estrogen, and more importantly, increased incidences of breast and uterine cancer, infertility, autoimmune disorders, and thyroid issues, as well as symptoms of PMS and menopause. The revolution was started to gather intel to arm women with accurate information instead of rumors. Repeat a statement enough times and it magically becomes true. An uneducated woman is a sitting duck to these propaganda and mantras. An educated woman is powerfully armed to protect herself and her family.

It is vital to understand the enemy or the cause so that it can be treated and defeated. Estrogen increases stimulation of breast cells. This is how breasts mature during puberty. Presently, around 80 percent of breast cancers are estrogen-driven. Estrogen does not cause cancer, but acts as the fertilizer that feeds the seed of cancer. It does not matter if the estrogen is considered weak or strong; excess estrogen increases risk because it may stimulate the cancer. Decreasing our cancer risk is actually simple: reduce exposure to estrogen.

Synthetic estrogens stimulate breast cells and increase risk for breast cancer. Examples include HRTs, estrogen patches, estriol a.k.a. the "healthy" estrogen, estrogen vaginal cream, birth control pills (BCPs), IUD with hormones, estrogen rings, and injections.

Phytoestrogens, or estrogens derived from plants, attach to the estrogen receptors in breasts and increase risk for breast cancer by stimulating those receptors. These include bioidentical estrogens, flax, soy, black cohosh, and red clover.

Ecoestrogens increase breast stimulation and therefore raise breast cancer risk. These commercial-grade estrogens are used daily in everything from hair, makeup, skin, and body products; cleaning products; bedding; furniture; clothing; and plant pesticides found in "natural" body products and nonorganic foods. Ecoestrogens are also present in commercial products such as paint, carpeting, food cans, plastic products, estrogen given to livestock, and drinking water, including tap, reverse osmosis, filtered, and bottled.

To reduce the risk of breast cancer, decrease exposure to exogenous (outside the body) or environmental estrogens such as synthetic estrogen, phytoestrogens, and ecoestrogens. Join the revolution to promote the reduction of these environmental estrogens that are found in almost everything.

In 1971, Judah Folkman discovered that tumors caused neoangiogenesis, or new blood vessels. He later demonstrated that angiogenesis was necessary for the formation of new, abnormal growth of tissue– or neoplasia – to move from in situ (inside duct) to an invasive cancer. Interestingly, Dr. Folkman, who is now praised for his research and work, which is referenced frequently f, was once ostracized from the medical community for his preposterous theories.

Reduce risk of breast cancer with early detection through breast thermograms, which analyze blood flow or vascular patterns in the breasts. In breast thermography, stimulation of the existing blood vessel is referred to as vascularity. Chronic vascularity from estrogen stimulation has the possibility of promoting new blood vessels growth which is evidence of neoangiogenesis. Thermograms monitor vascularity and the growth of blood vessels, or neoangiogenesis, in the breasts and can alert an at-risk woman to make lifestyle changes to correct the vacularity before it escalates. This is the essential purpose of breast thermography. Many people believe it is to screen for breast cancer, but more imperative is its ability to detect those at risk for preventive treatment. This is true early detection.

Breast thermography was *not* created to replace any other imaging modalities, but to send high-risk women on for further study with mammography. This way, many women decrease their exposure to unnecessary radiation. Breast thermography is a vital tool for breast cancer screening, but it is actually much more integral to reducing risk. The images used in the book are to educate, and most importantly, to *show* the reader what increases and decreases breast cancer risk.

Thermography is not being used properly in the majority of breast thermography clinics. The minimum standard requirements set forth by thermographic studies are clearly spelled out in this book so women can find certified breast clinics. Unfortunately, there are only a few nationwide. One of the purposes of this book is to educate the masses so that they can demand the highest-quality thermography for their breasts!

Theromography will never be accepted by the medical establishment if it continues to be performed incorrectly and if unfounded rumors and false claims persist. This book simply and clearly explains the correct approaches to breast health and reducing breast cancer risks through scientific studies coupled with thermographic evidence. Thermographic images offer an incredible way for women to literally see the results before their eyes! No guessing involved. This is an educational picture book for methods of breast cancer reduction. Explanations are very easy to follow, as each argument will feature an image.

> At Johns Hopkins Hospital in 1898, Dr. Halstead reported his five-year survival rate of 48 percent with radical carcinoma of the breast. The survival rate, as now judged some fifty years later at the same institution with all the new modalities… have not provided the female any increased safety in being cured from this malady."
>
> William Hobbins, MD, "To Mammogram or Not," 1969

In 1969, with all the "modern medical technology" available, Dr. Hobbins saw that the best treatment was still a mastectomy and the five-year survival rate was still around 48 percent. In 120 years, breast cancer treatment has only improved marginally! Ladies, our health is literally in our own hands. We have to educate ourselves and change our lifestyles to reduce our risk.

Dr. Hobbins and I recognize that every woman is a dynamic individual and will respond to the effects of estrogen differently. That is why monitoring breast health risk with thermography is so important. Each woman's vascular pattern is examined. Then her individualized treatment protocol for breast health, and more imperative, breast cancer, is scrutinized and evaluated for the utmost effective treatment.

*Reduce breast cancer risk with prevention.*

Reduce the risk of breast cancer by balancing hormones with progesterone and testosterone. Estrogen deficiency is actually very rare. What are considered to be signs and symptoms of estrogen deficiency are actually side effects of estrogen excess or progesterone and testosterone deficiency. Unsupported rumors have perpetuated risk, clearly evidenced by the increase in breast cancer rates. Balance hormones correctly and you will not only find relief, but you will also improve your breast health.

Cancer requires a large amount of sugar to survive. Decrease the risk of breast cancer by reducing intake of processed food, sugar, or anything that breaks down to sugar including carbohydrates and alcohol. Avoid or limit bread, pasta, cereal, crackers, white or brown rice, candy, chips, dressing, health bars, and powdered health shakes and juices even if they are organic! Avoid all products processed with "whole grains"; these are still carbohydrates and convert to sugar which causes weight gain, inflammation, and feeds cancer. Anything in a bag, jar or box has been processed and usually contains sugars and carbohydrates. Reduce breast cancer risk by only eating whole foods, which includes meat, fruit, vegetables, nuts, and dairy.

Reduce risk of breast cancer by decreasing usage of body and household products that are not organic. Nonorganic products including "natural," are toxic and contain petrochemicals that are dangerous to the body. These products also contain ecoestrogens, commercial-grade estrogens that increase risk.

Reduce breast cancer risk by limiting use of supplements and vitamins; they are toxic due to preservatives and processing. Some supplements are acid or alkali; others are oil-based or water soluble, antagonistic elements. When purified and combined together, they do not mix well and become toxic. The processing of supplements increases risk of external contaminates. Supplementation is not medicine and should only be used as a treatment therapy by ill individuals, not healthy people. Recent studies have found that cancer risk increases with supplementation and vitamin usage.

Reduce risk of breast cancer by seeing a holistic doctor to prevent illness. Holistic doctors can diagnose and treat an imbalance or illness before it manifests a disease. This is medical prevention and true anti-aging medicine. Holistic physicians include Chinese medical, Ayurvedic, and homeopathic.

Be forewarned, being healthy takes work. Personal responsibility must be taken. Most doctors believe health is found in pharmaceuticals or supplements, but it is not. Breast health is attained through prevention, which is mostly achieved through nutrition, removing all estrogens to balance hormones, good sleep, and moderate exercise. Most women are reluctant to change their belief systems. If taking a handful of pills, including supplements, is your idea of health, this book and information is not for you. If you are tired of being overweight, fatigued, cranky, and worried about breast cancer, then this boot camp challenge is for you. Only you can be the champion of your health.

This book is for brave women who will question the propaganda fed to the masses for decades. It will question the efficacy of the medical establishment with evidence gathered from studies and thermograms. It will reeducate women and doctors on how estrogen truly works and affects the body. Most women and doctors are misinformed on how hormones affect breast health and cancer, which perpetuates and proliferates misinformation. They are so programmed in the false promises of estrogen, that even when hundreds of breast thermograms or their own thermogram is directly in front of them, they still deny the evidence.

The battle will not be easy. Standing up and shouting out the truth is met with harsh resistance. It is socially challenging to argue that environmental estrogen is harmful, but the truth is scary. This book is a reminder of how healthy people used to be when common sense – rather than a pill – was used to solve a disorder.

Dr. Hobbins started his medical practice in 1946. In 1974, after ten years of mammographic and thermographic research, to his utter dismay, he realized that the medical establishment was a blockade to creating healthy patients and removed himself from the American Medical Association (AMA). Dr. Hobbins stood by his research and questioned everything. We encourage you to do the same; don't be so accepting, especially of your health. We even encourage you to question us. Questioning leads to answers. Be personally responsible for you and your families' health. Find your truth using logic and evidence.

This book will clearly show the reasons for the increase in breast cancer and breast health risk while identifying simple treatments any woman can implement to decrease her risk. Don't focus on a cure to an illness; focus on strengthening health to prevent illness.

Don't wait for defeat. March towards victory.

# 3. Artillery

## Hormones: Understanding the Weaponry

In order for us to fight against an enemy of our body, we must first understand our body. Otherwise, we will continue to shoot for solutions we have no ability to hit. "Know thyself" could not be more accurate a motto in this battle, and "know thyself" we shall. To understand the enemies of your body, you must first understand how it works.

Do you ever wonder why women have such gorgeous curves? This is due to the amazing hormone estrogen. Developing girls need this hormone for the fallopian tubes, vagina, uterus, breasts, and skeleton, as well as for fat content. Estrogen causes cells to develop rapidly, which increases stimulation of the breasts. This stimulation is completely natural during a young woman's developmental stage, but as fully matured women, overstimulation of the breast by estrogenic factors can be quite harmful. This is the basis of this book, but there is plenty of "intel" that needs to be reported along the way.

Let us not neglect another equally important hormone: progesterone, the "yin" to estrogen's "yang." Once a woman is sexually mature, these two hormones ebb and flow with one another, creating the beautiful dance known as our "cycle." Beautiful dance? Well, many of us experience some difficult symptoms, and therefore, see it more as a horrible existence on the battlefield. Unfortunately, this is due to the exogenous or environmental estrogens that are attacking our bodies—*not* the *body's* estrogen, as this is not the culprit. These environmental estrogens consist of synthetic pharmaceutical estrogens, phytoestrogens (plant-derived estrogen) and ecoestrogens (commercial synthetics), all of which contribute to hormonal imbalances. This is termed as "excess estrogen" or a "progesterone deficiency."

These imbalances contribute to infertility as well as symptoms of both menopause and PMS. While these symptoms are experienced by a large portion of the female population, they are not normal. These are pathological conditions that will be discussed in greater detail throughout the book. For now, it is more important for us to understand what happens as these partnered elements decrease in our body that starts at around the age of thirty-five, during the premenopausal stage.

Imagine a perfect world, where all women are hormonally balanced with no external factors influencing their delicate systems. Our healthy functioning body would perform like this: during the premenopausal stage, the production of eggs declines. When we no longer produce eggs, our body will no longer produce progesterone or estrogen. I will repeat that: *no* egg = *no* progesterone and *no* estrogen. To this day, many doctors believe you can still produce estrogen without producing an egg. This misconception will be explained in detail below and in the "Breast Canswers" chapter.

In a perfect world, where estrogen and progesterone decline equally in the body, there will be little to no symptoms of menopause, other than the change in frequency or quality of periods. Just like PMS is a pathology, so are menopausal symptoms. Night sweats, hot flashes, and weight gain are all caused by excess environmental estrogens infiltrating your body and binding to your estrogen receptors.

There are some obvious questions that need to be addressed in regards to this. Why do doctors give women estrogen when both hormones are declining? Why do doctors still hand out hormone replacement therapy (HRTs) and "bioidentical" estrogens like candy? Taking estrogen and HRTs only increases hormonal imbalance, thereby creating a greater amount of estrogen relative to progesterone in the body. It makes no sense that estrogen is prescribed in such an irresponsible manner.

The idea that menopausal symptoms are caused by low estrogen is a complete farce not supported by facts or clinical studies. If someone spouts off about in vitro this and in vitro that, remember that women are not petri dishes nor test tubes, and that the human body is a diverse, dynamic operating system not to be reduced to such false claims. Many studies on estrogen are conducted in a controlled environment. When attempts are made to translate the use of estrogen into the human body, which is not a controlled environment, estrogen does not behave the same way it does in a controlled petri dish. Thermograms clearly demonstrate this appalling error.

So many women complain about the side effects of estrogen (weight gain, irritability, and insomnia) from birth control pills, hormone replacement therapies, and bioidentical estrogen. These physicians and other medical professionals think women are crazy, overdramatic, or making up these complaints—simply because a study conducted in a petri dish showed conflicting results. Stop letting these doctors tell you how you should feel. As physicians, it is our responsibility to provide medical information incorporated with our clinical experience to recommend a treatment plan—not deny that you are experiencing certain symptoms. Your body is your responsibility, and it's ultimately up to you to decide what is best for your health.

I tell all my patients, "Your breasts can't lie to you or to me. Now look at your thermogram!" Thermograms support what Dr. Hobbins has been saying for years: "Stop using all forms of estrogen." Excess estrogen stimulates the breasts, which increases the risk for both breast and uterine cancer. With all of the estrogen therapies available, why is breast cancer not cured? Why are its rates increasing rather than declining? As women, we need to educate ourselves and correct this horrific mythology thrust upon us by improperly educated doctors whose textbooks are written by pharmaceutical companies. It's time to pay attention to the facts—estrogen therapies continually show increased vascular patterns and neoangiogenesis which are considered risk factors for breast and uterine cancer.

## Traditional Perspective on Estrogen

Estrogen is a stimulant; in traditional Chinese medicine, it pertains to "yang," with progesterone being "yin" in relative terms. The common side effects of excessive estrogen include insomnia, agitation, and irritability among many others. This is due to excessive yang, or warm energy, overstimulating the body both physically and emotionally. Hot flashes, for example, can be described as yang rising in the body due to the inability of its yin counterpart to anchor it, much like a string does a balloon. When estrogen and progesterone are balanced, the body will tend to be closer to a systemic balance or homeostasis.

Chinese medicine regards menopause as a time for rest, reflection, and to pass wisdom on to the youth. Hopefully, we are not "old," but rather, have aged gracefully with experience. It is time to enjoy life, and to see this as a reward, not a curse. Excessive stimulation is not an answer for anything, for we are simply becoming more yin and less yang.

Older women are the target of so many jokes, often considered neurotic and "dried up." Take the term "hysterectomy" for example, which is derived from the word "hysteria." Well, no kidding—with all the symptoms that excess estrogen creates, is it any wonder one would be called that? Present-day menopause symptoms are actually a result of our diet and environment; they should be considered abnormal.

It's imperative to question why doctors would want us to increase estrogen or stimulation at this time in our life. We are not here to thrust upon you a belief or way of life, but rather to make you question the propaganda that has become "truth." We have to get out there in the trenches and battlefields of this war and seek out the facts. Not all good soldiers have to die for the causes of others.

## Breast Anatomy: Knowing the Lay of the Land

Our breasts don't complete their growth cycle until around the age of twenty-five, at which point, their composition is nearly 100 percent breast tissue and connective tissue. So for those women still under the age of twenty-five and worried, there is plenty of hope for your "breast friends." At around the age of thirty-five, and corresponding to perimenopause, the breasts begin to involute. This is a fancy term for the gradual shrinking or maturing of the breasts. Between the ages of thirty-five to forty, our breast composition is reduced by 50 percent. Involution continues until the ages of sixty to seventy, when breast tissue and connective tissue are reduced to a composition of about 35 percent. One of the reasons this happens is that as the estrogen declines in the body, so does stimulation from estrogen to the breasts. In addition, with age, the connective tissue in the breast becomes dehydrated and inelastic. Lastly, the breast tissue is no longer preparing to make milk every month, and thereby shrinks and loses shape.

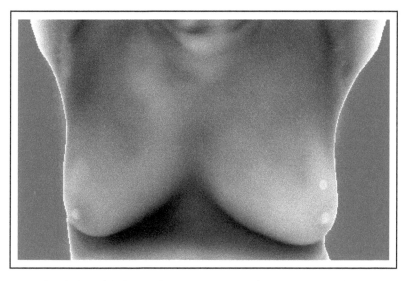

Correct involution of the breasts in a post-menopausal woman. Normal thermogram.

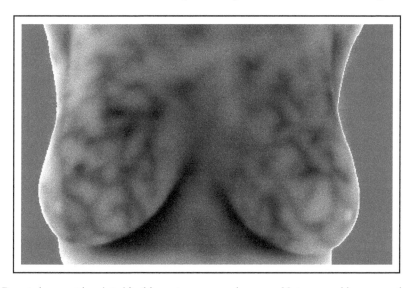

Breasts have not involuted in this post-menopausal woman. Note unusual hypervascular pattern. "At risk" thermogram. Severe progesterone deficiency imbalance.

# The Menstrual Cycle:
# A Reconnaissance Mission

For those who might not know, women are born with a predetermined supply of eggs. These eggs are stored within follicles that are influenced by the hormones the body produces. The pituitary gland can be seen as the "general," as it directs these hormones. Once we reach maturity, or puberty, we experience what is called the ovarian cycle. The pituitary alerts the ovary to produce an egg, which is then released with the goal of fertilization. If no fertilization occurs, a new cycle of egg development and release continues. This cycle should last about twenty-eight days and is divided into three phases: follicular, ovulation, and luteal.

During the follicular phase, the follicular stimulating hormone (FSH) increases and stimulates the development of three to thirty follicles in the ovary. Each of these follicles contains an egg, and as the FSH decreases, each follicle battles for dominance. The remaining dominant mature follicle then secretes estrogen, resulting in a mature egg. Remember this: estrogen is produced from the follicular cells. This is important because, during menopause, the general tells the ovary to cease egg production which also means no more estrogen secretion.

Approaching the end of this phase, another hormone called a luteinizing hormone (LH), surges to initiate the release of an egg from the follicle. As the follicle ruptures, the egg exits the ovary and moves into the fallopian tube—this is called "ovulation." We should now be at midcycle, entering the luteal phase. As soon as the egg is released, the follicular cells undergo a metamorphosis to become leuteal cells. These luteal cells transform into the ovarian scar, known as the corpus luteum, which produces progesterone. Let me emphasize this: *the corpus luteum produces progesterone.* This is very important, not only for reproduction, but for understanding the reasons behind hormonal imbalances, as this is the *only* source of progesterone the female body will ever have unless fertilization occurs.

The luteal phase has two participants: the egg and the ruptured follicle, now called the corpus luteum. This recently released egg has just twelve to twenty-four hours to become fertilized by the "Navy Seals."

With estrogen and progesterone now present, the formation of the endometrium, a thick layer of blood and nutrients on the wall of the uterus, makes it possible for the fertilized egg to nestle safely and securely. Progesterone also increases the fertile mucus in the cervix, which lowers vaginal acidity so that sperm can survive in this environment.

In regard to the breasts, estrogen and progesterone prepares the mammary glands for fertilization by widening the milk ducts, thus creating swollen and tender breasts. If there is no fertilization, progesterone decreases as the corpus luteum degenerates, while estrogen also decreases, resulting in the uterus shedding its lining. This begins day one of the menstrual cycle.

## Shell Shock

Explanations to some of our complications.

## Early Puberty: Why is it Increasing and the Age Dropping?

It's clear that estrogen is a vital part of reproductive growth, development, and fertilization. Estrogen allows for fat accumulation in the connective tissue, so when we reach puberty and our ovaries start to secrete estrogen, our breast cells become stimulated and start to grow. It is also at this time that our bodies transition from the primary growth cycle to the secondary growth cycle. Basically, we grow "up," and then we grow "out."

Many women experience cycles as short as twenty days or as long as forty. Some consider this normal, but this is "anything but," especially if you are trying to conceive. This is either a shortening or lengthening, respectively, of the follicular phases, as the luteal phase always takes place fourteen days from ovulation (egg released).

Another common abnormality today is the early age of menarche, the onset of first period. It is not uncommon today for girls to begin their periods at the age of ten to eleven or even younger. *This is not normal.* A woman should begin her period between the ages fourteen to seventeen.

There is mention of this in ancient Chinese medical texts that states that women are capable of becoming pregnant upon entering their second cycle, at the age of about fourteen. In traditional Chinese medicine, women are on seven-year developmental cycles, while a man's cycle lasts eight years. This may explain why the body "magically" changes at certain times of our lives.

Some may not find early menarche concerning, but think of the biological message that it presents. For thousands of years, girls became women when it was biologically time to have children. Look at a young girl of ten or eleven and ask yourself if they should be a "woman" at that age. Should they be conceiving children? They may look and dress like women at times, but they are not; rather, they are overly stimulated children prematurely thrust into the chemical world of a woman, due to environmental estrogen.

It's interesting to see the drop over the years in the average age of a woman's first period. During my generation, most girls got our periods around eleven to twelve. It was recently reported that some girls are getting their period as early as five. I have observed preteen girls who are as active as I was at their age, yet they have fatty tissue around their abdomen, known as "muffin tops." That slang term didn't exist when I was young—because no one had it! Guess what a side effect of excess estrogen is? Weight stored around the abdomen!

Symptomology has also changed in recent times. There is supposed to be a subtle change, an enlarging of the breasts, when a woman gets her period. Breast pain, cramps, and irritability are not normal. Just because everyone has PMS does not make it normal. Rather, it is another sign of excess estrogen, which unfortunately plagues the majority of women.

# Dense Breasts: The Covert Ops Exposed

Think of the blood vessels in your breasts as a garden hose. When you are hormonally balanced the blood vessels are normal, similar to the garden hose, and semi-soft. But what happens when you turn on the water? The hose becomes tense. What happens when the blood vessels in your breasts are exposed to excess estrogen? They become dense.

This is why women who are still menstruating have dense breasts, stimulation due to estrogen, and usually the reason your mammogram returns "inconclusive" due to density. A mammogram is only 48 percent accurate for a woman under fifty. Guess what? After menopause, you should have *no* estrogen, your body stopped producing it because estrogen is only for reproduction, it does *not* keep you young. This is the lie they told you to sell you hormones. Interestingly, a mammogram is 68 percent accurate for a woman between the ages of fifty and sixty.

Dense breasts are not caused by the tissue of the breast, which many people think, but the blood vessels, which have expanded and become tense. Any pregnant woman or nursing mother can testify to this: as the body prepares for milk, the blood vessels expand, causing dense, swollen breasts, which is normal. This is why breast thermograms of women with excess estrogen look similar to pregnant or nursing mothers.

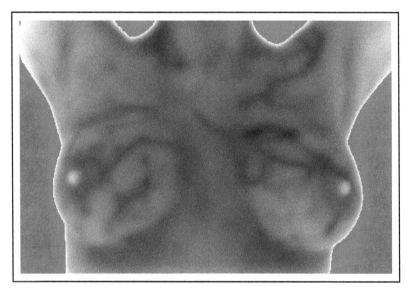

Normal vascularity during pregnancy.

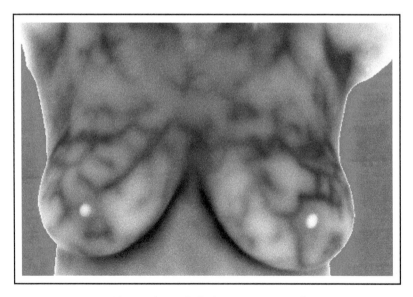

Abnormal vascularity in post-menopausal
woman due to estrogen pellets.

Estrogen is a stimulant, and when you have an excess amount, like most women do today, it stimulates the blood vessels, causing them to become tense, which is referred to as vascularity. Vascularity is stimulation of the existing blood vessels, resulting in dense breasts. You can't have dense breasts and be estrogen-deficient, estrogen stimulates the blood vessels.

Are you ready for another shocker? This is what causes breast pain. The blood vessels are actually smooth muscle and when they become tense or expand, it causes the breasts to be tender. Breast pain is caused by expansion of the blood vessels, not the tissue of the breasts. When you balance out your hormones, reducing estrogen, your breasts soften and pain dissipates. Yes, it really is that simple. Breasts are simple if you understand how they work. Now you can see why breast cancer is increasing - no one is heeding the warning signs. Instead, doctors, including alternative doctors, just suggest more estrogen. Does this make sense, ladies?

## Cramps: The Side Effects

Estrogen has a clotting factor, which is why when a woman is on The Pill she has to sign a waiver acknowledging that The Pill may cause heart attack, stroke, DVT (deep vein thrombosis) and embolisms. Do you know why? It's really quite fascinating. Estrogen is a stimulus to produce blood clots, during birth when the placenta is expelled you will clot and not bleed to death. This is why men bleed longer. Clots in our period are another sign of excess estrogen, since estrogen causes clotting.

Cramps have nothing to do with the ovaries. All pain is from the sympathetic nervous system which controls the smooth muscle. The uterus is smooth muscle and when pressure from blood is built up in the uterus it irritates the smooth muscle, causing pain. This usually happens when a woman is bleeding faster than the blood can exit, causing a buildup of blood and pressure.

What this also means is that estrogen causes fibroids or fibrocystic breasts. Another sign of excess estrogen, from any form synthetic or plant, is fibroids or fibrocystic breasts. Many women can dissipate their fibroids by reducing estrogen therapies or balancing their hormones with progesterone.

Premenstrual syndrome – or PMS – which includes cramps, is mostly due to excess estrogen. When you are balanced, you won't experience cramps or PMS. You can easily do this by removing all estrogen. Some women may use progesterone cream and I highly recommend a customized (no pills or ready-made prescriptions) Chinese or Aryuvedic herbal formula from a highly trained herbalist. Stop dealing with the pain, get treated, naturally, without estrogen.

## Why Estrogen Makes You Crazy

Another side effect of excess estrogen or being hormonally imbalanced is irritability. But, come on, let's call it what it *really* is—crazy! How many jokes do we have to hear about *monster*ating, er, I mean menstruating? Every time we get upset or cry, "it must be your time of the month" is thrown in our face.

But, how many times are they right? Let's face it – "our time" makes us irrational, unbearable and impatient. To add insult to injury, during this time, many of us feel as we have no control, only making the situation worse. We barely recognize ourselves. Then we have to live with the fallout by feeling horrible for hurting the ones we love. And this vicious cycle continues to repeat.

Want to know a secret? All of that "craziness" is *not* normal! Let me repeat that, PMS or "Crazy Time" is *not* normal! If you read one section in this book, make it this one, just for sake of vindication!

We have been brainwashed by doctors and media to believe that PMS and its symptoms, such as being crazy, are normal. Just because everyone experiences it now doesn't mean it's normal. PMS is actually a shallow form of depression. In fact, PMS is a result of excess estrogen, something that also causes weight gain, hair loss, fibroids, dense breasts, symptoms of menopause, breast pain, infertility, and an increase of breast and uterine cancer, just to name a few. PMS is not normal, but actually a side effect of excess estrogen. In fact, research is finally showing Birth Control Pills cause depression. That is why so often times middle age crisis is due to estrogen. If you mistreat menopause symptoms by adding more estrogen, then it can possibly create depression or what many call a mid-life crisis. Menopause is not normal; in fact, my great-grandmother had never heard of menopause and did not have any symptoms. Menopause and coincidentally, a mid-life crisis, are new and now you know why.

But here's the thing: We are *not* estrogen-deficient! If we want to heal ourselves, first we must face the brutal truth. Stop buying into propaganda that wants to sell products/supplements. Eighty percent of breast cancers are fed by estrogen. You know what that means? That means that if we were estrogen-deficient breast cancer numbers would be significantly lower.

Being healthy is balance – a balance between estrogen and progesterone.

When we are going through puberty the first 14 days of our cycle is estrogen-involved. Estrogen is a stimulator, it causes our breasts to grow, and that is why during this time you may feel a tingling sensation due to growth from stimulation. Then the follicular cells, which are creating estrogen, magically transform to luteal cells, which produce progesterone. This fact is key to your well-being! Your body will always make equal amount of estrogen and progesterone from this process. When you understand how your body works you can understand when there is an imbalance or *dis*ease! Progesterone is calming, it's the yin to the yang. It calms the breasts and stops their growth. Everything has a balance or opposite. If we didn't produce progesterone our breasts would continue to grow and we'd all have large breasts.

A normal amount of stimulation is healthy; like a cup of coffee, it gives us energy. But that's not what we're talking about. We're talking about continuous stimulation, we're talking six-Red-Bulls-and-vodka-a-night kind of stimulation, one that keeps you wired and anxious. That's what excess estrogen is doing to you, it's keeping you over-stimulated.

The good news is that we're not doing this to ourselves, at least our bodies aren't. What's causing excess estrogen is not our estrogen, but what is called exogenous, or outside or environmental, estrogen. Here is a quick explanation: Environmental estrogens are bioidentical. Bioidentical does not mean "safe" or "natural," it means same chemical structure. All environmental estrogens are bioidentical to our own.

Environmental estrogens include birth control pills. And we all know what happens when you start these synthetic pills, you go crazy and gain weight! Now you know why, excess estrogen.

When you hear about hormones in food do you think to ask, what hormone? Well, it is estrogen. Estrogen causes weight gain in livestock. Don't be a fat cow! Stop using environmental estrogens.

What many people are shocked to learn is that plants contain hormones, too. Certain plants are phytoestrogens or plant estrogens. The medical community wants you to believe these are weak and they are compared to synthetics. But, as discussed, they are bioidentical to our estrogen. Like the medical community tells us they attach to our estrogen receptors like a lock and key. But think about it, the plant estrogen is binding to our receptor, like a key to a lock. If it is attaching, then it is simulating it. If it couldn't attach, then it wouldn't simulate. That is why hundreds of studies on soy, a plant estrogen, are showing increased breast cancer risk. What our breast thermography research is showing, since the 1980s, is that all plant estrogens, including flax, black cohosh, red clover, sesame, hummus, and lavender, and some others, are also stimulating our receptors.

Estrogen is a stimulator and when it is in excess it causes irritability and anxiety. Do you realize how many relationships are destroyed by excess estrogen? How many couples divorce during menopause?

My mother and father were happily married for twenty-plus years and then my mother started menopause and her doctor put her on Premarin, or synthetic estrogen, and she became incredibly emotional. The full gamut of emotions for five years. After this horrific experience, she understands why men divorce their wives after twenty-plus years of marriage! My father loved my mother and he stood by her, which was very difficult on their marriage and come to learn, actually preventable!

It is heartbreaking to realize how this hormone is affecting our lives. To hear my patients' relief when I tell them crazy is not in their head, but due to excess estrogen, as seen in their thermogram – they appreciate, first that I acknowledge they "feel" out of control and second that I can confirm it with a thermogram! My patients are absolutely relieved to have this horrible side effect decrease with removal of estrogen from their lifestyle, and maybe an additional of progesterone cream to raise progesterone levels. Bad days due to a hormone imbalance are exhausting and now treatable.

When patients first start working with me they mention they feel calmer. That is a sign of hormone balance, ladies. It's tragic knowing women are walking around agitated every day and it is treatable. The best way to achieve hormone balance, decrease menopause symptoms is with testosterone and progesterone while removing all estrogen or following the Estrogen Free® Lifestyle. To treat PMS most women won't need testosterone, but will need to remove all estrogen and maybe supplement with progesterone cream.

Being estrogen-free® is not the answer to *all* your problems, but being hormonally balanced will make life a little easier, for everyone.

Congratulations ladies, you have just completed basic training. It has been clearly explained through physiology that PMS, symptoms of menopause, and early menarche (periods before age fourteen) are *not* normal and are a medical pathology. You now have a basic understanding of how the body should function properly. Throughout this book, I am going to show that when the basics are tampered with, use of estrogen therapies, breast health risk is increased. Reduce risk of breast cancer by avoiding all forms of estrogen. So let's march on…

# 4. Chemical Warfare

## Synthetics: Don't Be So Fake!

I hope that we have learned by this time that we should not add estrogen to our bodies, but rather balance it. Just in case someone needs a push to the other side, we're providing more facts that should be considered scare tactics by pharmaceutical companies and doctors. There is only a small amount of money to be made in promoting wellness or prevention, while there are billions to be made by keeping large amounts of people ill. I believe anyone who works hard or creates something should reap the benefit of their work, but without knowingly doing harm to others. I also believe that Western medicine has its place, especially as emergency medicine. However, within the scope of breast health, we have been fooled for too long and too many have died because of it. Please open your mind and seriously think about the information we've spent years compiling. Be in charge of your own health and your family's.

If women take anything away from this book, I hope at the least they will be compelled to avoid these synthetic hormones, in whatever form.

Avoid the following:

- Synthetic estrogens
- Estrogen replacement therapy (ERTs)

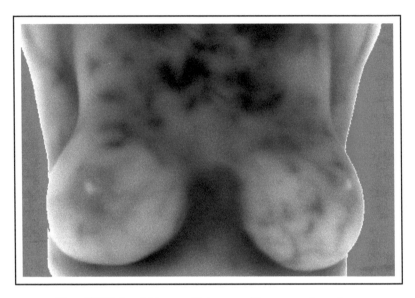

Use of HRTs for eight years. Note unusual hypervascular pattern.

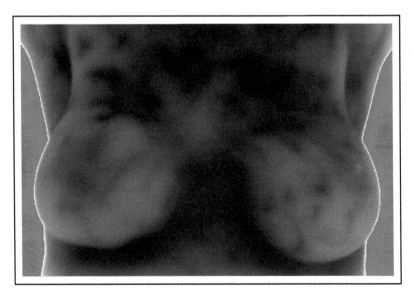

Repeat thermogram. Quit using HRTs. Right breast abnormal

- Hormone replacement therapy (HRTs)
- Bioidentical estrogen therapy (they are not "natural," but processed patches and pellets)
- Birth control pills (BCPs)
- Estrogen rings
- Estrogen injections/shots
- Estrogen vaginal creams
- IUDs with hormones
- Progestins

*Products' side effects by manufacturers are listed in "Collateral Damage."

Many women literally cry to me about aging; they take estrogen, thinking it will help them to stay young. The sad part is that the imbalance of excess estrogen actually accelerates the aging process, but more importantly, it increases our risk of many diseases. Women have literally been sold snake oil. We are brainwashed by propaganda stating that if we take more estrogen, we can avoid growing old. Ladies, it is simply not true—you have been lied to. It is a balance of estrogen *and* progesterone that keeps you healthy and hopefully young.

## Past Battles

Estrogen replacement therapy (ERT) was the first of these inappropriate approaches to women's health. The reason for this book and one of the causes for the rise in breast cancer stems from a *Newsweek* article published in 1964 entitled, "No More Menopause?" Dr. Wilson reported that the "change of life" in women was caused by a decrease in estrogen and progesterone. He promised that women could be beautiful forever with ERT. As it turns out, little to no research was conducted and therefore women served as guinea pigs. By 1975, research confirmed that women on ERT contracted uterine cancer four to eight times more than those who were not.

Such a large number of women died from heart disease, breast cancer, and uterine cancer, that these products were removed from the shelves. This is why many of you have not even heard of ERTs.

Historical evidence shows that unopposed estrogen was proven dangerous. Not to be discouraged, they came up with HRTs, synthetic estrogen, and a synthetic form of progesterone called progestin. They even claimed that HRTs would prevent osteoporosis and reduce heart disease. These are all-out deceptions. HRTs are incapable of any of these claims, but sadly, to this day, many older women are still convinced these theories are true. These lies were sold as truths that many women, including my mother, swallowed every day. Again, same results—too many women got uterine and breast cancer, and too many died.

One of the largest studies on the effects of HRTs was conducted by the Women's Health Initiative (WHI). The results were astounding—the study noted rising rates of breast cancer, heart diseases, strokes, and thromboembolism. In fact, the WHI had to terminate their mass study early due to the increased health risk of the participants. They concluded that HRT usage corresponded to increased breast cancer occurrences. Again, some younger readers may not even know what HRTs are because, after the results were published, prescriptions for HRTs dropped dramatically. Again, history repeated itself. Today, my generation is given bioidentical estrogen. This book will show that history will repeat itself once again when bioidentical estrogen is studied and data is finally collected. Right now, we are the lab rats; bioidentical estrogen is being tested on us.

The current generation is given bioidentical estrogen creams, patches, and pellets, which is just unopposed estrogen, similar to estrogen replacement therapy (ERTs). Bioidentical *does not* mean natural; it simply means biologically similar or same chemical structure. Any particle that is biologically similar or identical to estrogen will fit our body's estrogen receptors. Birth control pills and HRTs, which are synthetic estrogen, are considered bioidentical.

This book is meant to serve as a survival guide, to show you with actual images and facts, that these approaches are just as dangerous. In the same fashion as with the previous treatments (ERTs and HRTs), our system will be flooded with so much excess estrogen, our risk of breast cancer and uterine cancer will increase.

Did you ever wonder how women in the Victorian era or the Wild West dealt with PMS or symptoms of menopause? They didn't! This was not such a widespread occurrence as it is today. Sure, some women went through gynecological issues or pathologies, just as people get sick from time to time, but this was not the cultural norm. How common is it now to hear women complain about the discomfort, and sometimes complete agony, of their periods and symptoms of menopause? Why would we be culturally led to believe that this is natural and just part of being a woman? It is utter nonsense that we envy the rare friend who has no pain or problems with her periods, and accept that being a woman requires us to live a quarter of our reproductive life as a tolerated hell.

As mentioned previously, girls are not supposed to get their period until around the age of fourteen to seventeen, when the body is biologically ready to have children. The wave of preteen menstruation is relatively new. What we now consider normal is actually pathology or a disorder! When the body is hormonally balanced, these issues tend not to exist. Estrogen is integral to reproduction, but when unopposed or in excess, it throws our bodies off balance and causes many problems.

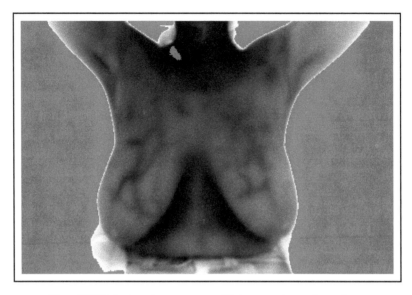

Use of HRTs for twenty seven years. Note unusual vascular pattern.

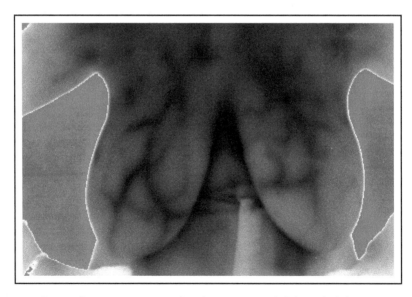

Repeat thermogram note continued progesterone deficiency imbalance.
"At risk" thermogram.

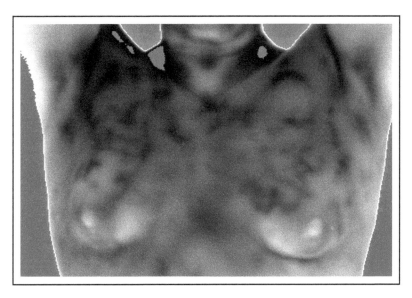

Use of HRTs for one year. Note unusual vascular pattern.

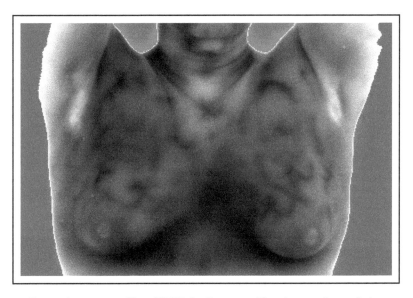

Repeat thermogram. Use of HRTs for four years. Note increased vascularity.
Right breast abnormal

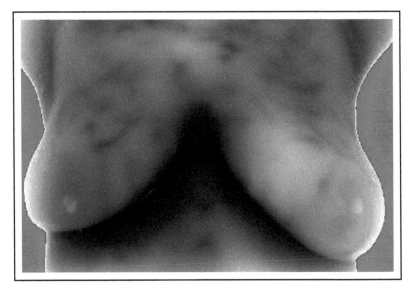

Diagnosed estrogen receptor positive breast cancer four years ago. Using HRTs for three years and bioidentical estrogen for two years. Right breast abnormal.

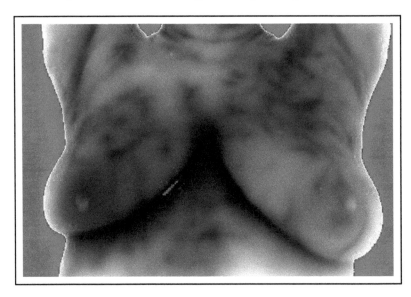

Repeat thermogram three months later. Right breast still abnormal.
Suspicious of possible recurrence.

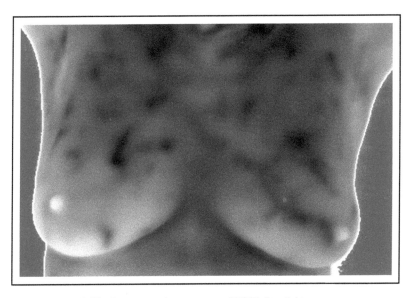

Use BCPs for twenty-three years and HRTs for eighteen years.
Note unusual vascular pattern.

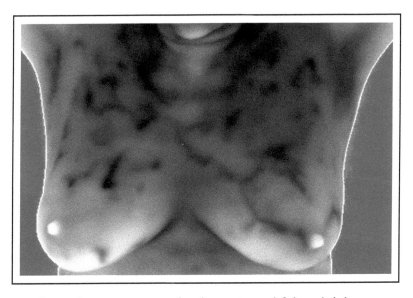

Repeat thermogram note continued progesterone deficiency imbalance.
"At risk" thermogram.

# Battle Wounds

Below is Dr. Lee's list of conditions that can be caused or made worse by excess estrogen. Dr. Lee coined the term *estrogen dominance*.

- Acceleration of the aging process
- Allergies
- Anxiety
- Autoimmune disorders
- Breast tenderness
- Breast cancer
- Decreased sex drive
- Depression
- Fat gain, abdomen, hips and thighs*
- Fatigue fibrocystic breasts
- Foggy thinking
- Gallbladder disease
- Hair loss, another complaint I see often
- Headaches
- Hypoglycemia
- Increased blood clotting and risk of stroke

- Infertility
- Insomnia
- Irritability
- Memory loss
- Migraines, especially premenstrual
- Miscarriage
- Osteoporosis
- Premenopausal bone loss
- PMS
- Seizures, related to menstruation
- Strokes
- Thyroid dysfunction mimicking hypothyroidism
- Uterine cancer
- Uterine fibroids
- Water retention/bloating

* This is my number one complaint in the clinic. These women say that no matter how much they exercise or diet they do not lose this fat. Now you know why—estrogen!

# Bioidenticals: What You Wouldn't Wish on Your Worst Enemy

Bioidenticals are covered further in "Biological Warfare," as estrogen creams are derived from plants. However, it is important to note that doctors use the term bioidentical to sell you pellets or patches, which are processed synthetics, under the title of "natural." What is "natural" about a pellet or patch? Bioidentical does not mean "natural," "plant," or "safe" – it means "same chemical structure" as estrogen; which means birth control pills and hormone replacement, or synthetic, are also bioidentical. It will result in excess estrogen in the body, creating an imbalance thereby increasing risk. That they are being sold as "natural" makes them quite dangerous.

Plants contain hormones, too. Certain plants are phytoestrogens or plant estrogens. The medical community wants you to believe these are weak and they are compared to synthetics. But, as discussed, they are bioidentical to our estrogen. If a plant estrogen can bind to our receptor, like a key to a lock, then it is simulating it! If it couldn't attach, then it wouldn't simulate. That is why hundreds of studies on soy, a plant estrogen, are showing increased breast cancer risk with soy use. What our breast thermography research is showing, since the 1980s, is that all plant estrogens, including flax, black cohosh, red clover, sesame, hummus, and lavender, and many others are also stimulating our receptors.

What many in the medical community want you to believe is that weak or "natural" estrogens block other environmental estrogens, but they don't. Scientists found that if you take equal amounts of estradiol and DES (synthetic estrogen) in the blood, more DES enters the cells than the natural hormone estradiol. What this proves is that our cells have an affinity for synthetic estrogen and actually produce more binding sites.

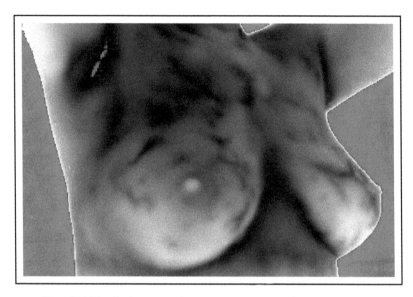

Use of bioidentical estrogen three years. Note unusual vascular pattern.

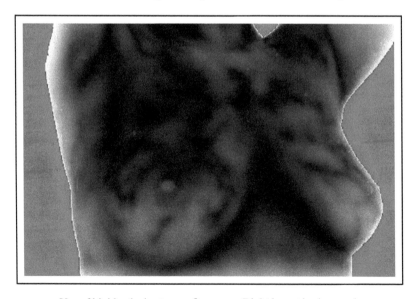

Use of bioidentical estrogen five years. Right breast is abnormal.

# Progestin: The Undercover Synthetic Progesterone

Progestin is a synthetic form of progesterone, and as we have learned, the molecule may be similar but the effects can be very different. Natural progesterone is used and eliminated as needed by the body, whereas progestin is stronger. Its effects are prolonged, and it competes for the same binding sites that natural progesterone utilizes. This will send different feedback information to the body in regards to its hormones and the body will react accordingly to the situation. The problem is that this information is false and unnatural.

Many patients report that their doctor says progesterone and progestin are the same, or that progesterone causes cancer. This is *not* true. Women who undergo infertility treatment are familiar with progesterone since fertility doctors use it instead of progestin to increase the viability of conception. So why do fertility doctors know and understand this important fact, but general practitioners do not? Start asking questions!

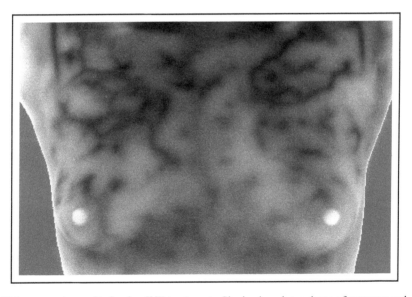

This woman is monitoring her IVF treatments. She is given large doses of estrogen and progesterone for fertility. Note progesterone deficiency imbalance.

Here are some such questions from Dr. Lee, a pioneer in hormone research.

If progesterone and progestin are the same:

- Why do fertility doctors use progesterone and not progestin?
- Why are progestins associated with birth defects, while progesterone is essential for a viable healthy pregnancy?
- Why don't synthetic progestins show up in blood and saliva tests for progesterone levels? In other words, why doesn't taking progestin raise progesterone levels in the body?
- Pregnant women produce 300 mg of progesterone. Why don't they have higher rates of breast cancer like women who do use progestins?
- Why doesn't progesterone cause the side effects of progestins?

Now remember, progestins are found in birth control pills (BCPs), hormone replacement therapy (HRTs) and some IUDs. Please read *all* about the adverse effects of progestin in the "Breast Canswers" chapter and "Collateral Damage" appendix.

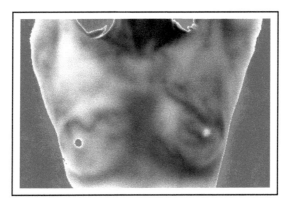

Use of BCPs for twenty five years and IUD with hormones for four years.
Abnormal thermogram.

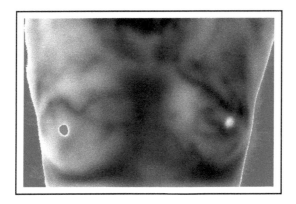

Repeat thermogram with continued IUD use. Note hypervascular pattern in left breast.

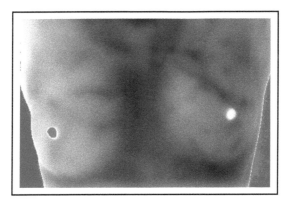

Repeat thermogram. Removal of IUD for six months plus use of progesterone cream. Note decrease in vascularity, however left breast is still concerning.

# Birth Control Pills (BCPs): Being Safe Has Never Been So Dangerous

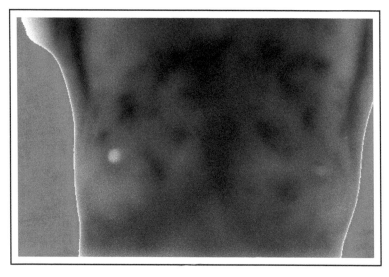

Twenty-six year old. Use BCPs for three years. Note unusual vascular pattern.

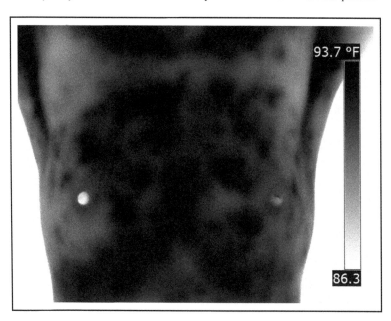

Repeat thermogram. Six years of BCPs usage.
Note increased vascularity. Left breast abnormal.

Before we dive into this topic, I must state that this book is not saying that young women should not have options for contraception. Rather, we should be informed of the risks and make educated decisions for ourselves. That said, here comes some scary stuff.

BCPs are handed out like candy for contraception or the treatment of menstrual pathologies, which is especially detrimental to developing women. Breasts do not fully mature until age twenty-five and are adversely affected by unopposed estrogen. A teenage girl who is on BCPs increases her risk of breast cancer by as much as four times—the younger the start, the higher the risk. Sadly, we live in a society that claims to be fighting a "war on drugs," but at the same time, "drug czars" deal out pills that potentially cause cancer. How did we get to this state of affairs when, as parents, you fear that your children may experiment with drugs when, in reality, they already are, under the euphemism of a pharmaceutical? Many women my age were put on BCPs in their teenage years for severe menstrual pain because doctors were incapable of treating this medical disorder. In actuality, this condition is easily treated with holistic medicine and the removal of all estrogen from women's lifestyles.

Most forms of BCP have either synthetic estrogens, progestin (synthetic progesterone), or both. These are released to provide a steady stream of hormones that inhibits the feedback for FSH and LH production. No FSH means there is no egg production, while no LH means there is no egg release; and therefore, no corpus luteum. The creation of the corpus luteum is the only direct supply of natural progesterone that the female body has.

"But the pill gives us estrogen and progesterone. So isn't everything balanced?" First of all, if everything was balanced, why wouldn't we produce an egg? Second, these are not *our* estrogen and progesterone, but rather synthetic mimics of our own. This is not the same. Molecules have been added or subtracted so that they can be patented and sold. Since these hormones are an imperfect copy, it simply does not work exactly like our own and has a negative effect on our body and breasts. These synthetics are strong and toxic, with many linked to cancer and other serious side effects.

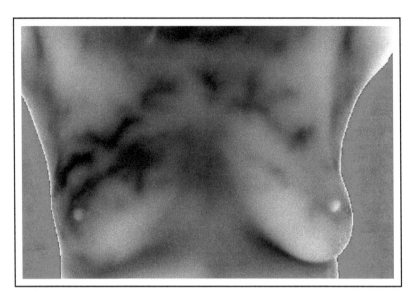

Use BCPs for twelve years. Estrogen receptor positive DCIS right breast.

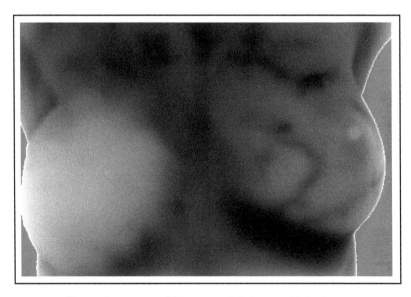

Repeat thermogram. Mastectomy right breast with implants.
Note unusual vascular pattern left breast.

Many girls experience endometriosis or other serious gynecological issues. Unfortunately, most western doctors lack the knowledge to treat these pathologies so they prescribe BCPs to mask the symptoms. Often times, this will lead to a hysterectomy because the underlying issue was never treated. Holistic medicine can successfully treat endometriosis and many other stubborn gynecological issues quite effectively.

So how does all this affect our breasts? As we learned before, breast tissue does not fully mature until age twenty-five. The cells of the breast receive information, like all other cells in the body, when molecules, including hormones, come into contact with their outer surface. This contact sends a message throughout the cell that influences the genetic material, DNA. As these synthetic estrogens communicate with the cells, they alter a genetic response. BCPs deplete the body of B6 and folic acid, which protects DNA. Those cells then replicate exponentially with the genetic material holding on to its previous programming. As an example, imagine an old Xerox machine. You make the first copy, which is pretty good, and copy that copy, which is still okay but not quite the same. Now repeat this a couple hundred or thousand times, and what do you end up with? Definitely not the original.

Keep in mind that all of this is happening in a young developing woman with a metabolism that is working overtime and breasts that are most likely just beginning to grow. In addition, progesterone is the protective counter to estrogen, and since the pill has eliminated this protection, our "breast friends" have lost their defense.

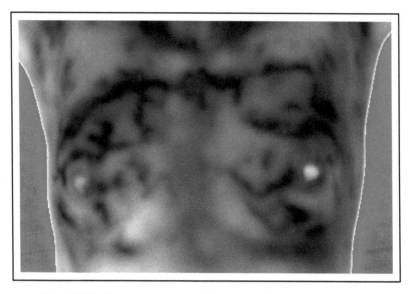

Use of BCPs for twenty two years. Note unusual hypervascular pattern.
Abnormal Thermogram.

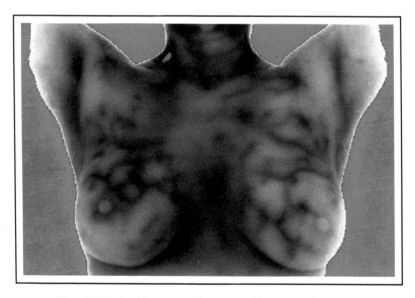

Use of BCPs for thirty years. Note unusual hypervascular pattern.
Abnormal thermogram right breast.

## Other Contraceptives: Same Mistakes

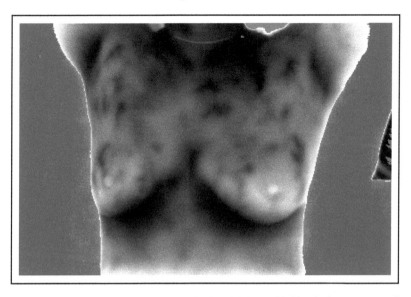

This woman is currently using an estrogen ring in addition to bioidentical estrogen patch and bioidentical cream. "At risk" thermogram. Progesterone deficiency imbalance.

The birth control shot or injection is a synthetic form of progesterone, and as we have thoroughly covered by now, synthetic hormones are not the same or the equivalent to our natural hormones. In addition, the shot alters your cervical mucus and uterine lining, creating a harsher environment for sperm to reach the uterus and minimizing the ability for a fertilized egg to attach to the uterus. The shot is administered into the muscle or beneath the skin via injections that are performed at various frequencies, some every week, others every three months. Variations in the frequency of administering this drug are based on the intended use of the drug, as it is not only used for contraception. Many accounts of sterility are believed to be caused by the use of this contraceptive. There is currently a class action lawsuit against the companies that produce these shots, with claimants seeking damages for their side effects.

The ring is a form of contraception containing both estrogen and progestin (synthetics) in a ring that is placed within the vagina, allowing the hormones to be absorbed into the bloodstream. These elevated levels of both estrogen and progestin send a chemical signal which inhibits the release of the hormones needed to initiate egg maturation, and therefore, halting egg production. After three weeks, the ring is removed, triggering a shedding of the endometrium, at which time the period occurs. A new ring is then inserted on the twenty-ninth day to restart the cycle.

The side effects of synthetic estrogen and progestin are too numerous to include in this chapter, so they are listed in the appendix, "Collateral Damage." Brand names of products were removed, but all the side effects are taken straight from the manufacturers. It should be noted that many of these companies are involved in class action lawsuits.

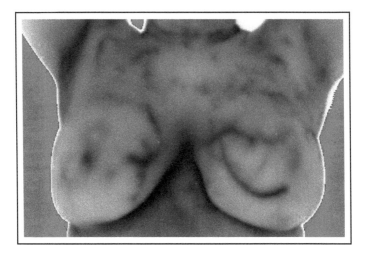

Use BCPs for eighteen years. Note unusual vascular pattern.

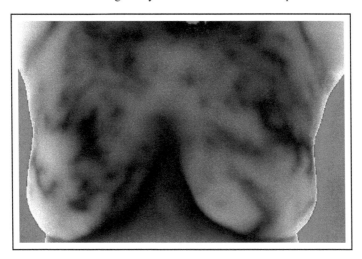

Repeat thermogram. Right breast abnormal.

# Safety First: Copper IUD

Dr. Hobbins wants this to be very clear: the only safe and effective form of birth control is the copper IUD—just the copper non-hormonal IUD, *not* the IUD with hormones. The copper IUD is not only incredibly effective, less than one out of one-hundred women who use it will get pregnant each year, but it doesn't raise the risk of damaging your fertility in the future. Rest assured you can't be poisoned by the copper and it can last up to twelve years with no side effects.

The copper works two ways: First, copper alters the thickness of the mucosa in the cervix so that the sperm can't penetrate it. Second, copper is an effective spermicide not just with women, but men as well. The sperm are killed before they can penetrate or fertilize an egg. Copper safely works by releasing copper ions that cause sperm phagocytosis, which means the sperm is killed - the ions actually detach the head of the sperm from the tail and then leaves it to be devoured by other cells. The copper ions remain local and won't affect the rest of your body.

To be crystal clear, you want to avoid the IUD with synthetic hormones, it increases risk of breast cancer and increased vascularity in the breasts. The non-hormonal copper IUD is safe for all ages and begins working when inserted. I personally use it as well and suggest it to all my patients.

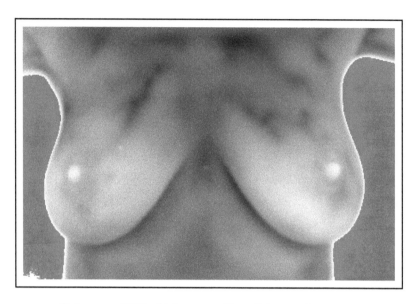

Before use of IUD with hormones. Note slight vascular pattern.

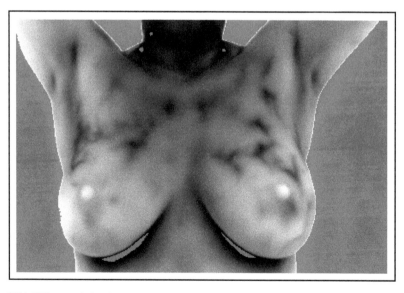

With IUD containing hormones. Note increased vascularity. Abnormal thermogram.

"Chemical warfare" plainly exposes that synthetic estrogen use increases many health risks. A couple of women imaged in this book are currently participating in class action lawsuits against the pharmaceutical companies that produced these dangerous forms of "medicine." Medicine is meant to treat, not increase disease.

Breast cancer rates increased in correlation with the introduction of estrogen therapies! When are you going to stop walking for a cure and realize that if you want to decrease breast cancer, stop taking estrogen? Around 80 percent of all breast cancers are estrogen driven. Remove the product that is increasing breast cancer, estrogen! It is that simple! We would see breast cancer numbers drop dramatically, if women realized this simple truth. Don't become a statistic—educate yourself and join the battle for truth.

# 5. Biological Warfare

## Phytoestrogens: Natural Disasters

Phytoestrogen is a term used to describe estrogens that are derived from plants. They are similar in structure and function to the body's estrogens, but nonetheless, these are not natural occurring hormones; they are environmental estrogens. Furthermore, the reason for this book is to show that the majority of women are progesterone deficient with excess estrogen.

The number of women adding these substances to their diet is of enormous concern. Every little bit of estrogen, especially exogenous estrogen, that we can limit will benefit us greatly. Unfortunately, due to propaganda, misinformation, and rational ignorance, few women are aware of the extent that they are in contact with phytoestrogens or their harmful effects. Soy and flax contain plant-based estrogens that have the exact same effect on the body as commercial-grade synthetic estrogen injected in farm animals—therefore, eating soy and flax is as harmful as consuming nonorganic beef, poultry, and pork products with regard to hormones.

Soy and flax contain phytoestrogens and do *not* reduce the risk of breast cancer. They actually stimulate the receptors in the breasts which results in vascularity in the breasts, therefore increasing the risk of breast cancer. It is important to realize that estrogen feeds or stimulates a large percentage of breast cancers, and this includes estrogens from plants. There is no difference in environmental estrogens-synthetic estrogens, ecoestrogens or phytoestrogens. *All* these forms of estrogen stimulate breast cells or increase vascularity, which may lead to increased neoangiogenesis, the process that causes breast cancer to become invasive. In the early 70s, Dr. Judah Folkman published an article that hypothesized that tumors caused new blood vessel growth or neoangiogenesis. He later demonstrated that angiogenesis was necessary for neoplasia to move from in situ (in its original place ducts) to an invasive disease.

We will walk you through the validity of soy and especially flax studies. Keep in mind, a medical theory needs to be implemented in the body with success in order to be considered valid and not just hypothesis. Studies showing success with soy and flax have not successfully been completed when transferred into a human being. We are showing the reader that these hypotheses are invalid when transferred into the human body as years of thermographic imaging shows increased risk.

Studies can be manipulated and are often done so to sell a product. Two prominent editors of two highly prestigious medical journals have revealed to the public that as many as half of medical studies are at best unreliable, and at worst simply false.

Dr. Richard Horton, editor-in-chief of the Lancet, published a statement in 2015 finally proclaiming that an appalling amount of research is unreliable if not completely false. "Much of the scientific literature, perhaps half, may simply be untrue. Afflicted by studies with small sample sizes, tiny effects, invalid exploratory analyses, and flagrant conflicts of interest, together with an obsession for pursuing fashionable trends of dubious importance, science has taken a turn towards darkness."

Dr. Marcia Angell, a physician and former editor-in-chief of the New England Journal of Medicine, has also made a similar statement. "It is simply no longer possible to believe much of the clinical research that is published, or to rely on the judgment of trusted physicians or authoritative medical guidelines. I take no pleasure in this conclusion, which I reached slowly and reluctantly over my two decades as an editor of the New England Journal of Medicine," she has stated.

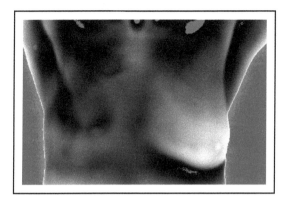

Woman is monitoring breast cancer treatments. Normal thermogram.

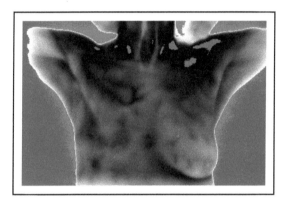

Repeat thermogram after use of soy and flax supplements for three months. Note unusual vascular pattern. "At risk" thermogram.

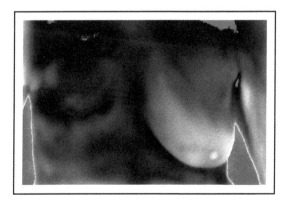

Repeat thermogram after removal of flax and soy supplementation for one year. Normal thermogram.

# Avoid All Phytoestrogens

Numbers below were obtained from "Implications of Phytoestrogen Intake for Breast Cancer," *The Cancer Journal of Clinicians*, 2008.

| *Phytoestrogens to avoid* | *Total PE (phytoestrogens) units per ¼ cup* |
|---|---|
| Flax | 163,133 |
| Tofu | 8,688 |
| Soy Milk (8.5oz) | 7,390 |
| Veggie burger | 484 |
| Hummus/garbanzo beans | 605 |
| Sesame seed | 2,722 |
| Multigrain bread | 2,207 |
| Dried apricot | 165 |

| *Phytoestrogens to limit* | |
|---|---|
| Almonds | 48.5 |
| Cashews | 41.5 |
| Garlic (tbsp) | 103 |
| Alfalfa sprout | 45 |
| Black Tea | 21 |
| Green Tea | 32 |
| Wine, red (6oz) | 95 |

Other phytoestrogens to avoid:

- Soy products including soy cheese, soy meats, soy cereals, and soy crackers
- Supplements or vitamins with soy added
- Flax-containing products including flax milk, flax crackers, flax cereal, flax seeds, and flax oils
- Beer

More popular phytoestrogens to avoid:

- Any women's supplement starting with "Est" for estrogen or "Phyto" for plant or "Meno" for menstruation or menopause.

  - Aloe (A. barbadensis Mill)
  - Ashwagandha/Indian ginseng (Withania somnifera)
  - Asian ginseng (Panax ginseng, Ren Shen)
  - Astragalus/Huang qi (Astragalus membranaceus)
  - Black Cohosh (Cimicifuga racemosa, Sheng Ma)
  - Burdock root (Arctium lappa)
  - Chasteberry (Vitex agnuscastus)
  - Dong Gui/Dong Quai (Angelica sinensis)
  - Fo-Ti/Ye Jiao Teng (Polygonum multiflorum)
  - Hops (Humulus lupulus)
  - Kudzu root (Pueraria montana)
  - Lavender (Lavandula angustifolia, L. officinalis)
  - Licorice (Glycyrrhiza glabra, Gan Cao)
  - North American ginseng (Panax quinquefolius, Xi Yang Shen)
  - Milk thistle (Silybum marianum)
  - Mistletoe (Viscum album)
  - Red Clover (Trifolium pretense)
  - Rhubarb (Rheum rhabarbarum)
  - Turmeric (Curcuma longa)
  - Xiang Fu (Rhizoma Cyperi Rotundi)

Avoid these estrogenic essential oils:

- Aniseed
- Basil
- Chamomile
- Cinnamon
- Clary sage
- Coriander
- Cypress
- Evening primrose
- Fennel

- Geranium
- Lavender
- Oregano
- Peppermint
- Rose
- Rosemary
- Sage
- Tea Tree
- Thyme

For updated and detailed list: estrogen-free.com

Breast thermography evaluates the health of the breasts and monitors changes due to phytoestrogen use. Below are thermograms showing increased risk from using flax, primrose oil and black cohosh.

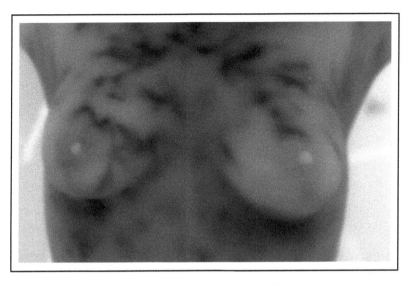

Initial thermogram in young woman in early thirties. Note unusual vascular
pattern in right breast. Abnormal thermogram.

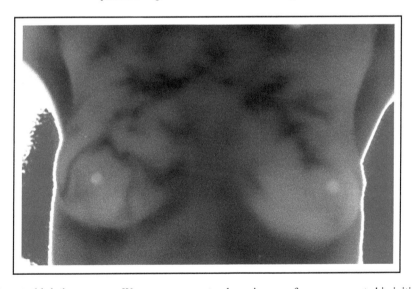

Repeat, third, thermogram. Woman *now* reports a lump in area of concern reported in initial
thermogram. Note increase in vascularity in right breast. Physician had recommended flax
as a "weak" estrogen and DIM a "natural estrogen blocker" for breast health after initial
thermograms. Abnormal thermogram.

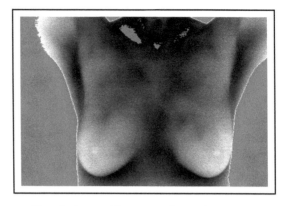

Use of primrose. Note unusual vascular patterns.

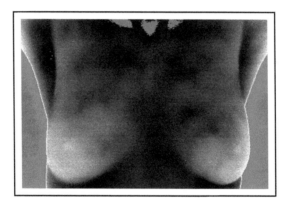

Repeat thermogram four years later. Still using primrose oil. Note increase in vascularity. Severe progesterone deficiency.

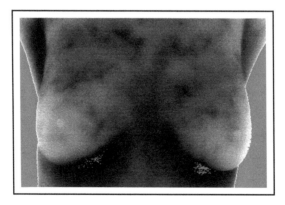

Repeat thermogram one year later. Still using primrose oil. Note unusual hypervascular pattern. Severe progesterone deficiency.

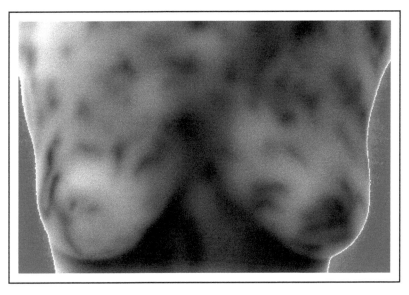

No hormones. Note unusual vascular patterns. Progesterone deficient.

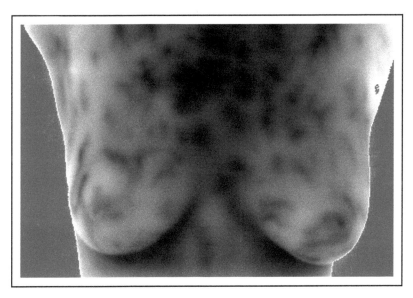

Repeat thermogram four years later. Use of black cohosh.
Note increase in vascularity. Severe progesterone deficiency.

Listed above are the majority of phytoestrogens you should avoid or limit. Notice flax is nineteen times more potent than soy! Although many substances contain estrogenic properties, our focus is on the largest and most heavily consumed, namely, soy and flax. Yes, these are your enemy, though many of us have heard quite the opposite. If soy and flax are supposedly beneficial to women's issues and breasts, and these substances are now, more than ever, consumed in higher quantities, why do women still experience PMS and symptoms of menopause? Why are so many women infertile? Why girls are starting their periods at extremely low ages like seven? And though somewhat rare, why are more men getting breast cancer?

The following excerpts from a study based article in *The Cancer Journal of Clinicians* (2008) titled "Implications of Phytoestrogen Intake for Breast Cancer" sheds further light on, and support of, this position:

> Interest in phytoestrogens has been fueled by data that suggests a decreased risk of breast cancer in women from countries with high phytoestrogen consumption. Women with a history of breast cancer may seek out these "natural" hormones in the belief that they are safe or perhaps even protective against recurrence. Interpretation of research studies regarding phytoestrogen intake and breast cancer risk is hampered by differences in dietary measurement, lack of standardization of supplemental sources, differences in metabolism amongst individuals, and the retrospective nature of much of the research in this area.
>
> Data regarding the role of phytoestrogens in breast cancer prevention are conflicting... In several placebo-controlled randomized trials among breast cancer survivors, soy has *not* been found to decrease menopausal symptoms.
>
> There is very little human data on the role of phytoestrogens in preventing breast cancer recurrence, but the few studies conducted do *not* support a protective role.

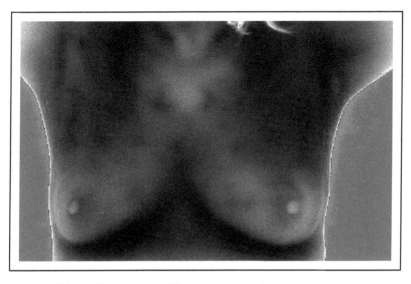

Use of bioidentical estrogen with progesterone and testosterone seven years.
Note unusual vascular pattern.

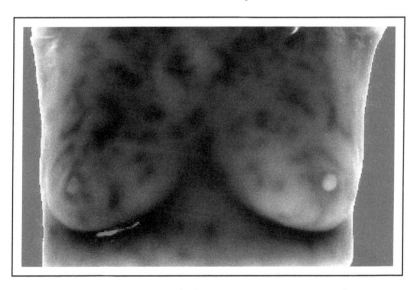

Repeat thermogram. Use of bioidentical estrogen with progesterone and testosterone
ten years. Note increased vascularity. Right breast abnormal

Ladies, be aware of propaganda and what they want you to believe versus what you actually see happening with your friends and family. If we consume more and more of these so-called beneficial estrogen-rich foods, why does breast cancer continue to rise? In fact, why are other developing countries who have adopted our "western diet" showing increases as well?

> "Discovering Dr. Wendy Sellens on YouTube and then purchasing this book are two of the most valuable finds in my adult life, in the search for clarity and direction about how to achieve breast health, and to gain peace of mind. Dr. Wendy clearly explains fifty years of thermography research, facts and truth as originally brought forth by Dr. William B. Hobbins, a pioneer in Breast Thermography. She expresses the truth in a concise and thorough manner, with the purpose of helping women emerge from the estrogen overload quagmire that we find ourselves in through consuming processed foods, supplements, estrogen-laced cosmetics, bath and body products, and even the water we drink. Our foods and environment are saturated with estrogens, synthetic and 'natural'. The book is filled with images of breast thermography results, which clearly show the connection between estrogen overload and increased vascularity in the breast. Dr. Wendy teaches us about hormonal balance. She writes about natural progesterone, how to use it properly, and the best sources to assure it does not contain any phytoestrogens.
>
> It is very disconcerting that 'famous' natural doctors, nutritionists, and so-called holistic health experts have continued to promote soy and flax as health foods, and specifically for breast health! They claim phytoestrogens are weaker estrogens, which block the estrogens that can cause breast cancer. Thermography results as illustrated in this book show that the increase in vascularity in the

breast is the same whether natural or synthetic estrogens are used.

In chapter 12 there is a section 'Become Estrogen Free'. Included in this section are lists of Phytoestrogens to avoid, and ones to limit. As I evaluated the foods and products I regularly consumed, I was literally shocked to discover how pervasive these phytoestrogens are in supplements, processed foods, bath and body products (even those that claim to be organic!). I was also alarmed to realize the eggs advertised as containing omega-3 could be estrogenic, even those that are advertised as 'pastured' or 'free-range', because many farmers give their chickens supplemental feed containing flax and soy. Thankfully, I found a local farmer who does not feed her chickens either one.

The valuable information in this book presented logically and with clarity is a wonderful gift, and one that gives me a solid direction with great hope that I can achieve breast health and lower my risk for cancer. My only regret is that I did not find this information years ago. I will continue to follow the work of Dr. Wendy Sellens, and recommend this book very highly to every woman."

Maire

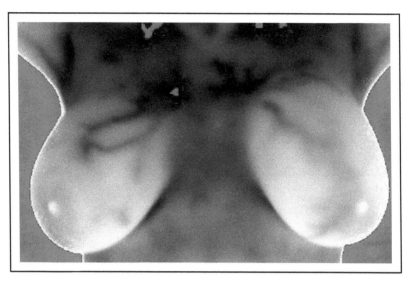

Use of bioidentical estrogen with progesterone and testosterone eight years.
Note unusual vascular pattern.

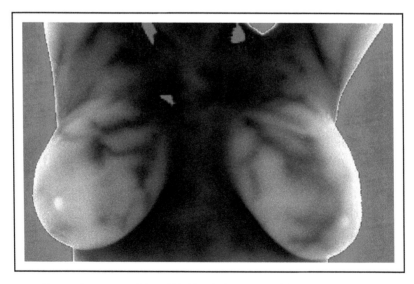

Repeat thermogram. Use of bioidentical estrogen with progesterone and
testosterone nine years. Note increased vascularity.

## Soy: Nature's Way to Tag 'Em and Bag 'Em

If you are still eating soy, I urge you to wake the heck up. Since the '80s, Dr. Hobbins has advised women to stop using soy due to the estrogenic effect it has on our breasts. Soy contains phytoestrogens, including fermented soy and isoflavones. As discussed earlier, phytoestrogens are plant-derived estrogen and do *not* reduce the risk of breast cancer but rather increase risk. Through the use of thermograms, we can see that soy stimulates the breasts, resulting in increased vascularity and neoangiogenesis in the breasts, thus increasing the risk of breast cancer. Even plant estrogen feeds or stimulates breast cancer.

If soy was "healthy" for the breasts, women who regularly consumed it would have nonvascular breasts that would be evidenced by a lack of stimulation, and therefore, no increased risk. This is just not the case. Since the '80s and the introduction of soy, Dr. Hobbins has noticed an enormous increase in vascular breasts. Stop and think about the correlation of the predominance of soy in our food products since the '80s with the continuing rise in breast cancer plus the earlier age of menarche (first period).

Like most legumes, soy is a toxic plant. It must be processed several times to reduce its toxicity for human consumption. The process of making temph and tofu is considered an art in some countries due to the ability to naturally reduce the toxicity of the soy bean. The process and amount of petrochemicals used are so toxic that some speculate that eating soy is as harmful as smoking. You can read more about this in *The Whole Soy Story: The Dark Side of America's Favorite Health Food*, by Kaayla T Daniel.

After the first edition of this book was published Dr. Daniel, former vice president of Weston A. Price Foundation, read our book and reviewed our research and included our soy and flax thermographic research in her blogs and in the fall 2014 publication of *Wise Traditions.* In addition, an RN and breast cancer survivor included our flax thermograms and research in the fourth edition of her book, *Cancer Free? Are You Sure?*

# Stealth Soy: It's Hiding throughout Your Cupboard

"But I don't eat much soy." I hear this from my patients all the time during their nutritional consultation. What they do not know is that soy is used as an emulsifier in nearly all processed foods. In the '80s, Dr. Hobbins found a correlation between three important factors in regards to what he saw repeatedly with breast thermography images: (1) there was an increase in the stimulation or vascularity or neoangiogenesis in the breasts of the female population, (2) that there was a rise in the occurrence of breast cancer, and (3) it was at this time that soy was introduced into all processed foods as an emulsifier, a glue that holds food particles together.

What these patients are instructed to do, as I suggest you do, is go into the pantry and read every box, bag, or bottle ingredient labels. If something has soy in it (look for the word soy, soya, soy emulsifier, soy lecithin), which most do, place an "X" on the container so that when this item runs out there is a marker to find a nonphytoestrogen containing alternative. By doing this, the patient doesn't have to throw everything out of their kitchen all at once, but rather slowly shifts to an estrogen-free diet. Most processed foods, including organic, have soy in it—bread, cereal, infant formula, health shakes, protein bars, crackers, peanut butter, cookies, cakes, salad dressings, pastas, candy bars—basically anything in a bag, box, can, or bottle. Also, most supplements and vitamins contain soy, so these have to be replaced as well if one wishes to continue using supplements.

Childhood obesity is becoming a national concern. It's probably no surprise that children nowadays eat too many processed foods. I believe that the addition of soy into these products since the '80s has contributed to the rise of childhood obesity. The supplementation of soy in processed food seriously needs to be addressed. I grew up in the '70s and '80s. Processed foods were very prevalent in our diet—we are the microwave frozen dinner generation. But we didn't have too many issues with our weight. I truly believe the soy that is found in all processed foods increases the risk for childhood obesity. This is no different than the use of hormones to fatten livestock, which is estrogen!

A reduction of soy and processed foods will decrease the risk of child-hood obesity. Just follow the tips in the nutrition chapter to reduce estrogen in your family's diet.

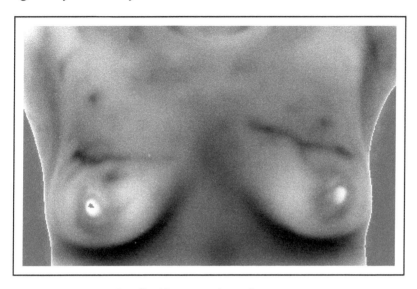

Soy diet. Note unusual vascular pattern.

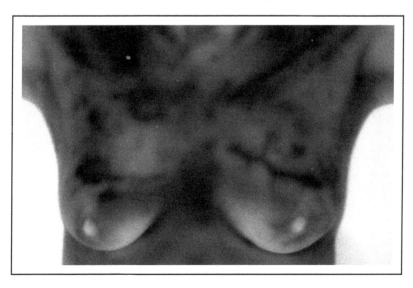

Repeat thermogram one year later. Soy diet. Note increased vascularity.

War Story:

A sixteen-year-old girl came in and told me she was losing her hair. She was a vegan who consumed large amounts of soy. The developmental years are the most important years in a child's life. In Chinese medicine, it is possible to treat children zero to seven years with great results. They are more responsive, and it is easy to alter their constitution if there is an illness or a family history of one, and change the future of their condition or health. Therefore, it is imperative to nourish and strengthen during the developmental years, until around twenty-one years of age.

This particular girl damaged her foundation by not consuming healthy animal fats, protein, and blood, which are the building blocks of the human body. In Chinese medicine, hair is an extension of blood. When blood is full in the body, our skin, hair, and nails flourish. As we age, blood is shunted to protect the organs and hair, skin and nails become brittle.

As a result of this health choice, she consumed large amounts of a toxic plant (soy) that is highly processed, sprayed with pesticides, and is a genetically modified food. Furthermore, she overconsumed a plant estrogen, so she is not hormonally balanced. A side effect of excess estrogen is hair loss.

If you are still eating soy and clinging to the belief it is "healthy," I strongly urge to read the groundbreaking book, *The Whole Soy Story: The Dark Side of America's Favorite Health Food* by Kaayla T. Daniel, PhD, CNN. You will never eat soy again. Below is a summary of how unhealthy soy is, taken from *The Whole Soy Story* by Kaayla Daniel and *Cinderella's Dark Side* by Sally Fallon and Mary G. Enig, PhD.

> Soybeans and soy products contain high levels of phytic acid, which inhibits assimilation of calcium, magnesium, copper, iron, and zinc. The soybean has one of the highest phytate levels of any grain or legume.
>
> Soaking, sprouting, and long, slow cooking does not neutralize phytic acid. Diets high in phytic acid

have been shown to cause growth problems in children. Trypsin inhibitors in soy interfere with protein digestion and may cause pancreatic disorders.

Test animals showed stunted growth when fed trypsin inhibitors from soy.

The plant estrogens found in soy, called phytoestrogens, disrupt endocrine function, which is the proper functioning of the glands that produce hormones, and have the potential to cause infertility and promote breast cancer in adult women.

Hypothyroidism and thyroid cancer may be caused by soy phytoestrogens.

Infant soy formula has been linked to autoimmune thyroid disease.

Circulating concentrations of isoflavones in infants fed soy-based formula were 13,000 to 22,000 times higher than plasma estradiol concentrations in infants on cow's milk formula.

An infant exclusively fed soy formula receives the estrogenic equivalent, based on body weight, of at least five birth control pills per day. By contrast, almost no phytoestrogens have been detected in dairy-based infant formula or in human milk, even when the mother consumes soy products.

A study of babies born to vegetarian mothers who ate a vegetarian diet during pregnancy had a fivefold greater risk of delivering a boy with hypospadias, a birth defect of the penis. The authors of the study suggested this was caused by greater exposure to phytoestrogens in soy foods popular with vegetarians.

Rats born to mothers that were fed an isoflavone called genistein had decreased birth weights and onset of puberty occurred earlier in male offspring.

Participants who consumed tofu in mid-life had lower cognitive function in late life and a greater incidence of Alzheimer's disease and dementia and "looked five years older." White and his colleagues blamed the negative effects on isoflavones—a finding that supports an earlier study in which postmenopausal women with higher levels of circulating estrogen experienced greater cognitive decline.

Soy has been found to increase the body's need for vitamin B12 and vitamin D.

Fragile soy proteins are exposed to high temperatures during processing to produce soy protein isolate and textured vegetable protein, making them unsuitable for human digestion.

This same process results in the formation of toxic lysinoalanine and highly carcinogenic nitrosamines.

The potent neurotoxin MSG, (also called free glutamic acid), is formed during soy food processing. Many soy products have extra MSG added as well.

Soybeans also contain haemagglutinin, a clot-promoting substance that causes red blood cells to clump together.

An interesting note is that in the last few years, soy-based foods (milk, cheese, pseudo-meats, etc.) have been imported into Asian countries. It will be interesting to see the outcome if soy foods become popular in these nonsoy dominant countries.

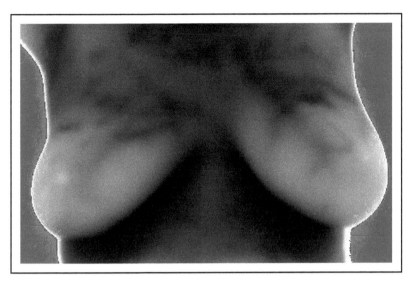

Soy diet. Note unusual vascular pattern.

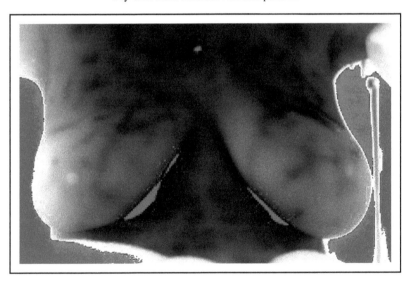

Repeat thermogram one year later. Soy diet. Note increased vascularity.
Left breast abnormal.

## Flax: Friend or Foe

In this section we will demonstrate the harmful effects of flax, a popular "health" supplement that is affecting women's risk for breast and uterine cancer. Take your time, read the evidence, look at the thermograms, and then make an educated decision about the effects of flax on you and your family.

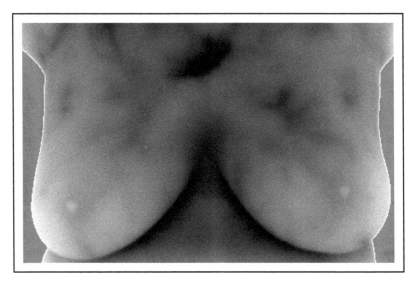

Before flax. Note mild vascular pattern.

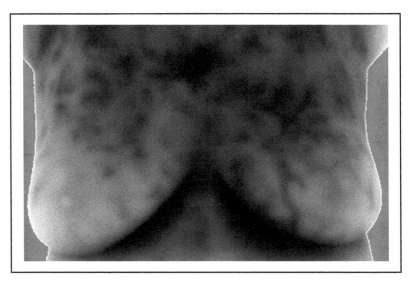

Repeat thermogram. Two years of using flax. Note major increase in vascularity.

Flax pilot study performed by Wendy Sellens April 2010.

> To demonstrate that flax, a phytoestrogen, increased risk by increasing vascularity or neoangiogenesis in the breasts. Thermographic monitoring was to be performed for six months, every thirty days. Patient consumed manufacturers' daily suggested amount of flax oil. After four weeks, patient reported inability to perform work requirements, gained ten pounds, and experienced severe mood swings, including anger, crying, irritability, breast tenderness, abdominal bloating and severe cramps. Symptoms were so adverse that patient believed she was pregnant. Due to increased health symptoms and breast health risk, patient discontinued study after six weeks.

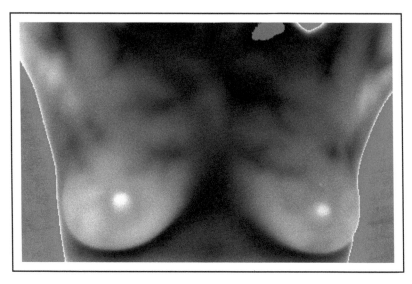

Before use of flax.

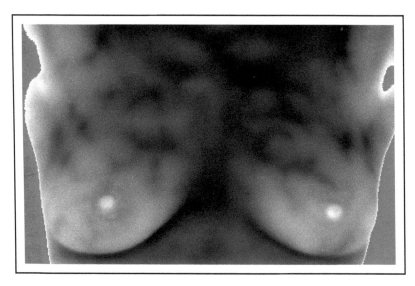

Repeat thermogram six weeks after flax use. Note increased vascularity.

Below is an article Dr. Hobbins and I wrote following my pilot study on flax.

## The Flax Myth
## Published September 2010

Breast cancer is on the rise. The American Cancer Society estimated that the number of women diagnosed increased from 175, 000 in 1999 to 211,300 in 2003. Not only are the numbers increasing, but the women afflicted with breast cancer are getting younger.

One of the reasons for this increase is due to the rise in environmental estrogens found in our food, water, air and household products. Phytoestrogens, one type of environmental estrogen, are derived from plants. They mimic estrogen in the body, but because they come from a plant, the effect is different. Soy, flax and bioidentical products contain Phytoestrogens.

When estrogen becomes dominate in the system, it creates a hormonal imbalance, often seen as PMS and symptoms of menopause, along with an increased risk for breast cancer. Estrogens, as well as Phytoestrogens, cause breast cells to grow rapidly, so if there is a cancer cell present, it has the possibility of being stimulated as well.

Stimulation of breast cells in breast thermography is referred to as "vascularity." Vascularity is stimulation from all types of estrogens and produces an increase in blood flow. In normal, healthy, balanced breasts there is no vascularity. With the Bales Tip infrared image analysis, an integral element of breast thermography, measurement of an increase or growth of vascularity can be monitored. Hormone levels of estrogen and progesterone can be determined with accuracy because the analysis measures the effects of all estrogens, including environmental.

Most women who are analyzed are estrogen stimulated or relatively free of adequate progesterone to reduce the effects of estrogen. Again, these symptoms are seen as PMS or the side effects of menopause. If a woman is hormonally balanced, she will not experience either. We recently conducted a pilot study to prove that flax, which contains Phytoestrogens, would increase breast cell stimulation, or vascularity, thus putting the breast at risk. It was challenging to find a subject who was relatively balanced to proceed with the study.

The pilot study was to last for six months. Due to the fact that we added an exogenous estrogen, flax, to a relatively hormonally stable system, the subject had such adverse side effects she refused to continue. Her side effects are similar to those caused by the synthetic estrogens found in birth control pills: severe mood swings, breast tenderness, weight gain around the abdomen and severe cramps. As seen in the accompanying images, six weeks was enough time to prove that flax, which contains Phytoestrogens, increases vascularity in the breasts, thus increasing risk.

There is a misconception that women need more estrogen—women are bombarded all day by environmental estrogens. Most women are actually progesterone deficient due to this environmental stress. We rarely see women who need estrogen. At one time, flax may have been a great health supplement, but now, due to the prevalence of environmental estrogens, this is simply not true—it actually increases the risk of breast cancer.

Try it yourself! Remember, most of you are estrogen dominant or progesterone deficient, so you may already have these complaints. If you add flax to your diet, watch the symptoms increase. Conversely, if you are taking flax, stop and see what happens. When we have our patients remove flax from their diet, they notice a decrease in weight, breast tenderness, hair loss, hot flashes and PMS, with an improvement in sleep, energy and mood.

Of course, many people are surprised by our findings, even angered. But these findings are the result of thousands of thermograms and talking with thousands of our patients. For obvious reasons, those associated with the flax industries do not wish to believe our findings. We have had owners of flax seed/oil companies send in their rebuttals, which are discussed below, to explain their false claims to the readers. We will walk you through each of the studies to clarify the study's deception about the benefits of flax for breasts.

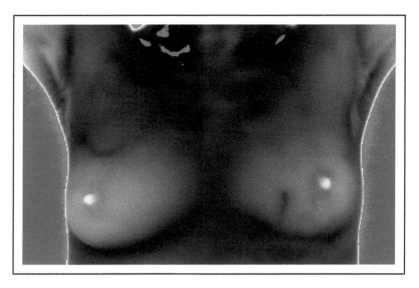

Before use of flax. Note slight vascular pattern.

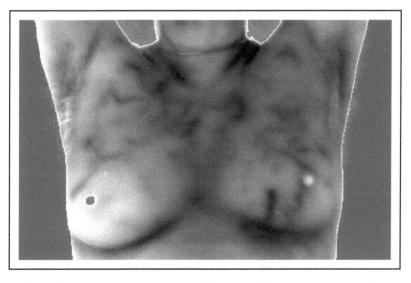

Repeat thermogram after six months of flax use. Note increase in vascularity, nipplar delta T and possible neoangiogenesis of neoplasia is suspected in left breast.

"This is hands-down the BEST book I've read on breast thermography. Every woman and every thermographer needs a copy! Thermography is such a great adjunctive tool to evaluate overall breast health risk, but it needs to be done properly within certified clinics by certified technicians, taking the images in both gray scale and colored images with a high quality, cleared camera and then read by experienced, certified interpreting doctors.

This book is beautifully illustrated with before/after images which clearly shows some of the physiological responses in the breast caused by various forms of estrogen especially from phytoestrogens, xenoestrogens, birth control, HRT, certain herbs and supplements. As a thermographer and nutritionist, I have personally seen the effects of these excess hormones on the breast and the health that can be regained by eliminating them. Wendy Sellens images of before/after flax seed use were of particular interest to me. Flax seed is extremely high in phytoestrogens, even higher than soy! At one point I had added 2 TBL of flax into my diet and within 4 weeks I experienced extremely tender breasts, hot flashes, and even skipped a period. After removing flax, within a few weeks the symptoms subsided. Hormones do affect our breasts!

Having breast cancer in my family history, this book brings incredible hope. One study on PubMed tells us that only 5-10 percent of cancer has a genetic link. The remaining 90-95 percent has its roots in environmental and dietary habits. This tells me that although we may not have 100 percent control, there is much we can do to prevent chronic diseases such as breast cancer. By utilizing all the tools available, including thermography, we can screen the breasts for changes. Then by changing lifestyle and nutritional habits, we can have a positive effect on our health.

I emailed Wendy Sellens to personally thank her for writing this book with Dr. William Hobbins. Within a day she responded and we set up a phone consultation. Her passion for women's health is amazing and her pursuit for thermographic excellence is extremely important. Breast Cancer Boot Camp is a must read. Wendy is definitely a soldier for breast health!"

Melissa

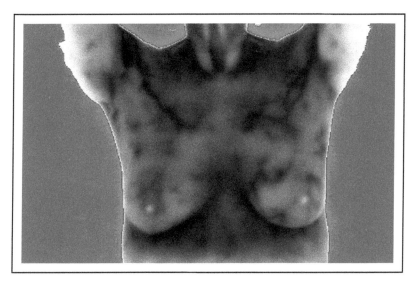

Using flax. Note unusual vascular pattern.

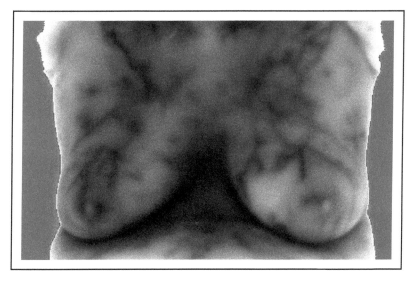

Repeat thermogram. Five years of using flax therapy.
Note increase in vascularity. Right breast is abnormal.

## Flax studies: War By Deception

Everyone thinks flax is healthy because a study *says* it is. We are going to reveal how misleading and deceiving flax studies are. We will demonstrate that flax studies are performed on organs and cancers that are *not* affected by estrogen because they have *no* receptors for estrogen, how studies conducted with female subjects are based on hearsay, testimonials or opinions and studies that are performed on estrogen receptor positive breast cancer are so convoluted that they are deceiving. Women have been duped. Look at the evidence presented in this section and then decide for yourself if flax is truly healthy.

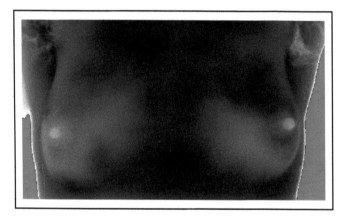

No Flax. Note slight vascular pattern.

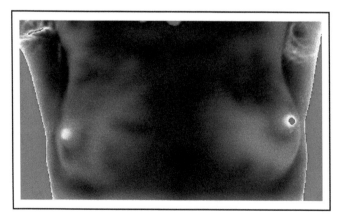

Repeat thermogram two years later. Two years of flax use. If flax "blocked" estrogen, breasts should be non-vascular. Note increase in vascularity. "At risk" thermogram.

The first rebuttal to our findings was a study sent in by a large popular manufacturing flax company. The study states that flax reduced colon or prostate cancer. The problem with this flax study, which was performed on rat colons, is that the colon *does not have* receptors for estrogen, so there will be *no effect* on the colon in regards to estrogenic factors. The breasts have estrogen receptors, so all types of estrogen (including phytoestrogens like flax) affect the breast; this is called bioidentical identity. There is no study showing that phytoestrogens affect the colon as there is no molecular biology similar to breast estrogen receptors, and therefore breast cancer, in the colon. One cannot draw conclusions from the study of a phytoestrogen-containing substance and its influence on an organ that does *not* contain estrogen receptors. This is either purposeful deceit or lack of education, but in any case, it's very misleading. And that is what they do to convince women that flax is healthy.

Our pilot study was looking at the effect of a phytoestrogen—flax—and how it stimulates the breast. We are concerned with excess estrogen and its effect on the breasts, not colons, as we are breast thermographers. Flax may have beneficial properties for the colon, but physicians then justify the use of these supplementations for *everyone* without consideration of how it will affect *other* areas of the body. General supplementation is not medicine. Each person should be treated as an individual.

If a patient comes to me with severe constipation, I could use a rhubarb root-based formula to treat this condition as directed in Chinese medicine (if it is indicated). If I were to draw the same conclusion that so many health practitioners get caught up in, that is "that rhubarb root is beneficial to the colon," I would place all my patients on rhubarb root. This is a huge no-no, as these patients would eventually become very ill. The problem is that medicine is no longer individualized for the patient. Propaganda spreads rampant throughout the medical community, after which these mantras become facts. For example, rhubarb is beneficial for constipation, now everyone should be using rhubarb. This is absolutely wrong, as the side effects for some people could be harmful. This is how supplements like flax, soy, and many others get abused.

145

For years, Dr. Hobbins has treated breast cancer with testosterone and prostate cancer with estrogen. This is an example of the use of what is called an endocrine antagonist. The theory is that when testosterone is reduced in a male with elevated PSA, and he is treated with estrogen (an antagonist to testosterone), PSA will drop to zero. Estrogen blocks the testosterone, so it becomes less influential on the cancer. Ironically, the rat study above supports Dr. Hobbins' principle of antagonistic endocrine treatment, as the study showed that the estrogen containing flax was beneficial to prostate cancer-afflicted rats.

In the case of breasts, Dr. Hobbins has used testosterone in metastasized recurrent breast cancer, and has successfully been able to shrink tumors. Just as estrogen blocks testosterone in the case of prostate cancer, the testosterone will block the estrogen in the breast. Therefore, testosterone is effective in decreasing vascularity in the breasts, while at the same time, the testosterone lacks the ability to biosynthesize into estrogen. This is evident in transgender therapy when a woman who wishes to become a man injects large amounts of testosterone in order to shrink their breasts.

Another interesting fact is that when men are treated for prostate cancer, estrogen is often used. As a result, the men experience a side effect of gynecomastia (enlarged breasts in men), meaning the male's breasts are stimulated from the excess estrogen and stimulation results in growth. This is what we see in breast thermography—estrogen causes activity which is seen as vascularity in the breasts.

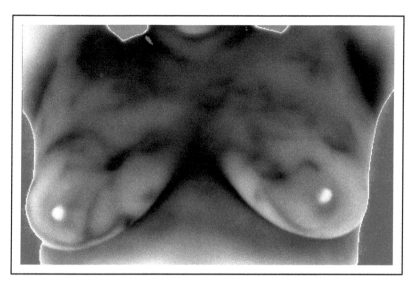

Using flax and progesterone pills. Note unusual vascular pattern.

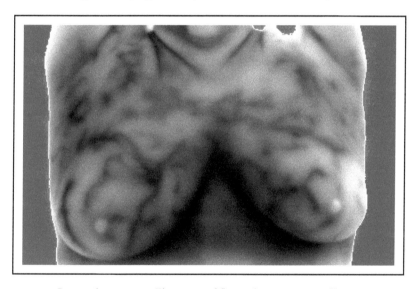

Repeat thermogram. Five years of flax and progesterone pill use.
Note increase in vascularity. Right breast is abnormal.

Another flax company didn't send us any studies, evidence or proof; just a link to their website, which only has articles stating flax is beneficial to women's health. One article states, "Our findings have implications," but right there is the flaw: assumption. What it actually means is that there is no scientific merit. There are no numbers, no blood samples, no urine samples, no tools of measurement (like a microscope), etc. Women have just related how they "felt" after taking flax. To get directly to the point, there is no scientific evidence to indicate this as proof to the benefits of flax. This is where we can find the misguided medical practices of what we call "therapy by association." In other words, if A is associated with B, and A has the end result of C, then B is the cause of C. But this is an illogical analysis, and again, this is how they mislead women in order to sell a product. The women questioned could have been doing many other things to affect the outcome, like improving nutrition, increasing exercise, sleeping better, etc. Do not believe hearsay. What works for one person does not always work for another. They later state, "Results regarding a 300 percent decrease." Where the heck are numbers coming from? This is especially unethical to print as proof that flax works.

This next study is also misleading. Many studies are conducted and paid for by companies who want to prove their product works. This actually happens quite often and leads to *many* conflicting studies on the effects of estrogen on women and causes a lot of confusion.

"Flaxseed and its lignans inhibit estradiol-induced growth, angiogenesis, and secretion of vascular endothelial growth factor in human breast cancer xenografts in vivo" by Jungestom, M.B., LU. Thompson, and C. Dabrosin. 2007 Clin Cancer Res:13:1061-1067 was a study conducted to prove flax was beneficial to breast cancer.

I would like to point out some very obvious flaws within this study and how making determinations from such studies are contributing to the medical incompetence we see today with regard to women's breast health. This study claims to support the notion that phytoestrogens, flaxseed in particular, are "potential compounds in breast cancer prevention and treatment." Let's see…

The experiment uses ovariectomized mice (mice with ovaries removed), divided into four separate groups. One group receives injections of an estrogen called enterdiol, another group injections of an estrogen called enterolactone, and a third group received no injections while all three were fed a basal diet modified to contain 20 percent corn oil. A fourth group was put on a modification of the basal diet with 10 percent flaxseed and received no injections. *All* groups are given a continuous supply of the same estrogen known as estrodiol, or E2. The mice are then implanted with breast cancer tumors (MCF-7) which are estrogen receptor positive (ER+) and have the ability themselves to process estrodiol.

First, the study states in their results that "this experimental model mimics breast cancer in *premenopausal* women" (emphasis added). Really? Do premenopausal women have functional ovaries? I would hope so. So how does removing the ovaries from mice somehow make them a "mimic" of a premenopausal women? Well they claim that because every mouse was given estrodiol (because this particular cancer requires estrodiol) that this is just like a premenopausal woman. Wow! Are we forgetting one little tiny thing here? Oh, yeah…progesterone. Somehow these medical researchers forgot that premenopausal women also produce the very hormone which balances estrogen in the breasts.

Second, the study is making determinations based off of measurements of VEGF, a stimulator of angiogenesis and therefore enabling cancer growth. They make the "suggestion" that because the groups given injections and flaxseed yielded less VEGF and less cancer growth, that they have antiestrogenic effects. In actuality, they are all estrogens, just different forms. The cancer masses they used for the experiment are stimulated by estrodiol, and these other forms may just be weaker estrogens relative to this model's conditions. That's it, they're just acting differently with this cancer, and this in no way should be concluding that these other estrogens have an antagonistic effect. They are just less potent, relatively. Just because one form of estrogen fails to produce equivalent results with regard to another, does not mean that either is antiestrogenic, and it would be even worse to take this information and apply it to the treatment of women.

Let's end with some quotes from the study's conclusions. The researchers state that "the rate of breast cancer differs…with highest incidence in countries with a Western lifestyle." They then continue to say that "this difference is largely attributable to lifestyle factors, such as a diet containing large amounts of phytoestrogens." And finally, they acknowledge that "cumulative exposure to estrogens is a risk factor of breast cancer" but then reinforce what seems to be their agenda by stating that "mechanisms by which phytoestrogens may protect against the disease are today poorly understood." So let's get this clear: Western diets rich in phytoestrogens have a correlation with higher incidence of breast cancer, and long term exposure to estrogens are a risk for breast cancer, but they can't understand why phytoestrogens may protect against breast cancer.

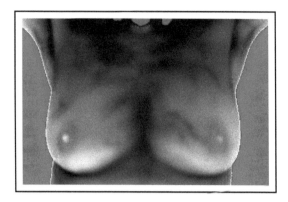

Using flax. Note unusual hypervascular pattern.

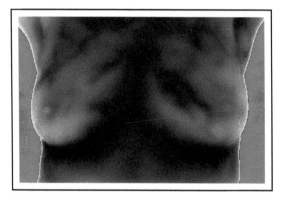

Repeat thermogram two years later. Still using flax. Note increase in vascularity. Left breast is abnormal.

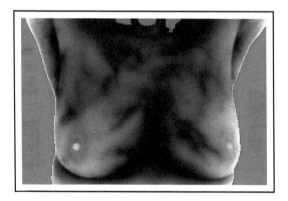

Repeat thermogram one year after previous thermogram. Still using flax. Left breast is abnormal.

Ladies, I hope you can clearly see how flax studies can be very confusing and convoluted. It is because of these studies, funded by companies, that "fudge" their evidence that women believe that flax is good for them. Who would take the time to read the entire study? What ordinary person could understand that study correctly? The author of the antiestrogenic diet book, where this study was found, obviously didn't. He trusted that the authors would produce honest work. Don't trust everything you read. If you want to truly understand flax studies, then get your hands dirty and start digging. Do your own research. Stop repeating rumors, find the truth yourself. I believe you will start to see the same flaws we pointed out.

Women can test flax out for themselves by megadosing for a couple of months and evaluating how they feel mentally, and more importantly, how their menstrual cycle presents. (I have to add a disclaimer that this is not medically advisable as it will increase vascularity and possibly neoangiogenesis) But remember, the breasts cannot lie, and a thermogram will show what you may not feel or see yourself.

Another popular study gathering quite a bit of chatter is the Budwig diet, which consists of cottage cheese and flaxseed. It appears this study was based on cancer that was estrogen receptor negative. Estrogen receptor negative means that there are no receptors for estrogen, and therefore, by definition, estrogen will not feed this cancer! When not presented properly by doctors and pundits, this information can be very harmful to breast health, especially since the majority of breast cancers are estrogen receptor positive. This treatment may be beneficial for some cancers, but we recommended avoiding this diet as it may stimulate the growth of estrogen receptor positive breast cancer.

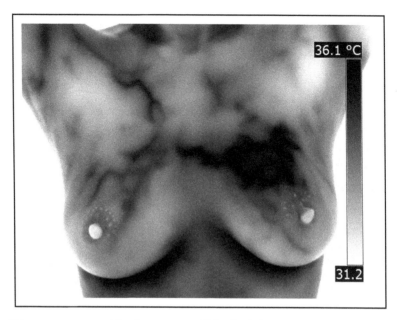

Estrogen receptor positive breast cancer. Using Budwig Protocol to "cure" cancer. Note cancer in right breast.

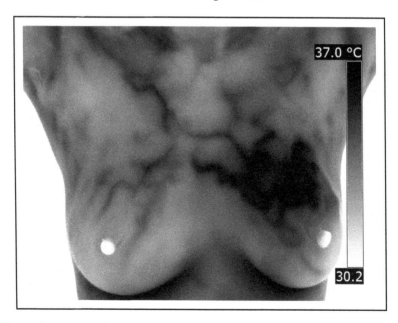

Repeat thermogram after six months on Budwig Protocol and tumor increased in size. Note possible neoangiogenesis of neoplasia is suspected in left breast.

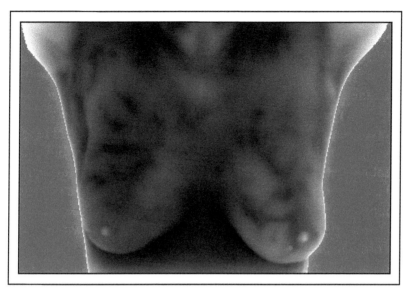

Estrogen positive breast cancer right breast two years prior. Currently doing Budwig Diet for prevention. Right breast abnormal.

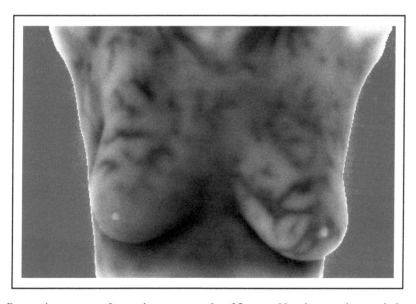

Repeat thermogram after twelve more months of flax use. Note increase in vascularity in left breast and possible neoangiogenesis. Right breast remains abnormal.

One clinic that I read thermograms for is an alternative cancer treatment center. I see thermograms of many women with estrogen receptor positive breast cancer who are using some form of phytoestrogen such as bioidentical estrogen cream, flax, and soy therapies. These therapies cause their breasts to become severely vascular, increasing risk. Estrogen "feeds" the cancer. Avoid all "health centers" using flax and soy treatment for breast cancer and breast health—they are increasing the patient's risk.

I have seen a few recurring breast cancers and the patient reports use of flax supplementation or bioidentical estrogen use. I believe flax and bioidentical estrogen could have possibly "fed" those cancers. Don't take the chance. If you had estrogen receptor positive breast cancer, do not supplement with any form of estrogen including flax.

It is important to monitor breast cancer treatments with thermography in order to observe the blood vessels in the breasts. This determines if a woman is being stimulated by any estrogen, increasing her risk, and also observes how cancer treatments are working, if they are effective or not effective. Many women use breast thermography to monitor breast cancer testaments. Look at these images of estrogen receptor positive breast cancer examples to see the amount of vascularity or neoangiogenesis in these women with breast cancer and consider the validity of some of these treatments.

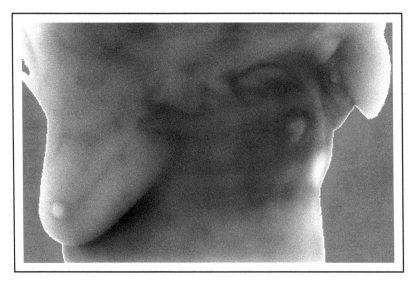

Recurrent breast cancer with history of flax use. Note neoangiogenesis in left breast. Abnormal thermogram.

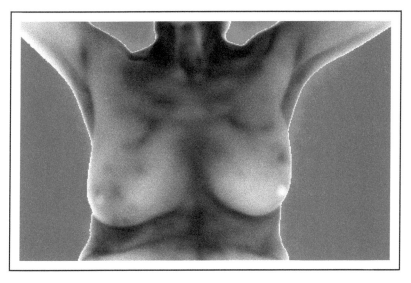

Breast cancer survivor with ten years of bioidentical estrogen cream use.
Note unusual vascular pattern.

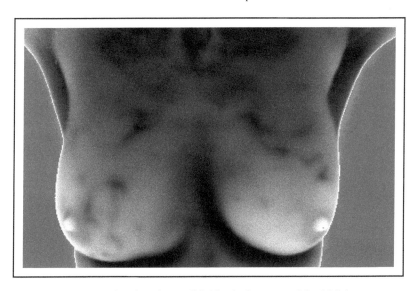

Repeat thermogram. Continued use of bioidentical estrogen. "At risk" thermogram.

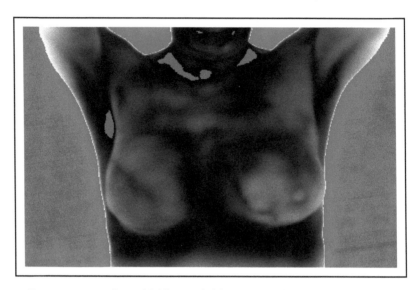

Breast cancer survivor with history of eighteen years of HRT use and currently using bioidentical estrogen. Note unusual vascular pattern.

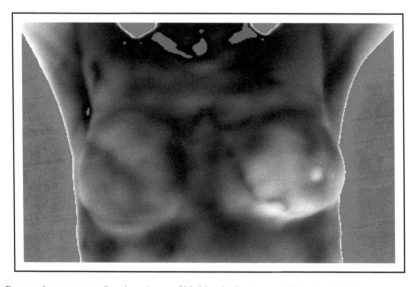

Repeat thermogram. Continued use of bioidentical estrogen. Note "at risk" thermogram.

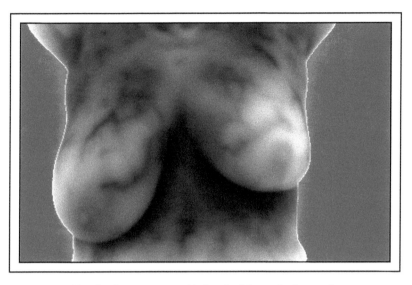

Treating breast cancer with flax. Left breast is abnormal.

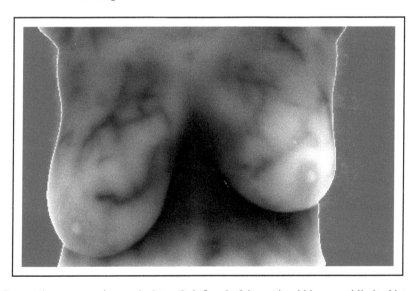

Repeat thermogram six months later. Quit flax. Left breast is within normal limits. Note unusual hypervascular pattern.

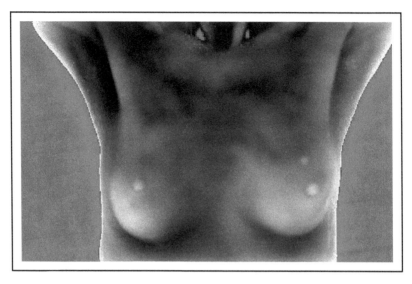

Before cancer. Bioidentical estrogen and flax use. Note unusual vascular pattern.

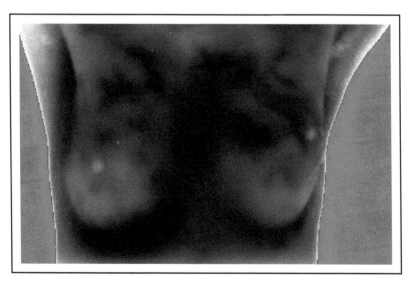

Repeat thermogram one year later. Diagnosed with breast cancer still using bioidentical estrogen and flax. Left breast is abnormal.

Most flax companies rely on the magic properties of lignans. But lignans are what contain the estrogenic factors of flax. Flax supplementation is a huge fad, especially among alternative health care providers. Many doctors oppose our evidence that flax increases risk because many of them have a large percentage of patients (male, female, and children) purchasing these flax products directly from them.

It is especially important *not* to supplement your children with flax or soy. It's the equivalent of giving them estrogen hormones found in nonorganic meats and poultry. These children become over-stimulated with unopposed estrogen, and this will affect their development. This includes foods like eggs and milk, even organic, with wording of "high in omega-3s," as this is may be achieved through feed that contains flax.

Dr. Hobbins and I have gotten thousands of women off flax. With their thermographic images, women can see objective (*not* influenced by personal feelings or opinions in considering and representing facts) changes in their breasts while they subjectively (non measurable opinion) experience changes in symptoms. Many of these women express their gratitude to us because of the reduction in symptoms like weight gain, heavy and irregular periods, PMS, breast tenderness, moodiness, irritability, insomnia, night sweats, and hot flashes. Excess estrogen causes severe mood swings, and women are amazed at how much calmer they feel when they get off of flax.

A study we advise our patients to read is "Implications of Phytoestrogen Intake for Breast Cancer," from *The Cancer Journal of Clinicians* (2008). Look at the table included in the study and also at the beginning of this chapter and see for yourself how high flax is in phytoestrogens. Flax is nineteen times more potent than soy; however, soy is more prevalent in our processed foods and supplements.

I encourage you to conduct your own study! Toss out all soy products and flax supplements. Then see how you feel.

"I have been so impressed with this book. I have learned so much about my health and how important it is to be mindful of what I put in and on my body. I was a lover of flax and truly enjoyed my soy milk lattes...daily! But it all changed after reading this book. So a little back story...I was tired of getting my breast radiated each year and decided to look at other options. My sister died from breast cancer five years ago and I was tired of worrying about being a statistic and decided that I would be vigilant about my breast care and cancer prevention. I heard about thermography some years ago, but decided that this year I would take a further look at it. After much research – and let me stress *much* – I found Pink Image Thermography clinic here in San Diego. The Pink Image is owned by Wendy Sellens, one of the authors of this book. I must say my thermography results changed the way my family lives and eats. The Thermography exam itself was quick and painless. I suggest anyone reading this book to get one; you will learn so much about your breast! A mammogram can't give you the details that this exam can. But please do your research on the first! Anyway, I saw this book there and thought I would check it out. Glad I did. This book goes into great detail on how to improve breast health which includes going estrogen-free, eating organic, omitting flax and soy from your diet amongst, other things. I gained so much knowledge from this book and I am truly grateful. Breast Cancer Bootcamp is must read! Order it now! In fact order extra copies to hand out to your love ones. You will not regret it!"

Monica

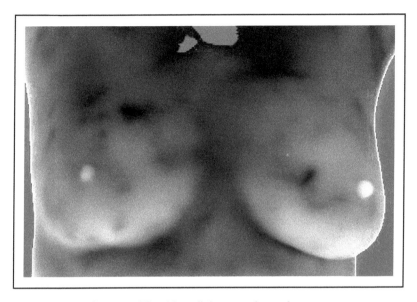

Before use of flax. Note slight unusual vascular pattern.

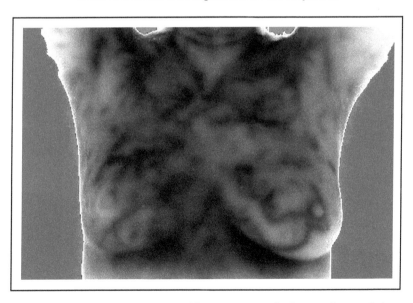

Repeat thermogram. Only one year of flax use. Note major increase in vascularity.

# Bioidenticals: Friendly Fire

Bioidentical estrogens have increased in popularity in the last few years. However, it is just a pretty name for the same ol' harmful estrogen. There have been no studies on the effect of bioidentical estrogen on women's breast health as of yet, therefore, women using it are literally guinea pigs. Bioidentical just means biologically similar. So any particle that is bioidentical to estrogen will fit the body's estrogen receptors. This means BCPs, HRTs, flax, soy, and bioidentical estrogen are all considered bioidentical.

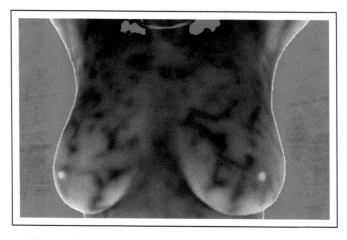

History of bioidentical estrogen. Note unusual vascular pattern.
Progesterone deficiency imbalance.

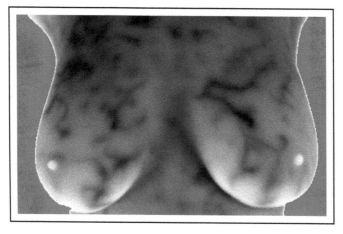

Repeat thermogram. Continued use of bioidentical estrogen. "At risk" thermogram.

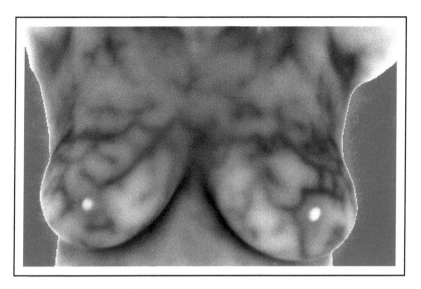

Bioidentical estrogen pellets. Note severe unusual hypervascular pattern. "At risk" thermogram. Severe progesterone deficiency imbalance.

War Story:

A patient told me that her nurse practitioner put her on progesterone and testosterone cream along with bioidentical estrogen pellets. So I asked her how she felt. "Well, kind of better," she stated, but then went on to say that though she had been menopausal for seven years, she was now experiencing continuous spotting. Big red flag, ladies! The estrogen was overstimulating her uterus. This is most definitely a problem, not just because it's a nuisance to bleed all month, but also because this increases the risk for uterine cancer. This is a side effect taken from the manufacturer of an estrogen cream—their warning states, "Vaginal bleeding after menopause may be a warning sign of cancer of the uterus." When you have gone through menopause, your body is done. It is now time for reproductive possibilities to cease, and therefore, bleeding is no longer normal. When the patient reported back to the nurse practitioner that she had gotten her period, the nurse practitioner said it was fine. Either doctors do not realize they are harming their patients or they just don't care. Whichever the case, this is completely unacceptable, as the Hippocratic Oath proclaims to do no harm to the patient.

However, there is more to learn from this case. Three months after the initial pellets were placed in the patient, she was tested with blood work, and the results indicated that her estrogen levels were still too low. At this time, the nurse practitioner doubled the dosage of estrogen pellets, thereby initiating the return of her period. In response to this information, Dr. Hobbins and I believe that when exogenous estrogens are in the body, they send a signal to the pituitary gland that says "Hey, there's plenty of us estrogen here. Let's shut down production." Now understand, blood and saliva tests can only test for the twenty-six naturally occurring estrogens that the body makes, and because the pituitary gland has received information to stop production, the endogenous estrogens levels are going to show up as low. In reality, levels are so high from exogenous estrogens that they have caused the period to return, even after seven years without one.

In response to this patient's presentation, I told her to apply progesterone cream on her breasts, as this is where the receptors are located, instead of on her abdomen, where she had been applying the cream. Within a few days she stopped bleeding. She then came in for breast thermography, and the images showed that she had the highest grade of progesterone deficiency possible, grade 3 (relative). We can now conclude that her body had been bombarded with estrogen, her progesterone levels could not counter the excessive estrogen the progesterone cream had been applied to the wrong region, and that her nurse practitioner was clueless to the practice she claims to represent.

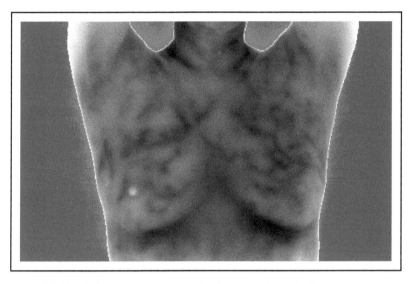

Bioidentical estrogen cream use for six years. Abnormal thermogram.

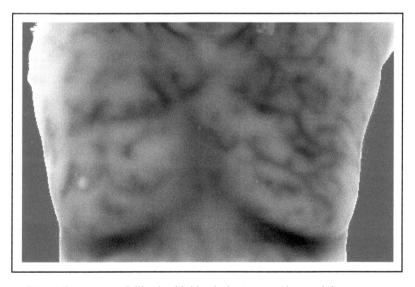

Repeat thermogram. Still using bioidentical estrogen. Abnormal thermogram.

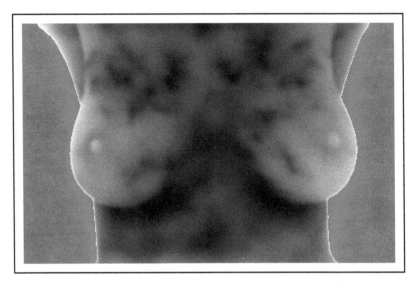

Reports use of Biest and Triest supplements which are bioidentical hormones. Note unusual vascular pattern. Progesterone deficiency imbalance.

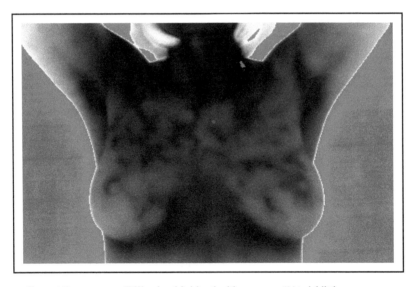

Repeat thermogram. Still using bioidentical hormones. "At risk" thermogram.

Please do not be fooled by the misrepresented title of "bioidentical," it's just a fancy term to sell the same ol' estrogen. Synthetic estrogens, ecoestrogens and phytoestrogens, flax, soy and bioidentical estrogen are *all* biologically similar to our body's estrogen. The term *bioidentical* was created to sell estrogen under the guise of being "natural;" it is *not* - it is the same as all estrogens mentioned above. Manufacturers and prescribing doctors are trying to convey that this product is just like what you create in *your* body and these health remedies are somewhat formulated just for you—another complete farce. Your bioidentical cocktail is hardly different from the next and is most likely given to you by a doctor who studied it in a one-weekend class. These cocktails are sold to us under the belief that this form of estrogen is a "natural" alternative treatment. What is natural about a pellet or a patch? These are still pharmaceuticals! Women were taken off of Premarin because of the increase in breast and uterine cancer, and now they have repackaged it under a new "natural" title. Bioidentical is estrogen. Stop the vicious belief system of deceptions!

Now let us look at a couple of interesting contradictions that occur with regard to these products in the treatment of women's health. Most women suspected of having estrogen receptor positive breast cancer are put on Tamoxifen, an estrogen blocker. Estrogen blocker drugs are used because estrogen stimulates breast cell receptors and may over stimulate those cells which are cancerous. Simply put, estrogen "feeds" the cancer. A cancer cell is basically an unchecked replicator—stimulation is the worst thing that can happen because it accelerates cancer growth. Isn't this a little odd that estrogen-based therapies are pushed onto women, yet the exact opposite approach is made when cancer is involved? Why are we surprised that women are getting breast cancer at a higher rate than ever before, even when medicine is supposedly improving? More surprising is the high amount of breast cancer survivors that are on bioidenticals. Their doctors are literally increasing their risk of recurrence.

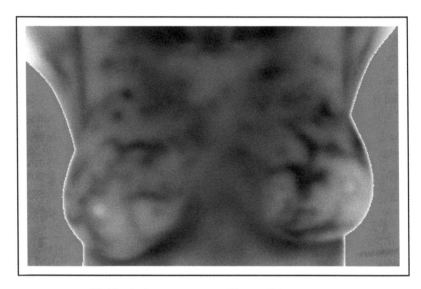

Bioidentical estrogen cream. Abnormal thermogram.

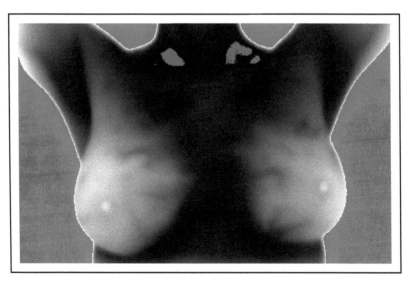

Repeat thermogram after decreasing bioidentical estrogen cream in half.
Note reduction in vascularity.

Strategic Operation: Decrease estrogen cream by half.

I had another patient who was progesterone deficient grade 3 (relative) with an abnormal report. I told her that she needed to remove all exogenous estrogens (soy, flax, bioidentical estrogen cream), but she was hesitant due to all the propaganda that said women needed to be on estrogen. She also reported that her doctor is "famous" for hormone therapy and told her to put it on every day. I showed her thermogram to her and said "your breasts can't lie." She compromised and reduced her bioidentical estrogen cream to every other day. The results shocked even me! By just cutting her dosage of estrogen cream in half, she decreased her report from abnormal to within normal limits, but "at risk" due to vascularity that is still present. Her hormone imbalance improved as well to a progesterone deficiency grade 2 (relative). The funny thing is, after all this, she still wouldn't remove estrogen from her lifestyle. She wanted to believe her physician, and therefore, the propaganda, even with proof right in front of her!

Your breast can't lie. Breast thermography evaluates the "health" of the breasts. Still believe plant estrogens are healthy? Several repeat thermograms to prove bioidentical estrogen is increasing risk of breast cancer and causing estrogen dominance, even when used with bioidentical progesterone and testosterone! Thermograms will show that it doesn't matter if estrogen is a pill, patch or cream, all delivery systems increase risk.

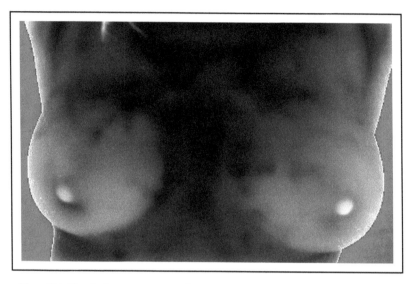

Use of bioidentical estrogen cream for ten years. Note unusual vascular patterns.

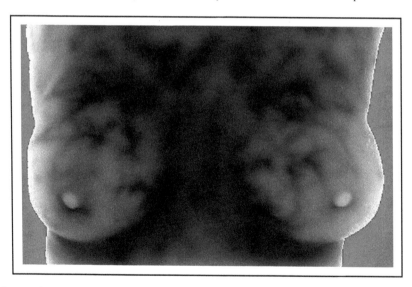

Repeat thermogram. Use of bioidentical estrogen for twelve years and added bioidentical progesterone and testosterone cream for two years. Note increase in vascularity. Severe progesterone deficiency.

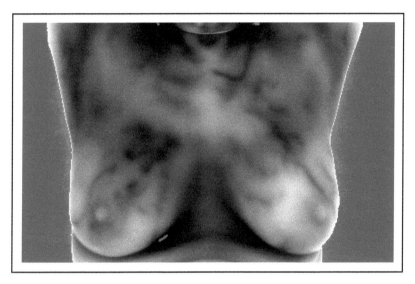

Use of bioidentical estrogen cream for twelve years. Note unusual hypervascular patterns.

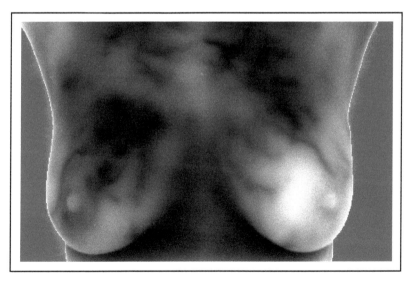

Repeat thermogram. Use of bioidentical estrogen for thirteen years.
Note increase in vascularity. Right breast abnormal.

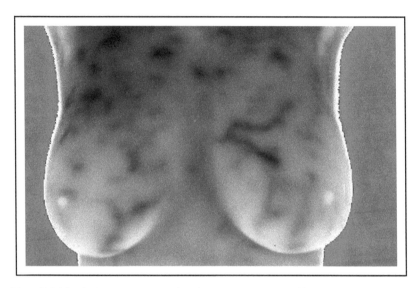

Use of bioidentical estrogen cream for six years. Note unusual hypervascular patterns.

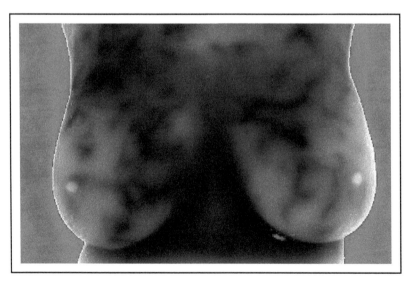

Repeat thermogram. Use of bioidentical estrogen for eight years. Suspicious of possible neoangiogenesis at three o'clock position of right breast. Right breast abnormal.

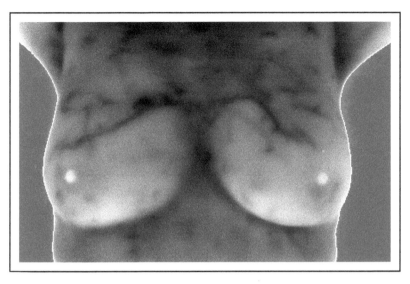

Use of bioidentical estrogen, progesterone and testosterone creams for four years. Note unusual vascular patterns.

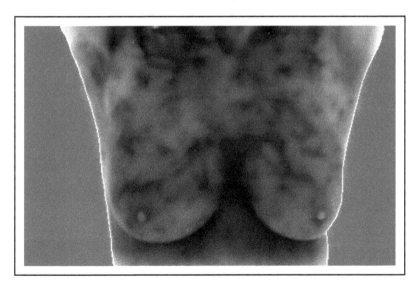

Repeat thermogram. Use of bioidentical estrogen, progesterone and testosterone creams for seven years plus started using black cohosh and primrose oil. Note increase in vascularity. Severe progesterone deficiency.

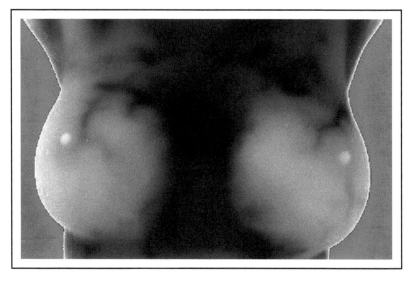

Using primrose and red clover. Note unusual vascular patterns.

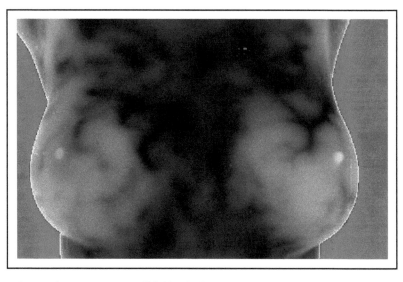

Repeat thermogram. Use of bioidentical estrogen, and testosterone creams with progesterone pills for last two years. Stopped primrose oil and red clover. Note increase in vascularity. Severe progesterone deficiency.

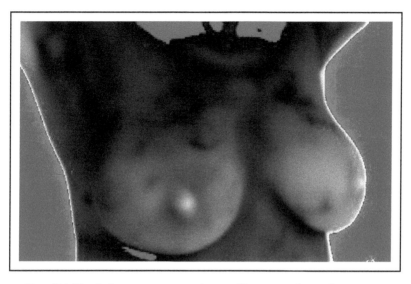

Use of bioidentical estrogen, years unknown. Note unusual vascular patterns.

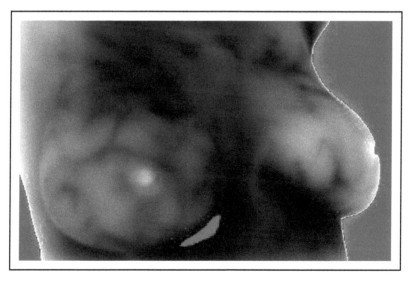

Repeat thermogram fifteen months later. Use of bioidentical estrogen and added
progesterone and testosterone creams. Note increase in vascularity.
Severe progesterone deficiency.

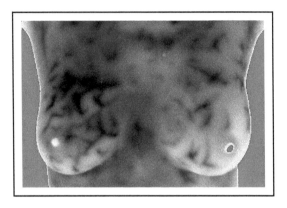

Use of bioidentical estrogen two years. Note unusual vascular patterns.

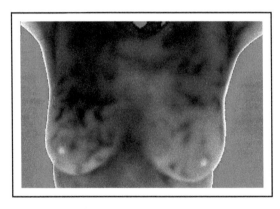

Repeat one year later. Use of bioidentical estrogen and added progesterone cream three years. Note increase in vascularity. Severe progesterone deficiency.

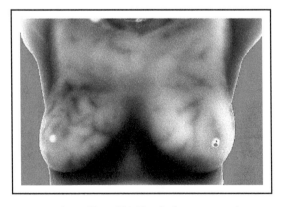

Repeat thermogram one year later. Use of bioidentical estrogen and progesterone creams four years. Note increase in vascularity. Severe progesterone deficiency.

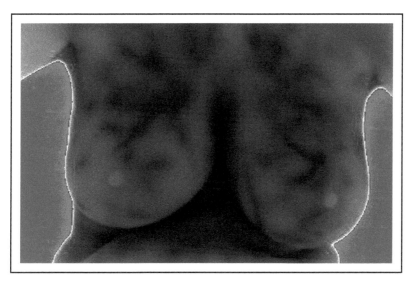

Use of bioidentical estrogen pills for ten years. Note unusual vascular patterns.

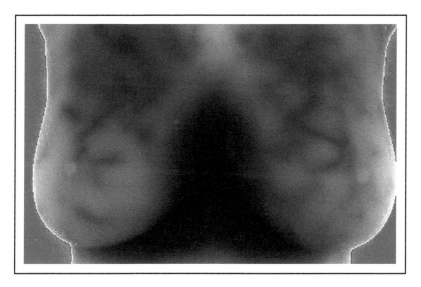

Repeat thermogram. Use of bioidentical estrogen and progesterone pills fifteen years. Note increase in vascularity. Severe progesterone deficiency.

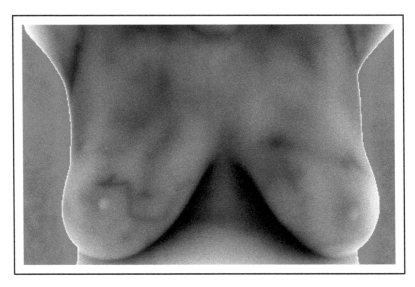

Use of bioidentical estrogen and progesterone pills for five years.
Note unusual vascular patterns.

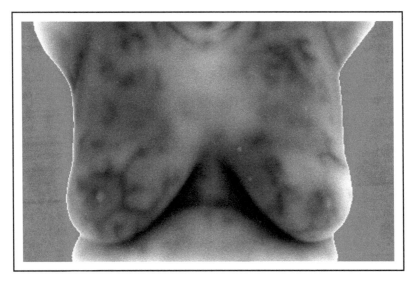

Repeat thermogram three months later. Use of bioidentical estrogen and progesterone pills.
Note increase in vascularity in just months. Right breast abnormal.

Many doctors believe that Biest™ or Triest™ is a more effective or a safer form of estrogen. After ten years of breast thermography research this theory cannot be proven correct. Biest™ and Triest™ both increase risk of breast cancer and estrogen dominance even when used in combination with bioidentical progesterone and/or testosterone.

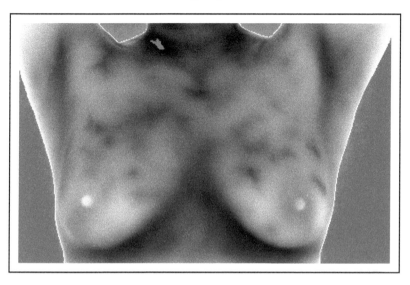

No hormone therapy. Note unusual vascular patterns. Progesterone deficient.

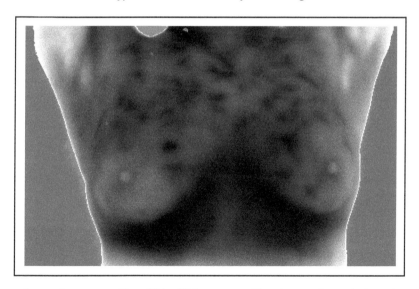

Repeat thermogram. Use of Biest™ for one year. Note increased vascularity and increase in progesterone deficiency.

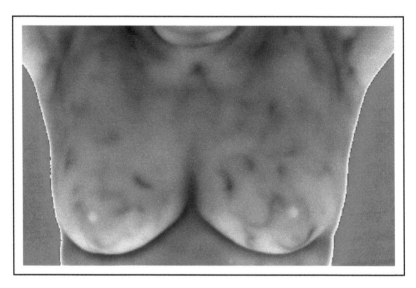

Use of Biest™ for nineteen years. Note unusual hypervascular patterns.

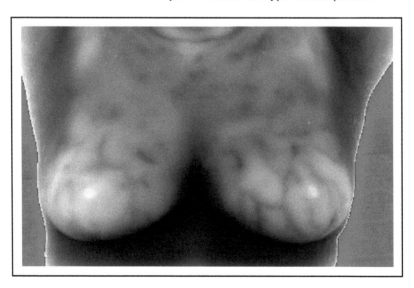

Repeat thermogram. Use of Biest™ for twenty years.
Note unusual hypervascular patterns.

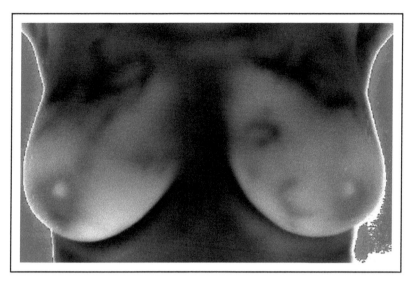

Use of Triest™ for nine years. Note unusual hypervascular patterns.

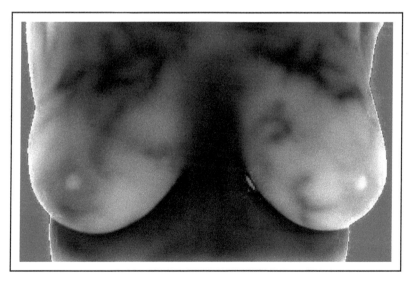

Repeat thermogram two years later. Use of Triest™ for eleven years. Note unusual hypervascular patterns.

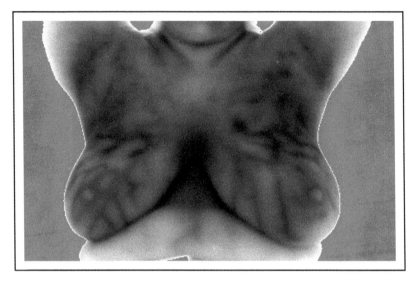

Use of Biest™ years unknown along with progesterone and testosterone. Note unusual hypervascular patterns.

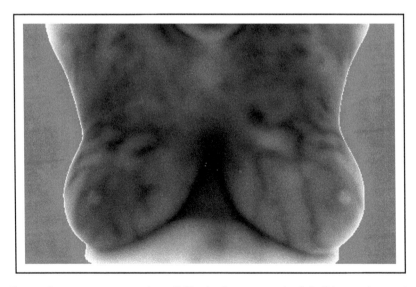

Repeat thermogram one year later. Still using hormone cocktail. Left breast abnormal.

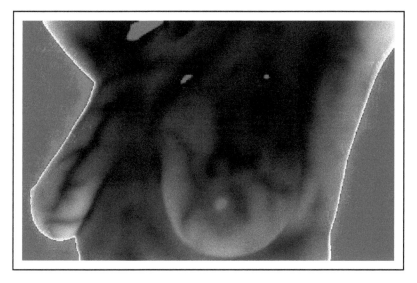

No hormone therapy. Note unusual vascular patterns. Progesterone deficient.

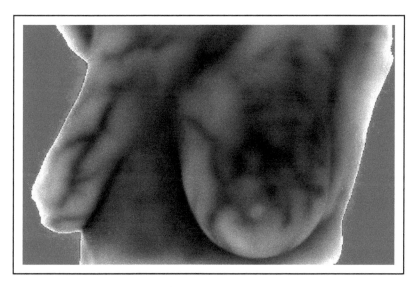

Repeat thermogram. Use of Biest™ for one year. Note increased vascularity.
Left breast abnormal.

Stop buying cancer. Most breast cancers are "fed" by estrogen. However, women continue to walk for a cure. If women just stopped walking and stopped buying estrogen products, soy, flax and bioidentical estrogens, breast cancer numbers would plummet. Stop believing flax, soy, and bioidentical estrogen are healthy because they come from a plant. Stop believing flax and soy are weak estrogens because they are "natural." Stop believing propaganda that estrogen keeps women young; it is killing us. Start investigating these facts for yourself and get educated.

# 6. Ecoterrorism

The rise in the incidence of obesity matches the rise in the use and distribution of industrial chemicals that may be playing a role in a generation of obesity, suggesting that endocrine disrupting chemicals may be linked to this epidemic.

The Endocrine Society, founded in 1916, is the world's oldest, largest, and most active organization devoted to research on hormones and the clinical practice of endocrinology.

Chemtrust

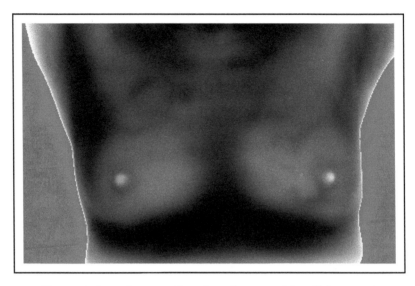

No reported use of estrogen therapies or hormones. Note slight unusual vascular pattern. "At risk" thermogram.

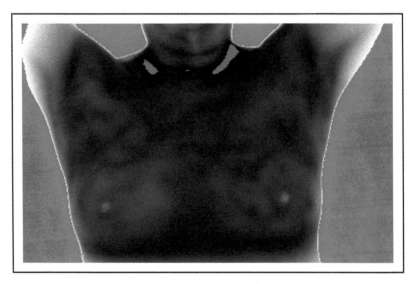

Repeat thermogram. No reported use of estrogen therapies or hormones. Note increase in vascularity pattern. "At risk" thermogram.

Ladies, we are the lab rats for the effect of environmental estrogens. Petrochemical estrogens (also known as ecoestrogens, xenohormones, and xenobiotics) are strong and toxic environmental estrogens that are bioidentical (similar chemical structure) to the body's estrogen. Ecoestrogens *are* estrogen, actually synthetic pseudo estrogens. Petrochemical estrogens are derived from petroleum-based products and are found in everything from laundry detergents to body lotion. Now keep in mind that, even though these particles are very small, it is not their size, but rather the accumulated daily exposure, often for years, that results in high levels of toxicity and estrogen.

Petrochemical estrogens are fat soluble, meaning they have the ability to pass through the skin layer. Once in the body, many of these *never* break down, actually sitting in the cells of the body *forever*!

Watch out for these prevalent ecoestrogens that are used in popular household products. BPA, PABA, paraben, propylparaben, butylparaben, phthalate, petroleum/petrochemicals and Triclosan. Also, avoid other carcinogenic chemicals found in household products, too.

Below is a synopsis on ecoestrogens taken from the 1996 *American Scientist, Volume 84*, by John A. McLachlan and Steven F. Arnold. John Mclachland has coined the term ecoestrogens —"estrogens found in the environment" and has been studying the effects of estrogenetic chemicals for over twenty years.

In 1938, Sir Charles Dodds produced a synthetic estrogen known as diethylstilbestrol (DES). For years, it was used to fatten cattle, but as you can guess, that's not all they used it for. It would seem in this crazy world that "If it's good enough for cattle, it's good enough for a pregnant woman." As such, women were given this synthetic estrogen to prevent miscarriages. The problem with this, outside the fact that women were megadosed with a synthetic hormone that they produce quite easily and naturally, was that DES became the first chemical documented in humans to be "transplacental." This means that the drug has the ability to cross the placenta from the mother to the fetus. Women taking DES to prevent miscarriage, breast cancer, and menopause had actually caused cervical and vaginal cancer, testicular cancer, infertility, birth defects, and a higher incidence of bisexuality or lesbianism *in their* children. Recently, the effects of DES have been shown to extend into the third generation, which is quite amazing and frightening. This is currently a rising concern as "transgeneration" pharmaceutical and commercial products are increasing.

Studies on male rats with DES showed "higher percentage of undescended testicles, testicular cancer, sperm abnormalities, and prostate disease." In 1992, Niels Skakkebaek reported a decrease in semen quality worldwide. Sperm count has dropped more than 50 percent since 1940, while testicular cancer has tripled in the US and Europe.

In the past few decades, scientists have noticed that some chemical pollutants are mimicking estrogen and affecting the DNA of humans and wildlife. For example, in 1975, the spill of a chemical called Kepone, which was used in a pesticide, resulted in low sperm count in the men exposed to it. What the research showed was that Kepone was a "weak estrogen, but an estrogen nevertheless," and in 1979, scientists surmised that this was a rare case but questioned how many chemicals could reproduce these effects? Sadly, the effects were considered, but there was no further study.

A chemical can alter the body's signals. That is amazing if you take a minute to think about it! Unfortunately, that can lead to a whole host of problems. Scientists found that if you take the equal amounts of estradiol and DES in the blood, more DES enters cells than the natural hormone estradiol! What this showed is that human cells have an affinity for chemical estrogen over the body's natural producing estrogen. Our bodies are so amazing they can even metabolize and alter the chemical so that it is even more potent. They have also seen that ecoestrogens (petrochemical estrogens) are more potent because they create more binding or multiple binding sites, versus just one lock and key.

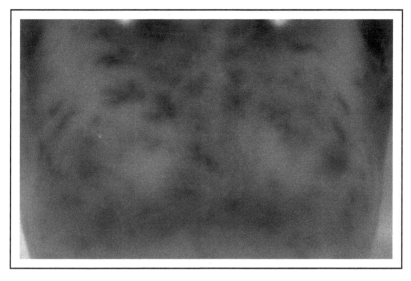

Thermogram of a man. Men should be non-vascular due to high levels of testosterone versus estrogen and why the rate of male breast cancer is lower. Note mild unusual vascular pattern.

Let's take a look at some of the effects on wildlife.

A study conducted at the University of West Florida found that female fish were masculinized after being exposed to pollutants. Lake Apopka was contaminated with DDT, resulting in many deaths, and the males had only half the "normal levels" of testosterone and smaller genitalia, which is referred to as feminization.

University of California Davis found that "seagull eggs exposed to DDT developed as females, no matter what their genetic sex." It has also been seen to cause birth defects.

At the University of Texas, turtle eggs exposed to estrogenic chemicals, such as PCBs and natural estrogen, became female.

Birds exposed to both waterborne or airborne pesticides showed female pairing, ovarian tissue in testes, failure to thrive, clubbed feet, crossed bills, huge thyroid glands and an abnormal amount of eggs with thinner shells.

Alligators exposed to pesticides had high estrogen and low testosterone levels. Male alligators in Florida exposed to DDT have smaller penises while the females have abnormal ovaries. The alligator population has been reduced by 90 percent and it is assumed to be caused by a failure to reproduce.

Adverse health effects found in sixteen troubled, top predatory birds, fish, mammals, and reptiles in the Great Lakes. Populations of these species had either disappeared or were in serious decline. Although the adult animals looked fine, their offspring, if they produced any, were not reaching sexual maturity and were incapable of reproducing. Information provided by The Endocrine Disruption Exchange.

The health effects that were causing the populations to crash included:

1. Obvious reproductive impairment or loss of fertility.
2. Eggshell thinning, a disturbance of endocrine-controlled calcium metabolism.
3. Metabolic changes that led to wasting and early death even before chicks hatched or fry could swim up.
4. Obvious birth defects, such as crossed bills and clubbed feet.
5. Abnormal thyroid and male and female sex glands in almost all animals examined.
6. Abnormal thyroid hormone production in almost all fish and birds studied.
7. Behavioral changes in birds, such as lack of parenting, nest inattentiveness, males forming fraternities rather than establishing territories and attempting to mate, and female/female pairing.
8. Immune suppression, evidenced by increased rates of internal and external parasitism.
9. The phenomenon of transgenerational exposure, where the maternal animals were passing the persistent organochlorine (DDT) chemicals in their bodies to their offspring before they were born, through their blood, or with fish and birds through the liver to their eggs before they were laid.

None of the above problems correlated with habitat destruction, lamprey eel parasitism, or overfishing, but they did correlate with the concentrations of organochlorine (DDT) chemicals in the maternal animals.

Examples below are provided by Chemtrust's protecting humans and wildlife from harmful chemicals.

- Fish—altered spermatogenesis (process of maturing sperm), eggs developing in testes, intersex genital apparatus, and poor reproductive success
- Amphibians—intersex features
- Reptiles—smaller penis in alligators and turtles, decreased hatching, and decreased post hatch survival.
- Birds—embryonic mortality, reduced reproductive success, including egg-shell thinning, and poor parenting behavior
- Rodents—reduced sperm, reduced testes weight, and reduced reproduction.
- Otters or mink—reduced penile bone length, smaller testes, and impaired reproduction
- Seals and sea lions—impaired reproduction, which includes implantation failure, sterility, abortion, and premature pupping
- Cetaceans—reduced testosterone levels, impaired reproduction, and hermaphrodite organs
- Polar bears—intersex features and deformed genitals, reduced testes and penile bone length, low testosterone levels in adult males, and reduced cub survival
- Black bears—undescended testes
- Florida panther—abnormal sperm and low sperm density, undescended testes and altered hormone levels
- Deer—antler deformities; undescended testes, testicular abnormalities including cells predictive of testicular cancer
- Antelope—abnormal testes including impaired spermatogenesis.

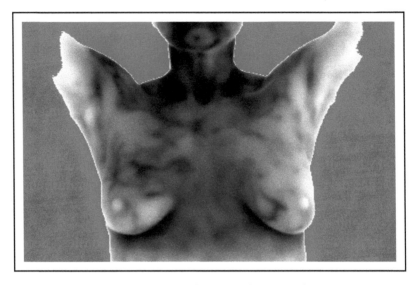

No reported use of estrogen therapies. Note slight unusual vascular pattern.
"At risk" thermogram.

## Ecoestrogens: Enemy on the Home Front

If these ecoestrogens can affect animals with such profound side effects, imagine what they are doing to us and our children. The research referred to in this chapter from the animal Kingdome should be strongly considered. We can see the effect on multiple generations in a few years, where as in the human species, it will take longer to see the adverse effects; nevertheless, the signs are already apparent – we must pay attention.

The feminization of the male species. Ask yourself why is low testosterone so rampant? Does anyone remember this being an issue twenty years ago? This is also exhibited in the rise in male breast cancer, a 0.9 percent rise a year from 1979 to 2006. One in 400 men are now being diagnosed with breast cancer. Testicular size has decreased by a third since the early 1900s along with a rise in sterility. Now, *mano-pause*?! Symptoms are low testosterone, low libido, increased body fat, loss of muscle and strength, decreased bone density depression, emotional, concentration and decrease in motivation or self-confidence. Sounds like menopause, which is actually caused by excess estrogen, not a deficiency, which was a lie. These are all red flags. Eco-estrogen along with popular phytoestrogens, like soy, flax and hummus are feminizing men, which is going to have an impact on our species, just like the animal kingdom, if it is not addressed.

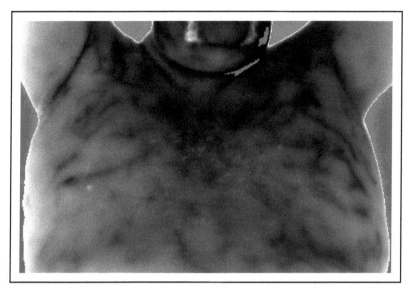

This man reports diagnosis of breast cancer twice, 1994 and 2009. Note unusual vascular pattern. Abnormal thermogram-left. Environmental estrogens are increasing incidences of breast cancer evidence is seen in the increase of male breast cancer.

Many diseases are now believed to be linked to commercial chemicals in our household products. These include cancer, infertility, birth defects, asthma, allergies, sterility, developmental issues, behavioral problems, cardiovascular disease, obesity, and diabetes.

We might even expect such results if we understand how accelerated the brain growth of a fetus is in the first three months of development. It is also believed that in these first three months, high levels of estrogen may affect the sexual development of children and increase risk of autism and ADHD. Research is ongoing.

Now think about these scary facts: a baby's blood brain barrier isn't developed until age two, and a baby's skin is thinner than adults. Nearly all baby products contain petrochemicals, which as we just learned, not only have estrogenic properties but also have toxins in them. These toxic products, which unknowing parents place in their children, wreak

193

havoc on their developing skin and respiratory system. If we are bombarding their fragile bodies with these chemicals, maybe it's no wonder that, since 1991, occurrences in autism are up 600 percent and one in 64 kids are now diagnosed with this disorder.

Have you noticed the increase in childhood issues? Why are so many children now diagnosed with ADD/ADHD? (There are obviously implications that this is over diagnosed and that many children excel in different environments). Why do countless children these days have so many allergies? Why are so many kids covered from head to toe with skin disorders? Why are learning disabilities and behavioral issues increasing? Think back to when you were in school, how many sickly kids were there? Maybe one. Nowadays, nearly all children are on a pharmaceutical routine with the school nurse.

This is further compounded by hypersensitivity caused by extensive anti-biotic use. The medical establishment has finally recognized the damaging affect caused by overuse and has dramatically pulled back prescriptions. But now, through propaganda the public believes it needs to sterilize everything! It is imperative to avoid all anti-biotic products, hand sanitizers and cleaning products, as it is the same as the pharmaceutical, with the same disastrous results. If we continue sterilizing every surface, we will eventually become sterile! Just look at the examples from the animal kingdom.

What we seem to have before us is a pattern of toxic mothers having toxic babies, feeding them toxic foods, and covering them with toxic products, with each generation resulting in weaker, sensitive, sicker children. People are looking to blame one cause like vaccinations, but there are many contributing factors.

I am not pointing the finger at any parents in particular. Rational ignorance is expected in a time when both parents are working and there is not enough time to research every little detail that pertains to their child. However, this remains the parent's responsibility, and there are more information sources available now, especially with the internet. This topic is much too important and enormous to be discussed in this book, but I urge you to do your own investigation into the damaging effects of petrochemicals on the human body and wildlife.

Only use organic or petrochemical free products on the skin and in the house. "Natural" is not healthy; it can still contain petrochemicals and phytoestrogens. Stop being seduced by the word "natural."

Ecoestrogens don't mimic estrogen they *are* synthetic pseudo estrogens. Avoid these popular prevalent ecoestrogens in your household products – BPA, PABA, paraben, propylparaben, butylparaben, phthalate, petroleum, Triclosan and all petrochemicals, look for chemical free labels.

The following products and practices should be avoided by everyone, but especially by pregnant women, babies and developing children:

- Processed foods, especially with soy as an emulsifier
- Nonorganic food (pesticides) Genetically modified organisms (GMOs) in food
- Pasteurized and homogenized dairy products, milk, and cheese
- Phytoestrogens – flax, soy, sesame, hummus and multigrain
- Scented products, including perfumes and air fresheners (they readily reach the brain and lungs)
- Hand sanitizers, hand wipes and baby wipes – anything labeled "anti-bacterial" (Triclosan)
- Fabric softener and laundry detergent
- Cosmetics, including nonorganic makeup
- Skincare products (moisturizer, cleanser, serums, sunscreens)
- Hair care (shampoo, conditioner, hairspray, gels, waxes, mousse)
- Bath and body products (soap, bath wash, lotion)
- Pesticides (gardens, lawns, produce, bombings for homes)
- Out gassing of new clothes, paint, carpet, furniture, and fiberboard
- Spermicidal gels and condoms
- Hot liquids placed in plastic or Styrofoam cups
- Teflon pots, pans and grills (Teflon is carcinogenic)
- Canned foods, including baby formula
- Bottled water, tap water, and reverse osmosis
- Never freeze foods in plastic
- Microwaves (high heat destroys nutrients)

The skin is the largest organ—everything placed, rubbed, and buffed into it is absorbed and delivered directly into the bloodstream, bypassing the cleansing effect of the liver. Why eat organic and then place poisonous products on the skin? Save yourself and your family's health; only use organic and petrochemical-free body and household products.

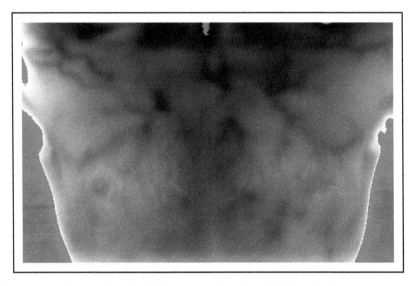

Thermogram of a man. Men should be non-vascular due to high levels of testosterone versus estrogen and why the rate of male breast cancer is lower. Note mild unusual vascular pattern.

We can no longer ignore the mounting research and evidence demonstrating that eco-estrogens are affecting our health. It is changing the human species, influencing our physiology and altering our reproduction, which is a dangerous evolution affecting our progeny and ultimately our future. Take a moment to observe the state of our world, our oceans, the animals, do you really think we are not affected? Do you really think we are truly healthy? Each species is a microcosm or a reflection of the macrocosm or world we live in. It is time to make a change and actually follow through! Stop saying and start changing ourselves and our world.

# 7. Breast Canswers to Estrogen Lies

No wonder women are confused about their hormones and health. Their doctors are so misinformed. We can no longer depend on the medical establishment to supply us with correct and evidence-based medical information because the majority of doctors are mis-educated in regards to breast health, do minimal to no research of their own, and they repeat medical rumor as medical fact.

Hormone therapy is big business. Women will do anything to stay young, and unfortunately, this trait is exploited. Misinformation spreads like wildfire as incorrectly educated doctors speak to colleagues at a weekend seminar, with the purpose of educating peers and medical professionals. They repeat that estrogen is the key to hormone balance and staying young, all based on erroneous rumors. The doctors attending accept these rumors as medical facts without question. These doctors now return to their clinic and "specialize" in hormones, selling women thousands of dollars of products that actually increase their risk of breast cancer.

Ladies, only *you* can stop this vicious cycle. You are the consumer who is creating the supply. *You* are the General to *your* health. A doctor is *your* health advisor, not your dictator. Educate yourself with the answers below so that *you* can make informed decisions.

Breast cancer is one of the easiest diseases to prevent, yet research into breast cancer receives more money than any other disease. It must be clarified again that estrogen does not cause cancer; it increases the risk because it provides an environment in which possible cancer may be "fed." If cancer was a seed, then estrogen would be the fertilizer that promotes its growth. Around eighty percent of breast cancers are influenced by estrogen. The more estrogen you use the faster the cancer grows. If you want to dramatically reduce your risk of breast cancer, stop using what causes it to grow, starve it! My question to you and the establishment…why are estrogen, birth control pills and bioidentical estrogen handed out like candy? We are *not* estrogen-deficient. If we were, then breast cancer would be significantly lower!

Below are the breast "canswers" to false claims concerning estrogens.

## Estrogen Therapies Are Healthy for Women.
## *False Intel!*

This beautiful chronology is from the book *Estrogen and Breast Cancer: A Warning to Women* by Carol Ann Rinzler. For the complete chronology, please refer to Appendix B.

1929:  The first estrogen (estrone) is isolated and identified

1931:  First American woman given first injection of estrogen

1932:  Estrogen injections produce malignant breast tumors in male laboratory mice

1937:  *The incidence of breast cancer in the United States is 67 cases per 100,000 (white) women*

1940:  The first oral estrogens for ERT (estrogen replacement therapy) go on sale
*The incidence of breast cancer in the United States is 59 cases for every 100,000 women*
*An American woman's lifetime risk of breast cancer in 1-in-20*

1950:  *The incidence of breast cancer in the United States is 65 cases for every 100,000 women*
*An American woman's lifetime risk of breast cancer in 1-in-15*

1960:  *The incidence of breast cancer in the United States is 72 cases for every 100,000 women*
*An American woman's lifetime risk of breast cancer is now 1-in-15*

1961:  800,000 American women fill their first prescription for an oral contraceptive

1963:  1.2 million American women are using the Pill

1969:  *The ACS predicts 29,000 female breast cancer deaths*

*The incidence of breast cancer in the United States is 72.5 cases for every 100,000 white; 60.1 cases for every 100,000 black women*

1970:  8.5 million American women are using birth control pills

*The incidence of breast cancer in the United States is 74 cases for every 100,000 women*

*An American woman's lifetime risk of breast cancer is now 1-in-13*

1972:  *Breast cancer is now the leading cause of cancer deaths among American women*

1973:  10 million American women are using birth control pills

1974:  5 million American women are using estrogen to relieve menopausal symptoms

*The ACS predicts 90,000 new cases of female breast cancer and 33,000 female breast cancer deaths*

1976:  22.3 percent of all fertile American women are using oral contraceptives

Approximately 6 million women are using ERT

1977:  *The incidence of breast cancer in the United States is 81 cases for every 100,000 women*

1980:  *The incidence of breast cancer in the United States is 90 cases for every 100,000 women*

*An American woman's lifetime risk of breast cancer is now 1-in-11*

1984:  *The ACS predicts 115,000 new cases of female breast cancer*

1985:  11.8 million American women age eighteen to forty-four are using the Pill

1986:  Nearly 12.5 million American women age fifteen to forty-four are using the Pill

*The ACS predicts 123,000 new cases of female breast cancer and 39,900 deaths*

*An American woman's lifetime risk of breast cancer is now 1-in-10*

1988:  Approximately 14 million American women age fifteen to forty-four are using the Pill

*The ACS predicts 135,000 new cases of female breast cancer and 42,300 deaths*

1989:  3.5 million American women are using ERT
*The incidence of breast cancer in the America is 105 cases per 100,000 women*

1990:  Incidence of ER+ (estrogen receptor positive) tumors among American women is increasing five times faster than incidence of ER-negative tumors
*The ACS predicts 150,000 new cases of female breast cancer and 44,300 deaths*

1991:  16 million American women aged fifteen to forty-four are using the Pill
15 percent of all post-menopausal American women are using ERT
*An American woman's lifetime risk of breast cancer is now 1-in-9*
*The ACS predicts 175,000 new cases of female breast cancer and 44,500 deaths*

1992:  *The National Cancer Institute predicts 180,000 new cases of female breast cancer and 46,000 deaths*
*An American woman's lifetime risk of breast cancer is now 1-in-8*

## Chronology continued by Wendy Sellens, DACM

2000:  *The AAFP predicts 182,800 new female cases of breast cancer and 48,800 deaths*

2005:  *The ACS predicts 211,240 new cases of female invasive breast cancer and 58,490 of in situ breast cancer and 40,410 deaths*
*The ACS predicts 1,690 cases of breast cancer in MEN and 460 deaths*

2011:  *The ACS predicts 230,480 new cases of female invasive breast cancer and 57,650 of in situ breast cancer and 39,520 deaths*
*The ACS predicts 2,140 cases of breast cancer in MEN which is about 1 percent of breast cancers and 450 deaths*

2017:  *The ACS predicts an estimated 252,710 new cases of female invasive breast cancer with approximately 40,610 deaths.*

*The ACS predicts 2,470 cases of bresat cancer in MEN and 460 men are expected to die from breast cancer in 2017.*

## Women Are Estrogen Deficient. *False Intel!*

Breast Canswer:

Estrogen deficiency is *extremely* rare. Only a small percent of menopausal women who have thermography performed are "normal," or nonvascular. Many will read this book and truly believe the information does not apply to them because they have been told countless times that they are estrogen-deficient. These are the woman I am writing this book for! I have seen only a handful of women who were taking estrogen and had a normal thermogram. The statistics are simply not on your side. I know you're shocked by this – I was, too, when my research led me to this conclusion. This is information you need to understand in order to share and save lives. Too many of our women have died because of this deception and will continue to do so until we unite T-O-G-E-T-H-E-R.

Eighty percent of breast cancers are fed by estrogen. If we were estrogen-deficient, like they want us to believe, then breast cancer would be significantly lower! Pause and think about that.

Let's start at the beginning.

In 1964 Newsweek published an article, *"No More Menopause?"* in which a New York gynecologist, Dr. Robert A. Wilson, reported that a woman's "change of life" was due to a decrease in estrogen and progesterone. That part is true - menopause occurs when women experience drops in both estrogen and progesterone. But in his book, *Feminine Forever*, Dr. Wilson discusses only discussed estrogen as treatment. Another enthusiastic writer, Anne Walsh, hopped on this bandwagon and in 1965 wrote the book, *Now! The pills to keep women young! ERT, The first complete account of the miracle hormone treatment that may revolutionize the lives of millions of women!* Both authors promised women would be beautiful forever. Well, it's been sixty years. Let's see if they lived up to the hype they created.

Unfortunately, we now know little research was done and the public, women, were used as the guinea pigs. By 1975 research confirmed that women on ERT, estrogen replacement therapy, were four to eight times more likely to get uterine cancer than women not taking ERT. Unopposed estrogen proved to be fatal. Not to be dismayed, they went back to drawing board and came up with HRT, hormone replacement therapy. What's the difference, you ask? They added synthetic progesterone, called progestin, which happens to be ... another carcinogen.

Not only did these researchers claim to find the fountain of youth, they also went as far as to vow that HRTs would prevent osteoporosis and reduce the risk of heart disease. These claims still can't be proven, but many of your mothers and doctors still believe them as medical facts. These were lies that were sold as truths that many women, including my mother, swallowed every day, literally.

The Women Health Initiative (WHI) initiated the largest study on PremPro™ (Hormone replacement therapy) to prove its effectiveness. However, in 2002 they pulled the plug after just three years due to the incredible adverse side effects. In 2010, further information was released that said that not only were users of PremPro™ more likely to develop breast cancer, that cancer would be more advanced and more deadly for those users than for non-users. To be sure, many women very likely would have died if this program had continued. Now keep in mind, to be in a study these women were the cream of the crop, healthy, with no history of breast cancer, heart disease or stroke.

HRT study - 16,000 women for five years Ages 50-79
29 percent higher risk of breast cancer
26 percent higher risk of heart disease
41 percent higher risk of stroke

Fortunately, HRTs aren't prescribed much anymore. However, the medical community hasn't let up on the so-called benefits of estrogen, promoting instead a "bioidentical estrogen" and touting it as safe and natural.

But here's the truth: When this book was first published, there no major studies, outside of the thermographic evidence in our first edition,

202

on bioidentical estrogen. No one else is testing the effectiveness, the side effects, the problems. Don't believe the hype – estrogen is estrogen.

The term bioidentical means "same chemical structure." It does *not* mean "natural," that's just clever advertising. Really, by this definition, HRTs and The Pill are bioidentical. Starting to see?

Believe it or not, your body is *not* trying to kill you! If estrogen truly was critical in keeping us young our body would produce it throughout our lives. Our body is designed to keep us healthy and alive for as long as possible, that is its primary function. Your body is perfect at maintaining your health, it's when we try to interfere, or "help" our bodies with pharmaceuticals or supplements that we start running into trouble.

The dangerous truth is most women are progesterone deficient.

Fact: Excess estrogen causes PMS. Hormonally balanced women do not have this disorder, and yes, PMS is a disorder. PMS is so rampant it is accepted as normal. How can pain, excess bleeding and irritability be healthy? It's the body's way of telling you something is out of balance.

Fact: Excess estrogen causes symptoms of menopause. If a woman is hormonally balanced she will not experience night sweats or hot flashes. My great-grandmother had no idea what these symptoms were nor did any of her friends. They did not have "book club" to covertly discuss these issues as they did not exist before or were not commonplace. Women who went through "the change" used to be revered and respected, now they are mocked on late night television as dried up and hysterical.

Fact: Estrogen has a clotting effect. This is why all forms of estrogen increase your risk of stroke. Fibroids are caused by excess estrogen. How many women do you know suffer from fibrocystic breasts?

Fact: Excess estrogen causes dense, swollen, painful breasts. These are so common we joke about our big boobs around the time of our periods.

Fact: Estrogen is used as a contraceptive, The Pill. All forms of estrogen, including plant estrogens, soy, flax and black cohosh, cause progesterone deficiency. And we wonder why infertility is increasing.

Fact: Menarche (first period) should begin at around age 14-16. I got mine at 11 and I've had four patients tell me their daughters started at age five – yes, you read that correctly, five.

When I suggest removing bioidentical estrogens or ceasing hormone replacement therapy on a woman who is progesterone deficient, first I get disbelief and then tears. I actually have women cry and tell me that they don't want to get old. This is how much propaganda has misinformed women—it's reached the point that they are actually willing to increase their risk of breast cancer in order to look young. When I explain that the excess estrogen is actually aging them, they start to listen. When you are hormonally balanced, your body performs optimally, while hormone imbalance creates a cascade of health issues.

Why do some women who stop using bioidentical estrogen say that they need it to feel better? I want to believe my patients, even when I am looking at their thermogram and thinking there is no way that this extremely progesterone-deficient patient needs more of what is causing her disorder. But I do know, I have been there; it took me months to adjust when I stopped taking BCPs after seventeen years. If I can do it, anyone can.

Here is a way to view this seemingly paradoxical presentation. When a woman has had too much estrogen from an outside source, just like a drug, she becomes dependent upon it. A junkie only starts to feel bad once the drug wears off, but as soon as they get their fix, they feel much better. Even though the drug makes them feel better, it certainly is not good for them. The majority of women do not need estrogen! Yes, it masks the issues, but it does *not* treat the underlying condition. If it treated hormone imbalance, then the other massive majority of women's thermograms would be nonvascular or normal. Unfortunately, this is not the case.

Stop believing the propaganda—excess estrogen ages women and increases risk for breast and uterine cancer. Numerous studies based on HRT usage show that excess estrogen increases the risk of cancer and *many* more health ailments:

Estrogens have been reported to increase the chance of womb (endometrial) cancer, estrogen containing products should not be used to prevent heart disease or dementia, estrogen given alone on in combination with another hormone (progestin) for replacement therapy may increase your risk of: heart disease (e.g., heart attacks), stroke, serious blood clots in the legs… or lungs, dementia, breast cancer. These risks appear to depend on length of time the patch is used and the amount of estrogen per dose. Therefore, the patch should be used for the shortest possible length of time at the lowest effective dose, so that you obtain the benefits and minimize the chance of serious side effects from long term treatment.

This was taken from the manufacturer's website of a popular name brand estrogen patch. Please refer to the Collateral Damage chapter for all other forms of estrogen, their side effects and cautionary warnings.

After reading the side effects of just one example, an estrogen patch, is this acceptable? When studies on bioidentical estrogen are finally performed, they will show an increase in breast and uterine cancer. All that needs to be done is to compare HRT thermograms to bioidentical estrogen thermograms, as the results of these images are the same. Interestingly, the quote from the manufacturers of the estrogen patch's website states: "Patch should be used for the shortest possible length of time at the lowest effective dose, so that you obtain the benefits and minimize the chance of serious side effects from long term treatment." Most women are treated for *years*, while dosages vary for each patient.

Women who have been on the pill, patch, and creams for a long time and are now quitting them will undoubtedly have some discomfort. It's called withdrawals! The pituitary has adjusted for the excess estrogen for a long time, and it will inevitably need time to readjust the entire system. The body will always strive for balance; just allow it to correct itself. For those ladies who are not confident enough to throw out their bioidentical estrogen, HRTs, or BCPs immediately, I have them slowly decrease their dosage, just as one might do with a drug dependency. Since your body is used to this excess, you have to let your body readjust.

I also suggest using a compounded progesterone cream and possibly a testosterone cream while decreasing estrogen, as this should decrease any discomfort. Once your body adjusts hormonally, you will learn what it feels like to not experience PMS or menopause symptoms. Being hormonally balanced makes a wonderful difference.

Remember the hypothetical model; if this was a perfect world and there were no environmental estrogens during menopause, we wouldn't have signs and symptoms like night sweats, irritability, weight gain, hair loss, etc. These are disorders and a product of our environment. Be easy on yourself when you remove *any* drug from your system.

Side effects of menopause can be successfully treated with progesterone and/or testosterone. Dr. Hobbins has researched and used bioidenticals since the '70s. As one of the original bioidentical researchers, he spent much time in France with the creators. Dr. Hobbins treated night sweats, hot flashes, irritability, and many more symptoms successfully with testosterone and progesterone. Try testosterone and/or progesterone to alleviate menopause symptoms. The correct application of progesterone is to apply a cream form *daily* directly to the breasts. The correct application of testosterone is by injections. If your doctor will not administer injections, apply the testosterone cream directly to the clitoris. Please refer to the "Breast Cancer Boot Camp" chapter for more details.

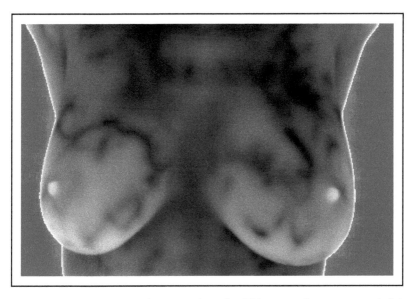

Average woman with no reported estrogen therapies. This woman is *not* estrogen deficient, but is actually progesterone deficient like the majority of women. Note unusual vascular pattern. "At risk" thermogram.

"I am so grateful this place exists and so close to me! The test is so easy and comfortable you just sit there with your shirt off while she takes pictures with the special equipment, nothing like the pain and agony of a Mammogram. I made an appointment for Thermography not really thinking I had any problems, I had just had a Mammogram ten months ago. Well, I did have a big problem and the doctor called me that night. I had a 30-minute consultation today and it was so informative! I am quitting my Estradiol™ today and hoping Kaiser will do an ultrasound right away. Everybody, this is so worth the money, it's your life!!! Thank you Pink Image for all you do for us, you are saving lives!"

Andrea

# Estrogen Is What Keeps Women Young.
## *False Intel!*

Breast Canswer:

As we have clearly proven, most women are estrogen dominant; therefore, they have an excess of estrogen to supposedly keep them "young." The truth is that excess estrogen actually *increases* the aging process. Estrogen does not keep us young, does not reduce wrinkles and is not the fountain of youth. If it was true then all the women who started taking it in the 1960s would still be here just as gorgeous, young and vital as they were then, sharing with us the fabulous benefits of this magical pill. Instead, many have become a statistic.

Estrogen doesn't make us feminine – that's our DNA. Estrogen is for reproduction. Period. That's why we go through puberty in our early to mid-teen years, and why the body stops production of it around age 50. Because we no longer need it. Very difficult to hear, but that is estrogen's purpose, that is the biological and physiological truth. If estrogen actually contributed to keeping us young don't you think our body would continue to make it? Believe in the simple wisdom of our bodies.

The majority of female physicians have the most difficulty believing that the above statement is a lie, as they personally use bioidentical estrogen as an anti-aging element. All of their thermograms show excess estrogen stimulation to the breasts, and yet most of these doctors cannot even accept their own thermogram as evidence! They have too much riding on the rumor that estrogen is anti-aging.

The truth is that excess estrogen increases the aging process. As stated above, most women already have excess estrogen. Again, if you experience PMS, signs and symptoms of menopause such as night sweats and hot flashes, infertility, migraines, weight gain, or the inability to lose the last ten pounds, insomnia, irritability, fibroids, anxiety, and memory loss, this may indicate that you have excess estrogen. Only when there is a balance in progesterone and estrogen will the body function optimally. Anti-aging is hormone balance—thermograms show that estrogen supplementation creates a hormone *imbalance*, which leads to an increased risk of cancer and an acceleration of the aging process.

Excess estrogen will confuse the pituitary, which governs many of the body's functions (think of the pituitary as the "general"). From birth, the body is in a constant battle to create homeostasis and the additional work by the body to restore this balance is what ages us. When the body is in balance, it has a surplus to add to its reserves. This is the true antiaging; not depleting oneself. If there is an imbalance or excess of estrogen, the body will react. First, it will try to restore balance, however, if the excess is long-term, it will lead to the body compensating by forming side effects including but not limited to the above mentioned signs and symptoms. Each woman's body will react differently. An imbalance in sexual hormones may disrupt other systems and eventually lead to more serious diseases. Autoimmune disorders, thyroid issues, stroke, heart disease, blood clots, dementia, high blood pressure and cancer have all been linked to hormone imbalance or excess estrogen.

As discussed in "Past Battles," women were given ERTs in the 1950s to 1970s. Please do not forget the disastrous results from just a few decades ago. By 1975, research confirmed that women using ERTs were getting uterine cancer four to eight times more than those not taking ERTs. Ladies, our grandmothers already experimented with estrogen therapy, why do you choose to be a guinea pig with bioidentical estrogen? As of yet, there are no studies on bioidentical estrogen. We are the study! Don't become a statistic, do your research on the increased risk of cancer associated with exposure to estrogen. Remember, bioidentical means biologically similar. So ERTs are bioidentical, as they are biologically similar to our body's form of estrogen. Don't be fooled by phrasing.

What about the millions of us who were on BCPs, birth control pills, which is just like following an HRT regimen? Shouldn't we still look 20? We don't. In fact, a woman who is put on BCPs before her first child will increase her risk of breast cancer by 400 percent. Another reason breast cancer is increasing: we are seeing the result of birth control pills (BCPs) on my generation. I strongly suspect the long-term use of BCPs is actually contributing to our generation's premature aging.

Our grandmothers already experimented with estrogen therapy, why do you want to keep the guinea pig cycle going? We *are* the study! Don't become a statistic, do your research on the increased risk of cancer associated with exposure to estrogen.

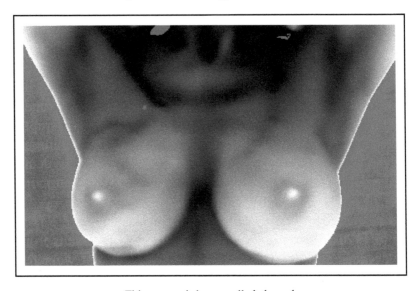

This woman is hormonally balanced.

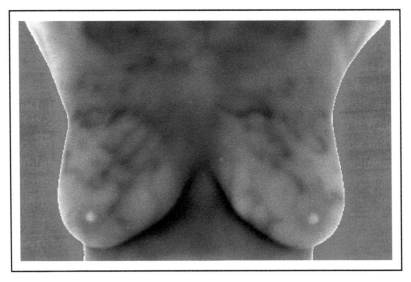

This woman has a progesterone deficiency. Does she look healthy? Do you think she is preserving her youth by using her bioidentical estrogen therapies? "At risk" thermogram.

# Estrogen Keeps Women's Skin Beautiful.
## *False Intel!*

Breast Canswer:

The vast majority of women are estrogen dominant; therefore, aging of the skin is not due to a decline in estrogen or estrogen deficiency. This medical fallacy will be explained further in this section.

The studies performed to demonstrate that estrogen decreased wrinkles or was beneficial to the skin were conducted with estrogen *directly* applied to the skin. Study results with women who ingested estrogen pills or HRTs are conflicting or inconclusive. For the purposes of the study, to effectively reduce wrinkles, estrogen had to be applied to the area of concern. I would argue that it is usually the other ingredients in the product to which these visible effects may be attributed to.

I've been a licensed esthetician since 2000, and never once was estrogen use taught or spoken about in relation to the skin. In fact, my Miladay's esthetician textbook only mentions estrogen as a hormone. There is no discussion whatsoever on its influence on the skin. This is because estrogen does not affect the skin directly. When women's hormones are balanced and the body is functioning properly, then the body has time to take care of other secondary tasks like the skin. It can effectively bring blood and nutrients to the skin for a healthy glow. Beautiful skin is usually a sign of a healthy person, while prematurely aging skin is a sign of an ill one.

There are products that include estrogen in their ingredients, but its use is a gimmick to attract aging women. If you look at any skin care line, lipid and vitamin C serums are a staple. Why? Lipids (fats) are the fundamental components for our skin and body. Use a lipid serum and eat healthy fats to maintain your beautiful foundation.

In Chinese medicine, you are what you eat. If you have digestion issues, you eat tripe or menudo, which represent stomach and intestines, respectively. If you want beautiful hair, skin, and nails, you have to consume animal products as they are composed of fat, blood, and flesh. As we age, the blood slowly leaves the appendages, arms, legs, and head, and shunt to the trunk to maintain the much needed internal organs. This reduction in blood and circulation creates wrinkles, dry skin, coarse grey hair, and brittle nails. To reduce the signs of aging, eat a balanced diet of animal products and follow a program of light exercise to promote blood circulation throughout the body. Plants are *never* a substitute.

Vitamin C is an antioxidant. When free radicals attack our skin, vitamin C attaches or forms a bond with them (remember high school chemistry?), preventing damage to the collagen or elastin in our cells. This is how antioxidants work on the skin and inside our body. They act like pawns in a chess game, protecting, guarding, and sacrificing for the king (and queen). Use vitamin C on the skin and eat healthy, vitamin C-rich foods to prevent aging.

Diseases usually appear first on the skin, as it is the first line of defense. If a disease isn't caught at the exterior, it moves inward. As an esthetician and Chinese medical physician, I observe ladies' skin all day. Of course, genetics plays a huge role in skin—many of us are very aware of those ladies who just use bar soap, eat whatever they want, and still look like supermodels in their fifties and sixties. There are always exceptions. Women who get daily sun for fifteen to twenty minutes, maintain a *balanced* diet of fruit, vegetables, meat, nuts, and dairy, perform light exercise and avoid grains, pharmaceuticals, supplements, and estrogen therapy are our healthiest patients. This is visible in their skin, hair, and nails.

Some women will argue and tell me their mother was on HRTs for twenty years and had beautiful skin. To become a strong, healthy adult, it is vital to have a balanced diet and limit exposure to toxins and pollution during the developmental stage of life, usually until age twenty-one. Our mothers and grandmothers were not exposed to the damaging environmental conditions that we were while maturing, so their constitution is stronger. The premature aging and increased cancer rates of our generation may be attributed to the rise in toxins in the food/water supply, pharmaceuticals, and the environment that has weakened our foundation.

# The Brain, Fat Cells, Adrenals, Stomach Can Make Estrogen. *False Intel!*

Breast Canswer:

Let's clear up some confusion about our hormones. Estrogen and progesterone are only made in the ovaries. Many people have been told that estrogen and progesterone are made in the brain, fat cells, and adrenals. This is completely and utterly *false*!

First, let us deal with the brain. There are no receptors for estrogen or progesterone in the brain. Just because many may "think more clearly" when using products containing these substances does not mean there are receptors for them in the brain. Dr. Hobbins is a surgeon and scientist who has taken biopsy slides of the brain looking for estrogen and progesterone manufacturing, as well as estrogen and progesterone receptors. They do not exist in the brain matter.

Second, the adrenals. The adrenals are situated on top of the kidneys and are considered the emergency hormone system; meaning, when the thyroid or ovaries are removed, the adrenals can assist and take over. Because of this, the adrenals do have the possibility to make progesterone, technically a bioidentical, but for most women, this is not evident as they are progesterone deficient (small amount or none). Dr. Hobbins believes that the human body is incredible and the adrenals could make a bioidentical progesterone, but no study has been found that proves this theory. If the adrenals were able to produce progesterone properly, the thermographic evidence would indicate this, and we would not be writing this book – and more importantly, if this was a fact, breast cancer numbers would be significantly lower.

However, the adrenals make DHEA. DHEA can change into estrogen or testosterone by removing an OH group. Under normal or healthy circumstances, the adrenals won't make these hormones, as the pituitary is in charge of the ovaries. In the absence of ovaries, or if there is a health issue, the adrenals *may* be able to produce estrogen and, possibly, progesterone. However, this is *not* an exact configuration of the original molecules, but an acceptable substitute. Making hormones typically produced in the adrenal are considered bioidentical. This may be shocking to most doctors, but only the original organ, the ovaries in this case, can produce the true hormone, anything else, made inside or outside the body, is considered bioidentical.

This reproductive mechanism is similar to a man who is castrated but can still grow a beard. The body is a wonderful machine and has the ability to treat itself or find balance in order to survive, but keep in mind that each of us is very different from one another. Though most human bodies tend to follow basic guidelines that most physicians follow, and this book is generalizing conditions as well, there are always women who don't "fit the mold" and are considered "miracles."

After menopause, there is a false claim that the adrenals continue to produce estrogen. The body doesn't contradict itself, it is a well-oiled machine. If the body has decided that you are no longer capable of having children the pituitary, The General, will stop sending signals to the ovaries to release an egg, estrogen and progesterone, or all of our eggs have been used. If the body has decided to stop producing sex hormones, why would it tell the axillary organ to produce it? It doesn't. After menopause, the adrenals will not make estrogen as the body is no longer creating life.

It should be noted that certified breast thermography can monitor DHEA and progesterone treatments and their effects on the breasts.

And third, we come to fat cells. All toxins are stored in fat cells, as this is where excess material is stored in the body. It is not stored in our organs due to the fact organs can't store. This is why most liver and kidney cleanses are a gimmick—*stop wasting your money and time*.

One of the nationally accepted risks of breast cancer is obesity. This is because of the "storing" function; fat cells are similar to a sponge in this sense. Excess estrogen is stored in your fat cells, but fat cells *cannot* produce any hormones. This is absolutely impossible as they do not have the complex mechanics needed to manufacture a benzene ring, which is how hormones are formed. Endogenous estrogen is only made by follicular cells in the ovaries.

Finally, the stomach is not an endocrine gland and does not produce sex hormones. Each organ has a specific duty, the body is an efficient machine, and the stomach's it to digest food. Saying the stomach does another task like creating hormones is the same as saying the ovaries digest food. The body is not built like this, it is well organized and each organ has a specific purpose.

You can't magically wave off physiology and that is what the medical community attempts to do with these false claims. Once again, it is the environmental estrogens that are dramatically increasing breast cancer, infertility, low testosterone and hormonal disorders in our children.

## Testosterone Can Biosynthesize into Estrogen. *False Intel!*

Breast Canswer:

Testosterone, like estrogen, is widely misunderstood by the majority of the medical community, and that's why low-T is being called a "new" health disorder and is currently on the rise. *Time* magazine has reported that the testosterone market is now a $2 billion industry. Breast cancer numbers are rising, but did you know they're rising in men? Breast cancer in men is a rare disease with less than one percent of all breast cancers occurring in men. In 2018, about 2,550 men are expected to be diagnosed and the lifetime risk of being diagnosed with breast cancer is about 1 in 1,000. The American Cancer Society has noted a 0.9 percent rise in male breast cancer from 1975-2006 and cite the reasons as "unknown." Well, the reasons aren't unknown, read on.

Here's a frightening statistic: Testicles have decreased in size by one-third since the early 1900s. Add that to the rising incidences of sterility and testicular cancer, and you really should be wondering what is happening? Why are these numbers increasing?

It is all tied to the rising levels of environmental estrogens. Breast cancer is theoretically rarer in men than in women, simply because men have higher levels of testosterone than women.

There is a medical theory the male hormone, testosterone, can biosynthesize (a process during which an enzyme converts a product into a complex product) into estrogen. Testosterone can theoretically be biosynthesized into estrogen. This is achieved with manipulation, usually in a lab. Testosterone cannot turn into estrogen and estrogen cannot turn into testosterone within the human body.

215

Think of a fork with three tines. The handle or source of all the sex hormones is cholesterol. From the source, each of the sex hormones are created: one tine is estrogen, the second is progesterone and the third is testosterone. All are similar and all from the same source, which is an alteration of the cholesterol molecule. It is possible to manipulate these similar hormones by removing or altering an OH group in a lab. However, the universal hormone DHEA has the ability to create hormones in an emergency situation. Does it do this on a daily basis? No, and below is the evidence why not.

Dr. Hobbins treated thousands of menopausal patients with large amounts of testosterone for libido, night sweats, and hot flashes. Never has any thermogram shown an increase in stimulation or vascularity to the breasts as a result of testosterone therapy.

The argument that testosterone can change into is estrogen is due to an enzyme called aromatase. There is a drug for breast cancer patients designed to block this enzyme. This was taken from breastcancer.org: "Aromatase inhibitors stop the production of estrogen in postmenopausal women. Aromatase inhibitors (AIs) work by blocking the enzyme aromatase, which turns the hormone androgen into small amounts of estrogen in the body. This means that less estrogen is available to stimulate the growth of hormone-receptor-positive breast cancer cells."

Since we specialize in monitoring breast cancer treatments with thermography we have *never* been able to prove this drug, AI, works at decreasing vascularity or risk in the breasts. We've had many patients try this drug with no change in their vascularity. And now you know why, because testosterone can't change into estrogen naturally in the body.

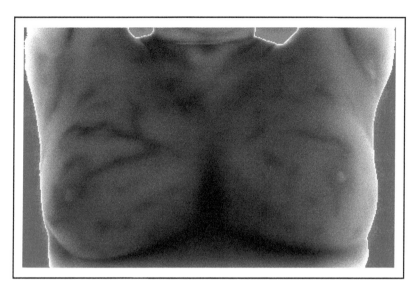

This breast cancer patient is being treated with the pharmaceutical AI or Aromatase inhibitor. Note breast cancer in right breast along with unusual hypervascular pattern. In theory AIs should block estrogen and return the breast to a healthy non-vascular state.

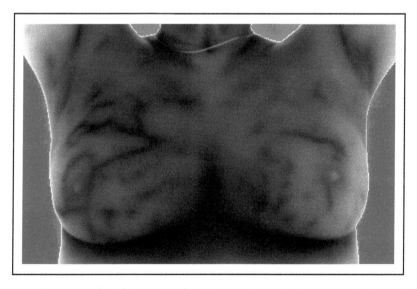

Repeat thermogram just three months later increased vascular structures, which may be evidence carcinoma appears unresponsive to treatment and currently suspicious of possible neoangiogenesis in right breast, which may allow cancer to spread.

In fact, Dr. Hobbins has used testosterone to shrink breast cancer tumors since the '70s. Only just recently has testosterone treatment for breast cancer become more "popular"—years after Dr. Hobbins' research was conducted. Dr. Hobbins has treated breast cancer with testosterone as well as prostate cancer with estrogen. This is an example of the use of what is called an endocrine antagonist. The theory is that, when testosterone is reduced in a male with elevated PSA and he is treated with estrogen (an antagonist to testosterone), PSA will drop to zero. Estrogen blocks the testosterone to diminish its effect on the prostate. Now in the case of breasts, Dr. Hobbins has used testosterone therapy in metastasized recurrent breast cancer and was able to shrink the tumor. Just as in the same approach of using estrogen to block testosterone in the case of prostate cancer, the testosterone will block the estrogen in the female breast in the case of breast cancer.

An interesting fact is that, when you treat prostate cancer with estrogen, the men experience a side effect of gynecomastia (enlarged breasts in men). Essentially, the male's breasts are stimulated from the excess estrogen, which results in breast tissue growth. In breast thermography, we can see that estrogen causes activity that is seen as vascularity in the breasts. This is clearly evident in transgender supplementation and most doctors who specialize in these procedures can substantiate the fact that testosterone cannot biosynthesize into estrogen. Testosterone reduces vascularity in women's breasts and can actually shrink them. When women want to become men, they inject extremely high amounts of testosterone to shrink their breasts. The opposite is true when men want to become women, as they inject high doses of estrogen for breast growth.

How to treat Low T: Application is key. Creams must be applied to where the receptors are located. The receptors for the sexual hormones are only located in the corresponding organs: breast, ovaries, uterus, testicles or penis. There are no receptors for sex hormones in the arms, thighs or abdomen.

If you have low T the easiest way to raise it is with bioidentical testosterone. Apply it directly to the shaft because this is where testosterone receptors are located. There are no receptors in your thighs or abdomen. Applying it to these areas is a waste of your time, product and money, since only a small amount will travel and reach the receptors. Since you are applying it directly to the sex organ you will notice results sooner and may not have to use as much product. Don't stress, as we've already explained, it won't change into estrogen. Then cut out all estrogen to increase testosterone levels naturally.

However, for men using testosterone *it is vital you monitor your levels*. Use of testosterone therapy in men increases risk of prostate cancer.

The major symptom of low testosterone in the ladies is low or loss of libido. Women need to apply testosterone cream directly to the clitoris; just like men, there are no receptors in your thighs or abdomen. It is easier to control the amount of testosterone with a cream versus pellets, which can't be removed. Now, most ladies require differing amounts. I suggest staring daily for a couple weeks, see how you feel and then adjust your application. Just like the men, since you are applying it directly to the sex organ results will be noticeable sooner than if applied elsewhere. Some women need daily application, some only need a couple times a week. Trust me, you will know, just listen to your body. Your passion will increase, along with your energy, while night sweats and hot flashes will decrease dramatically.

## Estrogen Is a Precursor for Progesterone in Hormone Supplementation. *False Intel!*

Breast Canswer:

Some doctors will tell women that they need estrogen as a precursor for progesterone to work. This is absolutely false. Healthy cholesterol is required to produce all of our sex hormones. As we have already gone over in a simplistic fashion, cholesterol becomes pregnenolone, which in turn, becomes progesterone and estrogen. Healthy cholesterol is found in organic butter, meat and eggs. Women who have avoided these healthy forms of cholesterol due to misinformation and appalling propaganda may have suffered hormonal imbalances.

Think of our sex hormones as a fork with cholesterol being the handle and our three sex hormones a separate and unique tine: the first is estrogen, second is progesterone, and final third is testosterone. All the sex hormones are produce from an alteration of the source, cholesterol, but can be independent of each other. Raising levels of one will decrease the levels of another. That is why breast cancer is continuing to rise due to rising levels of environmental estrogen in popular foods and supplements.

The answer is no, ladies, you do not need estrogen to make your progesterone cream to work. Many women use progesterone and testosterone together or alone, without the aid of estrogen, and have great success at hormone balance, which is evident in our 50 years of combined treatment with our patients proven with thousands of our breast thermograms, which is seen in our books.

## Estrogen and Progesterone Must be Combined Together for Hormonal Balance.
### *False Intel!*

Breast Canswer:

Many doctors believe they should combine estrogen and progesterone to keep women young. This theory sounds reasonable. However, women should *not* require the use of hormones after menopause as the body has stopped producing hormones for a reason. Such practices do not promote youth, but rather increase health risks! The reason that these, and most women, do require progesterone is due to the prevalence of excessive estrogen.

Women who are still menstruating should not use estrogen either, as this creates an excess, or imbalance, and may thereby increase risk. Women who use BCPs before their first child have four times greater a risk for breast cancer. Knowing this fact, why would a menstruating woman in her forties want to use estrogen? Stop believing in medical rumors.

The use of progesterone with estrogen rarely works. The estrogen stimulation is too strong. Estrogen is not required to make progesterone work properly; it is extremely effective on its own. Estrogen and progesterone are not an effective combination for hormone balance. Most women need only progesterone to decrease the exposure from environmental estrogens.

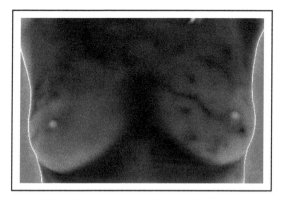

Bioidentical estrogen and progesterone pills, years unknow. Note unusual hypervascular pattern. Progesterone deficient.

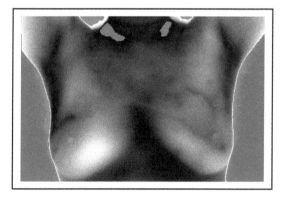

Repeat thermogram two years later. Bioidentical estrogen and progesterone pills for two more years. Note unusual hypervascular pattern. Progesterone deficient.

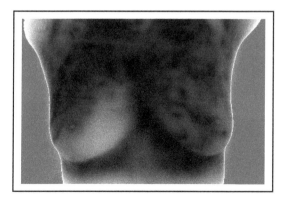

Repeat thermogram two years later. Bioidentical estrogen and progesterone pills for four more years. Note increased vascularity. Abnormal left breast.

# PMS Is Normal. *False Intel!*

Breast Canswer:

Just because most women suffer from premenstrual syndrome – PMS –does not make it normal; in fact, PMS is a sign of a health disorder.

That time of month again! How we all dread the cramps, the mood swings, the cravings, more cramps, heavy bleeding, having to sleep with a super size and a pad on a towel! No wonder we all dread this time of month! But what if I told you this is totally treatable?

Excess estrogen causes these issues and when you balance your body you will finally be that girl with a normal period.

Heavy or irregular bleeding is a surefire sign something is wrong and needs to be treated. Treating with more estrogen, like The Pill, will not resolve this issue, but actually increase your risk for breast cancer, by four times, uterine cancer, heart attack, stroke and DVT (deep vein thrombosis).

Heavy or irregular bleeding along with all the other symptoms of PMS can be treated by reducing estrogen, raising progesterone levels, under medical supervision, and if those don't resolve all your issues within ninety days, or if you want to jump start your treatment add a customized herbal formula, from a Chinese medical or Ayurvedic doctor, which is made specifically for your issues, should resolve the reaming issues. Endometriosis is more difficult to treat, but is possible with Breast Cancer Boot Camp too.

Your time of month is exactly what it means, *your time.* In many cultures most women leave the community, like the red tent, to relax and restore. This time of month is overlooked in modern times, but should also be revered.

This is your time to be easy on your body, since you are losing blood, that means no heavy cardio, as this will tax your body and age you or make you weak. No sex, which causes endometriosis. During ejaculation the force may push estrogen molecules out of the uterus into the body cavity from a small space between the ovaries and the fallopian tubes. In Chinese medicine you want to respect the flow of energy in the body. If the direction is down, then pushing it back up causes health disorders, including pain. Also, cold effects our periods and in Chinese medicine cold can travel up the feet to the uterus, so keep your socks on, literally. Warm feet – warm uterus. These tips will also increase fertility.

## Estrogen Studies Are Always Reliable. *False Intel!*

Breast Canswer:

Experts are finally revealing most studies are false, but is anyone listening? Studies can be manipulated and are often done so to sell a product. Dr. Richard Horton, editor-in-chief of the Lancet, considered to be another one of the most prestigious medical journals in the world, published a statement in 2015 proclaiming that an appalling amount of research is unreliable if not completely false. "Much of the scientific literature, perhaps half, may simply be untrue. Afflicted by studies with small sample sizes, tiny effects, invalid exploratory analyses, and flagrant conflicts of interest, together with an obsession for pursuing fashionable trends of dubious importance, science has taken a turn towards darkness."

Dr. Marcia Angell, a physician and former editor-in-chief of the New England Journal of Medicine, has also made a similar statement. "It is simply no longer possible to believe much of the clinical research that is published, or to rely on the judgment of trusted physicians or authoritative medical guidelines. I take no pleasure in this conclusion, which I reached slowly and reluctantly over my two decades as an editor of the New England Journal of Medicine," she has stated.

Read this section again, "Rely on the judgment of trusted physicians or authoritative medical guidelines." Maybe just one more time and let that sink in.

Here we have two prominent editors of two highly prestigious medical journals telling the public that as many as half of medical studies are at best unreliable, and at worst simply false, thus risking millions of lives. More evidence of this is apparent in the countless lawsuits against pharmaceutical companies. And since there are very few restrictions, the supplement industry is following the same dangerous path.

Reliance on supplements is not a "healthy lifestyle." A healthy person should not use supplements. Supplements should only be used as a treatment, like a pharmaceutical. Do you know who the healthiest people in the U.S are? The Amish have the lowest incidence of cancer, why? They are outside working six days a week growing their own food. They don't eat processed food, they don't vaccinate, they don't use pharmaceuticals, they don't smoke or drink and they don't use supplements!

Just because it is a plant doesn't make it "natural" or "safe." There is simply not enough research and review to see how conventional western vitamins and supplements combine with each other, not to mention to each individual patient. Compare western supplements to Chinese herbal formulas: Chinese medicine has been in existence for over 5,000 years versus just a couple hundred with conventional or western medicine. Each herb has been studied against every other herb for interactions and contraindications. They have reviewed which herbs are synergistic, or strengthen each other, which herbs reduce toxic properties, or which create toxicity together, but most importantly they were studied with how the patient reacts, which herbs are contraindicated for each specific patient. Yet here, in modern times, vitamins and supplements are sold over the counter for anyone and are believed to be beneficial to everyone.

These studies showing that certain estrogens are "good" for women simply do not apply in the real world. Isolated biochemistry studies are what they really are, and this is not representative of actual biological occurrences. These studies should be thoroughly analyzed, critiqued, and never taken as gospel from above. If the supposed evidence proclaims that these estrogens are "healthy" and this conclusion is transferred to a living animal, why do the findings not corroborate, but rather invalidate, such conclusions? (Please read ecoestrogens and in the "Breast Canswer" how "healthy" estrogen, when experimented with correctly on living dynamic animals truly affects animal growth and development!) Why do animals exposed to ecoestrogens in a toxic environmental accident have sterility problems, bear less male children or bear males with smaller testes or penises (feminization) and same sex pairing?

Doctors always tell me they research many studies, but what they fail to consider is that all of these studies take place in vitro. This means in a sterilized petri dish, in a very contained room with instruments, studied under the harshest of environments where scientists can watch and see what influences them. Believe it or not, your body is not contained in such a manner and is not sterilized, but lives in a variety of environments. It is a complex system that always astounds science, with enough amazement at times to utter the word "miracle." Also, no two women are the same. This is why a pill or medication may work for some but have a completely different effect or none at all, for others. Ladies, your bodies are not a sterilized, contaminant-free environment. You are a dynamic individual in an ever-changing environment.

Breast thermograms can and do show that estrogen stimulates and increases the vascularity in the breasts, on an *individual basis*. With that said, there are a few women who can metabolize high amounts of estrogen and have a normal thermogram, regardless of excessive estrogen. While this probably is primarily due to genetics, I might just call them a miracle.

I tell each of my patients, "Your breasts can't lie to you; they are your breast friends." Silly, but true. When patients look at the computer screen while they are being imaged, they can literally *see* the proof for themselves and determine which therapies are working. I challenge them to question why, if their doctor is so fabulous at hormones, do their breasts have an unusual vascular pattern that is considered unhealthy?

Since thermograms observe the blood vessels, women who take these supposedly "healthy" or "good" estrogens would be nonvascular. But nearly every woman who has taken these "good" estrogens has had an increased vascular pattern. If the theories taken from these studies were true, then thermography would support such claims. I'm going to repeat myself because it is vital you understand this. If estrogen supplementation was beneficial either with synthetic or plant then why doesn't 50 years of experience and thousands of breast thermograms support this theory? After all, a thermogram is a test of breast health. Why are breast cancer numbers continuing to rise? Because all types of estrogen stimulation is unhealthy. Another argument doctors attempt to use is that estrogen supplementation must be used with progesterone to balance it out. Sound reasonable, but the majority of those thousands of thermograms were with both hormones! The hormone cocktail rarely works, get off the band wagon and save yourself. However, evidence points to the opposite of their claims. Don't take my word for it, ladies, conduct your own studies; get a certified breast thermogram from an accredited clinic.

I encourage my patients to listen to their body, and together, we work out a treatment protocol; everyone is different so each treatment protocol varies slightly. We have been told for so long we aren't intelligent enough to know if we are sick. This is absolutely untrue. Many women know when something is wrong and it is important to trust our instincts. Remember, a doctor is educated to diagnose certain patterns and recommend treatment, but it is you who ultimately chooses which treatment. Always get a second opinion and find a doctor who you connect with and trust.

An argument which no one has ever been able to repudiate is this: if these studies are actually correct in their assumptions with regard to the healthiness of estrogen, then why do all "healthy" estrogen supplements list the side effects of estrogen as breast and uterine cancer? Please refer to "Collateral Damage" to view all side effects of estrogen supplements.

## Estriol Is the "Healthy" Estrogen. *False Intel!*

Breast Canswer:

If this is true then why does the manufacturer warn you that estriol causes breast cancer?

As we have mentioned, there are actually twenty-six estrogens that the body makes, with estriol being one of them. Estriol is considered "healthy" because it is the weakest of the estrogens the body produces. The estriol that *your* body makes is beneficial to *you*, but estriol that the pharmacy makes, and the doctor prescribed is not. Estriol may be the most beneficial of all the estrogens, but this does not negate the fact that the breasts are stimulated by such estrogen, and if progesterone is not present in sufficient levels, this estrogen will become a risk factor. Many doctors do not accept this view, but this is most likely due to their lack of knowledge in current estrogen-based studies or their stubbornness to accept the results of these studies.

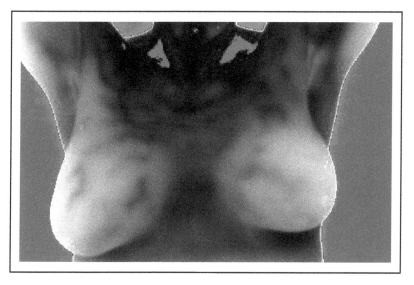

This woman has been using estriol therapy for seven years. Does she look healthy? Does she look hormonally balanced? Does estriol appear to be a "healthy" estrogen? She is progesterone deficient. Note unusual vascular pattern. "At risk" thermogram.

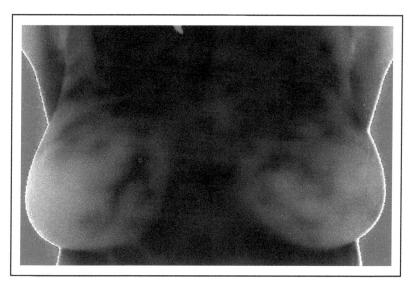

Repeat thermogram two years later. Nine years of estriol therapy. Increased vascularity. Severe progesterone deficiency. "At risk" thermogram.

One such study at the University of Texas exposed turtle eggs to "natural estrogen" and PCBs (a chemical ecoestrogen). Sexual development and differentiation in a turtle depends on the incubation temperature of the egg. Eggs incubated at twenty-six degrees Celsius become male, and at thirty-one degree Celsius, become female. Eggs incubated at twenty-six degrees Celsius (male developing temperature) and exposed to a "natural hormone" or PCBs resulted in all the eggs becoming female. "Natural hormones" and ecoestrogen have the same effect on animals. Scary study, huh?

Thermographic evidence shows that estriol and estradiol use after menopause increases stimulation in the breasts by causing an imbalance in estrogen and progesterone. As a result, women who used estriol and estradiol post-menopause are now at risk for breast and uterine cancer.

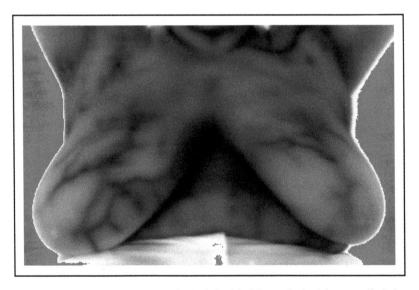

This woman uses estriol therapy. Does she look healthy? Does she look hormonally balanced? She is progesterone deficient. Note unusual vascular pattern. "At risk" thermogram.

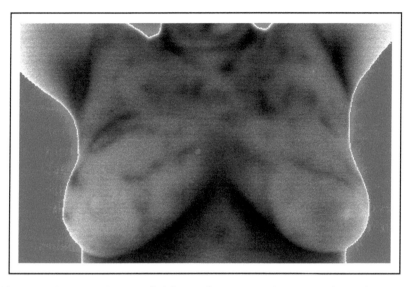

This woman has been using estradiol therapy for two years. Note unusual vascular pattern. "At risk" thermogram. Progesterone deficiency.

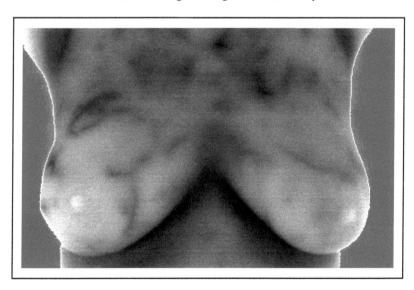

Repeat thermogram one year later. Three years of estradiol therapy. No change in vascular patterns. "At risk" thermogram. Severe progesterone deficiency.

# "Weak" Estrogens Are Beneficial. *False Intel!*

Breast Canswer:

Plants have hormones, too! The medical community wants you to believe because they are "weak" they don't stimulate. They may be "weak," as compared to synthetic, but they also stimulate our receptors. If a "weak" estrogen can attach to our estrogen receptors like a lock and key, then it is simulating it! If it couldn't attach, then it wouldn't simulate. That is why hundreds of studies on soy, a plant estrogen, are showing increased breast cancer risk with soy use. What our breast thermography research is showing, since the 1980s, is that all "weak" estrogens, including bioidentical estrogen, flax, black cohosh, red clover, sesame, hummus, and lavender, and some others are also stimulating our receptors.

What many in the medical community want you to believe is they block other environmental estrogens, but they don't. Scientists found that if you take equal amounts of estradiol and DES (synthetic estrogen) in the blood, more DES enters the cells than the natural hormone estradiol. What this proves is that our cells have an affinity for synthetic estrogen and actually produce more binding sites.

"Weak" estrogens usually refer to the estriol and phytoestrogens, flax, soy, black cohosh, red clover, evening primrose and xiang fu found in *most* supplements that are marketed to "restore balance." They claim these weak estrogens will occupy an estrogen receptor so a "strong" estrogen will not be able to. This theory is false as seen in most of the thermograms in this book. "Weak" or "strong," it is still excess estrogen causing an imbalance and increasing risk. Don't become a victim to this false theory.

If "weak" plant estrogens "blocked" harmful estrogen, then breast thermograms should be able to prove this theory and breasts should be non-vascular in breast thermograms. However, this is never the case. See with your own eyes if "weak" plant estrogens, flax, black cohosh and primrose can successfully block estrogen or if these plant estrogens actually simulate our estrogen receptors.

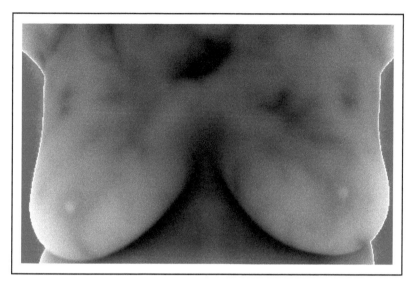

Using flax, years unknown. Note slight unusual vascular pattern.

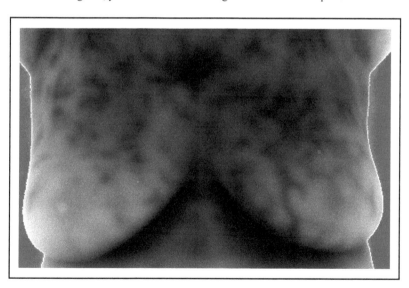

Repeat thermogram. Two more years of flax use. If flax "blocked" estrogen breasts should be non-vascular. Note increase in vascularity. Left breast is abnormal.

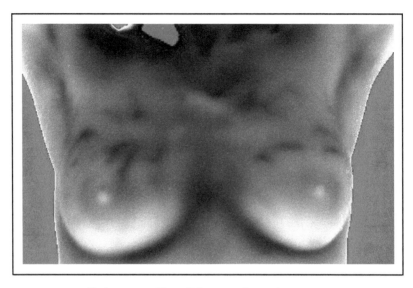

No hormones. Note slight unusual vascular pattern.

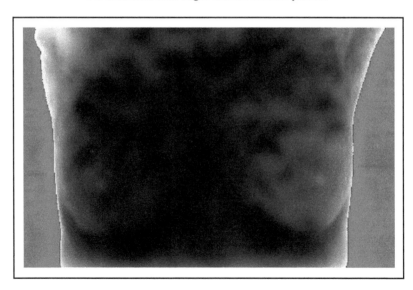

Repeat thermogram. Two years of black cohosh. use. If black cohosh "blocked" estrogen breasts should be non-vascular. Note major increase in vascularity. Right breast is abnormal.

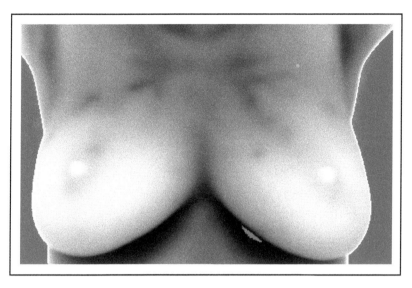

No hormones. Note slight unusual vascular pattern. Healthy breasts.

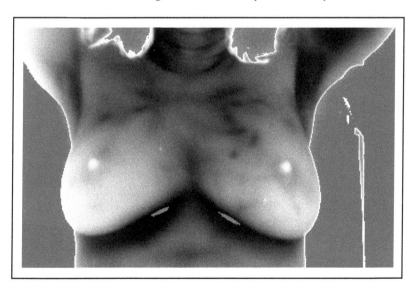

Repeat thermogram. Four years of primrose. use. If primrose "blocked" estrogen breasts should be non-vascular. Note major increase in vascularity in the left breast.
Left breast is abnormal.

War Story:

A woman who said she follows my Breast Cancer Boot Camp protocols finally came for a thermogram. We were both shocked at the hypervascular pattern evident in her breasts. She informed me she was told black cohosh was beneficial to her and her breasts. It was crystal clear this therapy was not working for her, as black cohosh is a phytoestrogen. I suggested she immediately stop using black cohosh and apply progesterone cream to her breasts daily. She returned three months later for a follow up, and instead of reducing her vascularity, she increased! When I asked what she had done, she replied that her nurse practitioner told her to use red clover, a "weak" estrogen, to block the estrogen receptors. Red clover is a phytoestrogen, and in just three short months, it increased her vascularity. She went from a potential "at risk" thermogram to an abnormal thermogram from red clover use. Now it should be noted she was using red clover, following the given directions of two capsules a day, for ninety days, *plus* she was applying a 10 percent progesterone for thirty days, and *still* had an abnormal thermogram. This shows how strong red clover phytoestrogen really is. After six months of no estrogen therapies, black cohosh, or red clover, her breast decreased in vascularity.

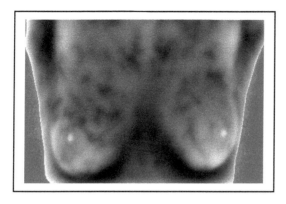

History of black cohosh use. Note unusual vascular pattern.

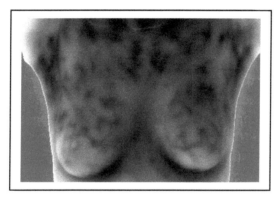

Repeat thermogram. Discontinued use of black cohosh for three months. However, three months of red clover use. Note increase vascularity around left nipple. Abnormal thermogram.

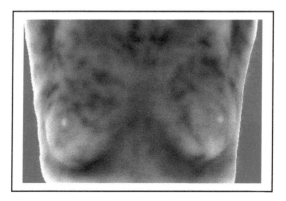

Repeat thermogram after six months of no estrogen therapies. Note decrease in vascularity around left nipple. "At risk" thermogram.

Essential oils are the hottest craze and many companies are expanding their popularity offering moms a small business while keeping it *au natural*. Love this natural approach to home remedies, however, remember plants are powerful and mastering these mixtures takes years of study. In the last couple years, I've had an influx of women applying these "breast" or "phyto" formulas directly to their breasts causing fibroids, breast pain, swollen breasts and irregular periods. *Never apply anything* to your breasts until it has been proven safe, which we do through our non-profit's research at The Pink Bow.

I stumbled across the effect of essential oils because I follow several alternative doctors who are using them daily on their patients. These physicians who had normal thermogram were progressing into atypical and worse abnormal thermogram. I started doing some detective work and realized it was implementing this new treatment, which exposed these practitioners to small doses, a few drops, of essential oils several times a day.

A small dose of just one of these for the everyday lady once a week may be fine, but keep in mind the majority of women are progesterone deficient: Don't consume or apply these plant estrogens in your essential oil collection if you are trying to conceive. Never use on children or have them ingest.

Allow me to repeat myself. *Never apply anything* to your breasts until it has been proven safe, which is basically nothing—maybe coconut oil.

- Aniseed
- Basil
- Chamomile
- Cinnamon
- Clary sage
- Coriander
- Cypress
- Evening primrose
- Fennel
- Geranium
- Lavender
- Peppermint
- Rose

- Rosemary
- Sage
- Tea Tree

I'm always updating information as more research comes in, for the latest list please visit estrogen-free.com

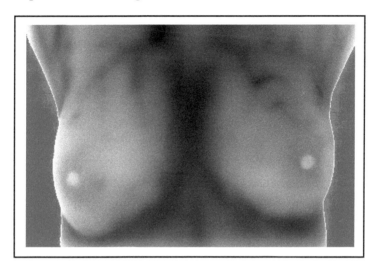

No use of hormones or essential oils. Note mild vascular pattern.

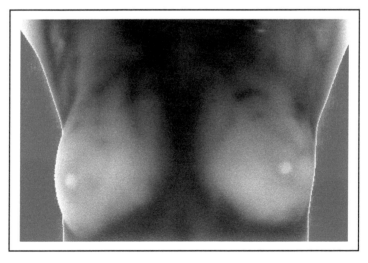

Repeat thermogram one year later. Use of many estrogenic essential oils applied directly to the skin for one year. Note increased vascularity. Abnormal left breast.

"Wendy Sellens is a phenomenal and one-stop-shop resource to women (and increasingly men) as it relates to hormone and breast health. I first found Dr. Sellens when I had a concerning palpable lump in one breast that had finally grown sizable over a short period of a few months. With two young children at home, I was panicked! I'd heard about the side affects and issues with mammograms and so was grateful when my community of healthy mamas introduced me to The Pink Image. Ironically, as I awaited the two weeks til my appointment time, I (still panicked) tried to be as 'healthy' as I could conjure up. I didn't know what that meant, except that I thought perhaps I should not be using my anti-perspirant. Instead I started using Tea Tree Oil (Essential Oil) directly rubbed onto my underarms morning, noon and night. The pain and size of my lump INCREASED SO dramatically that I was certain that a cancer diagnosis was the only possibility. As I spoke with Wendy a week prior to get details for my appointment, she reminded me not to wear deodorant the morning of, and I happily interrupted her to report that I don't even use deodorant, but use Tea Tree Oil. The pause on the other end of the voice told me something was wrong. She quickly and calmly explained to me that Tea Tree Oil is one of the highest phytoestrogen EO's available, and that by slathering it on my body I was adding greatly to my already disturbed hormone imbalance. I stopped using it from that day forward (and a few other items she mentioned briefly prior to my appointment), and within four days, the pain in that breast was gone and the palpable lump was gone within two weeks of seeing her. Her generous post-appointment phone consult was eye-opening and has impacted my total health as well as that of my daughter and son too. I'm convinced she is saving lives both through detection, but also through education. Don't delay, make an appointment with the Pink Image if you are even considering thermography or a mammogram!"

J.D.

## Blood, Saliva and Urine Tests Are Accurate for Measuring Estrogen. *False Intel!*

Breast Canswer:

Most women are estrogen dominant; therefore, demonstrating blood tests are unreliable and have contributed to one of the largest medical assumptions of all times, that women are estrogen deficient. This lie has led to an increase in breast cancer. According to The American Cancer Society the yearly death from breast cancer rose from 29,000, in 1969, to approximately 40,610 deaths in 2017.

Why do thermograms, a screening of breast health and estrogen stimulation, *not* correlate with blood tests. Why do the majority of breast thermograms show excess estrogen, which does correlate with the rise in breast cancer. Your breasts can't lie.

Let's make this one simple: You're going to have a lot of blood tests, and those blood tests are going to tell your doctor different things. Don't stress over them. Actually, take them all with a grain of salt. We have found that saliva and urine are absolutely unreliable and warn each of you to not have these procedures done. Hormones captured through blood, saliva and urine samplings do not accurately represent the actual circulation of these hormones throughout the body. These should be considered rough estimates, at best.

These tests can only attempt to check for circulating hormones. Any results being derived from such tests have neglected a major factor: progesterone and estrogen can be stored in the fat cells. Be careful in thinking hormones levels are the same throughout the entire body, blood, and brain versus the GI tract, muscles, or the liver. Is blood circulation even the same in the arm as it is in the breasts? All of these factors have to be considered when relying on blood test as a concrete measurement.

Another difficulty with obtaining correct results from blood, saliva, and urine tests is that hormones are measured in ratio with other hormones, as they all interact within the body together. Estrogen, progesterone and testosterone have to be measured relative to one another along with the thyroid and cortisol. Each woman reacts differently in this complex matrix, hence, each woman should be treated individually.

Blood tests: In order to even get just a suggestion of hormones by blood, several tests must be taken over a short period of time, as the body's hormones fluctuate daily, so one test done on one day is just a small part of the story. If you're *adding* hormones to your body, the blood levels are going to fluctuate even more.

Saliva and Urine tests: What is measured in saliva and urine tests is rarely the same as what is currently circulating in the blood. If this premise were true, then there should be tests that measure the hormones from sweat. This is absurd, as this test would never be accurate. Urine and saliva are unable to measure the ratios between the hormones, which is vital to hormone testing. What is circulating in your saliva and what is being excreted is not an accurate measurement of hormones, especially if you are currently using supplemental progesterone daily then it may test high in your urine or salvia. Some women will test high for progesterone with a saliva test and call me concerned. If you are using progesterone cream, which is fat soluble and accumulates, of course you will test high, but in ratio to estrogen levels in your body it may still be low.

How, you may ask? Well, let's first look at their thermogram: if progesterone and estrogen were in balance, then the thermogram would be non-vascular. Second, if they still have symptoms of menopause or PMS then their progesterone is still low. Just because it is circulating does not mean you are hormone balanced. The high amount is reflective of the hormone therapy, it still requires time to see a balance. Always listen to your body, if you have symptoms of excess estrogen, but your saliva test is reporting you have high progesterone this shows that this test is ineffective at correctly measuring hormones. These arguments should be a yellow flag that there is an issue with saliva tests. Saliva is not an accurate measurement of sexual hormones. If choosing between saliva and blood, always choose blood.

Think about testing water in the radiator for antifreeze—was it taken from the top of the radiator when it was filled up or out of the radiator drain? Where is the true concentration? How reliable does saliva or blood testing sound now? Be wary of any conclusions made from such tests; use these numbers only as a guideline.

What we believe is happening when a woman receives a report of low estrogen, especially while on bioidentical estrogen, is that when exogenous estrogens are in the body, they send a signal to the pituitary gland that says, "Hey, there is plenty of us estrogen here. Let's shut down production." Now understand blood, saliva and urine tests can only test for the twenty-six naturally occurring estrogens that the body makes, and because the pituitary gland had received information to stop production, the endogenous estrogens levels are going to be reported as low.

Another problem is that labs are not standardized, meaning each lab measures blood differently. This was demonstrated by researchers from New York Methodist Hospital, where they used blood samples from twenty-three patients who had a B12 deficiency. Three labs were sent a blood sample from each of the twenty-three participants. Each lab missed the B12 deficiency diagnosis, the first had a 26 percent error rate, the second a 22 percent error rate, and the third had a 35 percent error rate.

Take *all* blood tests with a grain of salt. Use them as only as an estimate, not fact. Just as with blood and saliva tests, urine test results should be used only as a guideline. These results are not absolute, each body metabolizes substances differently and it is, therefore, difficult to fit every person into the same model of "normal." In addition, it seems unlikely that these tests have the ability to measure environmental estrogens, so why waste the money?

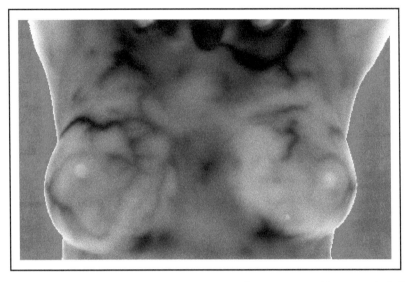

Many women test low for estrogen with blood and saliva tests. Does this woman look like her estrogen is low or deficient? She is actually progesterone deficient. Note unusual vascular pattern. "At risk" thermogram.

One patient (image below) told me her doctor wanted to do this test but that it wasn't covered by insurance. I told her to look at her thermogram. Does it look like your body is metabolizing estrogen? She replied "no." There is the answer. For those of you who do not have certified thermography clinics available to you, I would still avoid this test, unless insurance covers it.

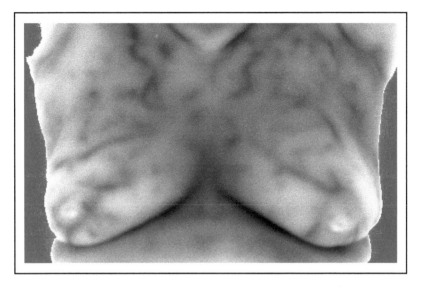

Doctor wanted to do a urine test to analyze estrogen metabolism. Does this woman look like she has excess estrogen? Would you pay for another test to tell you something you can see with your own eyes? Progesterone deficiency imbalance. Abnormal thermogram.

## Estrogen Therapy Treats Endometriosis.
### *False Intel!*

Breast Canswer:

The most popular treatment for endometriosis pain is synthetic estrogen with birth control pills. This is just a band-aid and does not resolve the root cause. In fact, women with a long history of endometriosis that were treated with synthetic estrogen eventually require a hysterectomy. If you want to treat a disorder you must understand physiology.

Endometriosis – how do you get it? Ever wonder how the cells got outside the uterus causing endometriosis? Answer: Sex during your period, trauma and surgery.

First, a quick review of our anatomy to understand how endometriosis is possible. There is a small gap between the ovaries and the fallopian tubes, which leaves access to the body cavity. When a woman would come in with fertility issues first thing Dr. Hobbins would check is blockage of the fallopian tubes, which is a very simple inexpensive procedure. He had a medical device that was similar to a turkey baster and would insert it into the vagina and blow air up. If there was no blockage the woman could feel pressure, from the air through her body on both sides and this was not issue causing her fertility issues. If one side was blocked she could only feel one side from the air pressure and blockage could possibly be her fertility issue.

Ejaculation is a vital biological process. The sperm must have enough force behind it to reduce distance in order reach the egg. When the man orgasms his muscles contract and he strongly ejaculates, pushing with the tip of his penis, which women can feel as pressure, up against the hole of the cervix, which hopefully from force pushes the semen up into the uterus close to the fallopian tubes. If a woman is still menstruating the lining, of blood and cells, which should be flowing downward, may get swept up too. Remember the gap? Sperm swim and they can leave the fallopian tubes and enter the body cavity at this point. That is why it is important when dating to have men wear condoms. It takes our bodies up to six months to get used to each other's bacteria through sex and kissing. To reduce exposure to multiple people's bacteria in your body cavity it is recommended to wear a condom. Some of you may be aware some women are allergic to their partners, this is the reason why.

Sex during your period causes endometriosis. The cells, not the tissue, may get pushed out the fallopian tubes and into the body cavity from ejaculation. These cells are what cause endometrioses because they have the receptors, including the estrogen receptor, which causes pain. When you have your period, the lining is sloughed off, but once these cells are outside they can't be dispelled monthly, just ask any woman suffering from endometriosis.

What about douching? The neck of the cap has holes on the sides not on the tip like a penis. The force of the spray is sideways into the vaginal barrel, not upwards into the hole of the cervix, like a penis. Also, women don't usually push the tip of the cap all the way to end of the vaginal barrel next to the cervix, it is comfortably inserted. However, to reduce possible risk of pushing cells out into the body cavity, by way of the fallopian tubes, don't douche until after your period has ended.

How to treat? Don't have sex during your period. If you choose to do so, then wear a condom or go old school and use a diaphragm to reduce the possibility of pushing cells out of the fallopian tubes. Once the cells are outside the body, it is very difficult to remove them if the body doesn't do so naturally, so you will have to treat the symptoms. As you have learned in this book excess estrogen stimulation causes pain. Keep in mind pain during your period it is *not* normal. Pain is your body's way of altering you to an issue, this case, excess estrogen. Balance your hormones by raising your progesterone levels to match your estrogen levels. Stop using all forms of estrogen. Women suffering from endometriosis can benefit from the estrogen-free® lifestyle. To immediately treat the pain of endometriosis Dr. Hobbins used 100 mg shot of testosterone. Testosterone is an incredible at treating pain of menses and symptoms of menopause.

In Chinese medicine sex during your period is strongly discouraged. The blood flow is moving downwards, with sex the energetics change to upward, causing stagnation, which in turn may cause irregular periods. In fact, some cultures for thousands of years women have celebrated the menstrual cycle. It is a time for self care, to spend time with other women and reflection for remembrance that our period or menses means life.

## Estrogen Therapy Treats Infertility.
### *False Intel!*

Breast Canswer:

Estrogen causes infertility, that is why women use birth control pills! Synthetic estrogen prevents ovulation, meaning, won't it produce an egg. Yes, progestin, which is the synthetic form of progesterone, is also included in the pill, but as discussed in this book, is not the same as progesterone and doesn't balance your hormones naturally. If it did birth control pills wouldn't work.

We've become a successful fertility clinic because many women are realizing their infertility is due to excess estrogen. They were using plant estrogens, black cohosh and flax are the most preferred, believing their issue was estrogen deficiency, instead they caused themselves to become more estrogen dominate and infertile. When they balance their hormones by raising their progesterone levels they happily became pregnant.

All fertility issues are not just due to hormones, but it is a simple way to attempt conceiving first. Remove all forms of estrogen and don't use any suggested "women's health" or fertility supplements as they usually contain more estrogen. Under the supervision of your doctor or alternative doctor, raise your progesterone levels with progesterone cream. Make sure you follow *our* progesterone treatments correctly! They are based off of 50 years of thermographic evidence! I get tons of complaints by women who have tired progesterone and didn't achieve the results we discuss, this is due to many factors. I cannot stress this enough, try again following *our* treatment protocols and specific progesterone creams. Read progesterone chapter or watch our videos.

If you are using IVF try this effective advice from Dr. Hobbins, who ran a very successful fertility clinic. Have sex or masturbate before IVF and don't wipe off the mucus or fluids. This is the body's way to simulate sex which moistens and prepares the body for fertilization with precious fluids. Vaginal mucus is created by stimulating the clitoris and vagina. There are two glands at the beginning of the vagina which excrete fluid. During the act of sex, the body will also produce cervical fluids. These fluids change the PH of the vagina barrel to alkaline, which is normally acidic and is hostile to sperm. The cervical fluid provides nutrients to the sperm. It's a long way to swim, and the mucus contains this substance, like Gatorade during a run. Fertile cervical fluid has a specific crystalline structure that creates a welcoming passageway for the sperm. Some women have what is called infertile cervical fluid, which is not formed correctly and looks like brambles. Do not simulate or have before IVF if the infertile cervical fluid is the issue the cause of infertility.

Sex before IVF will increase your chances of conception by producing vaginal and cervical fluids required for fertilization. Being dry during IVF is like trying to implant on cement.

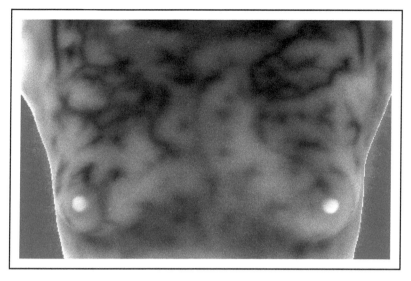

This woman is monitoring her IVF treatments. She is given large doses of estrogen and progesterone for fertility. Note progesterone deficiency imbalance.

## Estrogen Decreases Osteoporosis. *False Intel!*

Breast Canswer:

Many women coming in to see me stating they have osteoporosis have all been estrogen dominant? If the majority of women are estrogen dominate, how can estrogen influence bone density?

Why do men not suffer from osteoporosis like women? Are men's bones denser than a female's? Do men take hormone therapy, estrogen, for osteoporosis? No. Then why are we told *we* need it? Why are the few men who suffer from osteoporosis given testosterone, while women who suffer from the same thing are given estrogen? Doctors will say estrogen preserves bone density in both men and women and that all men normally convert testosterone to estrogen to build bone mass. But we have already proven that estrogen cannot become testosterone! Refer to testosterone section.

There is no real difference in male bones and female bones. Ask any surgeon who has done a bone graft, like Dr. Hobbins. While performing bone grafts on a male patient, Dr. Hobbins didn't ask the nurse whether the bone came from a female. Bone is bone. Our bones don't determine whether we're male or female, our DNA does that.

So why does the medical community claim we need to treat men and women with osteoporosis differently? The answer is, we don't. As we age our bones will get weaker; sorry to break it to you, but hearing the brutal truth is important for you so that you can begin treating yourself correctly. Men are generally more physically active over the course of their lives and are less likely to lose bone mass, since exercise has been shown to protect bone density. The medical community wants to provide a magic pill because there is no money in telling someone to walk.

The argument is that osteocalcin, a noncollagenous protein found in bone and dentin, is under the influence of estrogen, which contributes to indices of estrogen activity and tissue growth in bone. Listen up, you have cells that stop bone growth, otherwise you would keep growing. Osteoclasts break down old bone tissue, allowing osteoblasts to replace it with new material. Together, these cells facilitate bone mending and bone growth called osteogenesis.

If you want to increase bone density simply use it, when you use a bone cell by weight-bearing exercise, the old cell is replaced with a new one. Use it, lose it, replace it with a new one! Estrogen has nothing to do with this process. Even after you stop menstruating you still have bone cells, or osteoclasts, that will destroy old bone cells.

Think about it this way: Women don't make estrogen when they are pregnant. When you become pregnant, there is what is called the corpus luteum of pregnancy. The body naturally stops making eggs, preventing an already-pregnant body from the possibility of having a second egg fertilized. That could be extremely dangerous. The body knows how to take care of itself and won't produce an egg, saving the woman from this dangerous possibility. So consider this: If estrogen was in charge of osteogenesis, the formation of bone, then your bones would get weaker during pregnancy due to lack of estrogen. Pregnant women would be discouraged from participating in sports or even working out because their bones would be weak and at risk. All pregnant women would be on mandatory bed rest due to weak bones.

Guess what? *It's not true.* In fact, due to high levels of progesterone created during pregnancy after the first trimester, many women feel stronger and more powerful. When a woman is given a diagnosis of osteoporosis after menopause, this is a medical assumption that it is due to estrogen, when it is actually due to aging.

Let's take it a step further. Dr. Hobbins performed hysterectomies on women and didn't use estrogen therapy, ever, ever, ever! What's more, these women didn't suffer from osteoporosis until they were aging. A bilateral hysterectomy at a young age does not cause osteoporosis, osteoporosis begins post-menopause. It's assumed to be caused by a drop in estrogen and progesterone, but it is just the aging process.

Stop believing in medical association. Osteoporosis is happening because we are aging. Remember, the body knows best. If hormones were needed for bone density our body would produce it until the day we died. Our hormones are strictly for reproduction, that is why our body stops producing estrogen and progesterone, our bodies become too old to carry a baby. Brutal truth.

Much of the confusion is due to association studies. One group of post-menopausal women is given estrogen and a second group isn't. With these kinds of studies there is room for variables, lots of them. Some women walk, some do not, some will eat calcium and vitamin-enriched food, some will take supplements or pharmaceuticals. Then you need to take into account the fact that estrogen affects all women differently. Next they'll point to the X-rays and highlight darker areas, trying to prove bone growth from estrogen, when it's actually bone cells. As we age our bones weaken due to dead bone cells, which make the bones brittle and they appear dark on an X-ray. See, we're exposing all the ways they bend the truth to influence you.

If you are still convinced you need hormones for the prevention of osteoporosis, even after our wonderful explanation, at least take progesterone as well in order to not be overexposed to estrogen. In fact, The Pill is known to leach folic acid by lowering homocysteine, which aids in the prevention of osteoporosis. If birth control pills can contribute to osteoporosis, what about other forms of estrogen?

The only way to actually test if hormones actually affect the bones would be to take a test tube of bone cells and expose the bone cells to estrogen and see if it grows.

Unfortunately, as we age, so will our bones. Sorry to sound like a broken record, but I'm just trying to re-educate you. The best way to deal with osteoporosis is prevention from a young age. Trying to reverse the process when we're older will be much more difficult.

Here are some tips:

- It is vital for bone health to do weight-bearing exercise. This is the number one recommendation to increase bone growth. It's simple: just take a short walk every day. Web MD reported "a study of nurses found that walking four hours a week gave them a 41 percent lower risk of hip fractures compared to walking less than an hour a week." The goal is bone growth, which means replacing old bone cells with new ones. The only way to achieve this it to use your bones, which allows the old bone cell to die and it will be replaced by the new bone cell. Use it! Then lose it!

Low-impact, weight-bearing exercises include:

Dancing
Yoga
Pilates
Tai Chi
Golf
Elliptical machines
Brisk walking
Hiking

High-impact exercises include:

High-impact aerobics/dancing/Zumba
Running
Jumping rope
Stair climbing
Tennis

- Next, eat nutrient-rich foods and plenty of vitamin D and calcium. An easy way to get your calcium is from alkaline water, but you have to be careful when you are looking for it. There are only a couple alkaline water companies that infuse all the minerals into the water molecule while other companies use an additive or supplement. The mineral supplement will only keep the water alive for 48 hours whereas infused mineral water never "dies" – this is how you can tell the difference between the calibers of alkaline water companies. The key to vitamin D is to eat vitamin D-enriched foods, like fish, ham, eggs, and some mushrooms, and then you have to get sunlight to convert it. Some people may only do one of the requirements and not see any rise in vitamin D levels. If possible walk outside to get your weight-/bearing exercise and vitamin D at the same time.

- Avoid anti-nutrients. That means all forms of sugar, including grains. Grains are complex carbohydrates, meaning their composite is made up of a string of sugar. Fresh vegetables are also a complex carbohydrate, but unlike grains, they also have vital nutrients. Fresh vegetables are "alive" with enzymes, vitamins and anti-oxidants and fiber that are bio-available to our body. Grains are usually processed and actually are known to block nutrient absorption. The number one anti-nutrient product to avoid is soda, which has phosphoric acid and leaches calcium and other nutrients.

## Estrogen Is Healthy for the Heart.
### *False Intel!*

Breast Canswer:

Most women are estrogen dominant; therefore, they have an excess of estrogen to supposedly protect the heart, however research has proven estrogen increases risk of a heart attack. All types of estrogen supplementation should be terminated due to the fact that heart disease is the leading cause of death for women.

I had a doctor yell at me, in regards to my estrogen position, that he would not remove his patient from estrogen because it is "good for her heart." Look at the side effects chapter, "Collateral Damage," and you will see that one of the many side effects of estrogen is an increased risk of heart disease, as stated directly from the manufacturer of the pharmaceutical product. All the doctor had to do was read the side of the box to see that the estrogen he prescribed for the prevention of heart disease potentially increased his patient's risk for heart disease and heart attack. Estrogen enlarges the blood vessels while progesterone increases the elasticity of the blood vessels. It has been seen in studies that estrogen actually "increased the risk of coronary artery spasm whereas progesterone protected against it."

Estrogen has a clotting factor which increases risk for heart attack, embolism, stroke and deep vein thrombosis (DVT). This is why when your doctor prescribes The Pill or HRTs you have to sign waivers acknowledging the side effects of estrogen use so he is not held liable in case of a lawsuit.

The World Health Initiative (WHI) had to prematurely stop one of the largest studies on the effect of HRTs, due to the increased risks of cardiovascular disease and coronary heart disease.

> Although designed to yield appropriately powered risk estimates after 8 to 9 years, the trial was stopped at a mean 5.6 years of follow-up because of an increased risk of invasive breast cancer and the failure to demonstrate an overall health benefit. Based on outcomes adjudicated through a mean of 5.2 years of follow-up, women in the CEE plus MPA group had higher risk of cardiovascular disease (CVD), coronary heart disease (CHD), stroke, venous thromboembolism, and breast cancer...

This is quoted from "Health Risks and Benefits 3 Years After Stopping Randomized Treatment with Estrogen and Progestin" (from the Journal of the American Medical Association). Many of my patients comment they do not go to older doctors due to the fact they are not current on estrogen studies and still prescribe HRTs.

# Estrogen Therapy May Decrease Autoimmune Disorders. *False Intel!*

Breast Canswer:

Excess estrogen weakens the immune system. When the body is unbalanced, it has to take time away from normal daily functions, like stabilizing a strong immune system, to fix or alter the body to address the excess estrogen. Autoimmune disorders increase during menopause, perimenopause and puberty, with women suffering disproportionately to men. When women balance their hormones through the use of progesterone cream, testosterone, acupuncture, Ayurvedic medicine, homeopathy, personalized herbal prescription, meditative practices, nutrition, light exercise, and other forms of alternative medicine, the symptoms of their autoimmune disorder decrease or resolve entirely.

# Estrogen Is Healthy for the Thyroid. *False Intel!*

Breast Canswer:

Many women are experiencing symptoms of thyroid deficiency such as weight gain and lethargy, but when they get their thyroid tested, their T3 and T4 numbers are normal. Excess estrogen confuses the pituitary and the effect cascades to other areas of the body, like the thyroid. Even with normal test results, many patients shared their frustration with constantly feeling sick. One reason, but *not* the only, is that excessive estrogen inhibits the thyroid, which is involved in numerous hormonal functions.

Patients have reported that when they begin using progesterone to balance out their estrogen, their thyroid deficiency complaints decrease or disappear. Notice the rising trend in women diagnosed with hypothyroidism in the last few decades and the correlation in the rise in estrogen use, both in therapy and diet (soy and flax). Women who balance their hormones with progesterone cream and by drinking fluoride-free water (iodine and fluoride are in the same family and the thyroid uptakes fluoride), along with other holistic medical approaches such as acupuncture and herbal prescriptions, see their symptoms of hypothyroidism decrease.

## A Mastectomy Will Ensure No Recurrence of Breast Cancer. *False Intel!*

Breast Canswer:

Even after having a mastectomy, it is still possible to get breast cancer. A mastectomy will not stop breast cancer; it will reduce the percentage of recurrence. Around 15 percent of breast cancers are located in the Tail of Spence and the chest wall, which are not removed with a mastectomy. Many women have come in extremely upset with breast cancer recurrence after a double mastectomy. They believed they could not get breast cancer, but this is simply not true. Be aware that, with a double mastectomy, you are only reducing your percentages, not eliminating the possibility of breast cancer.

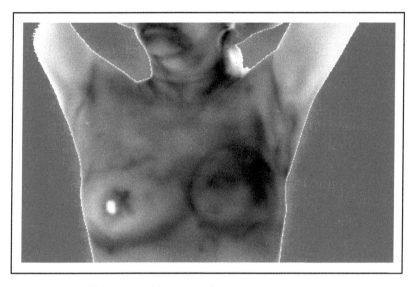

Mastectomy of left breast with recurrent breast cancer. Note neoangiogenesis in
left breast. Abnormal thermogram.

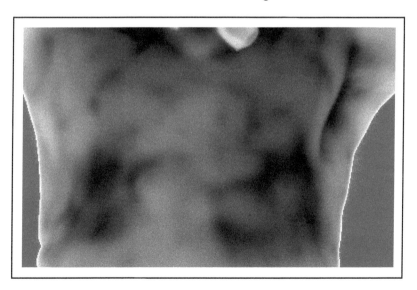

Double Mastectomy.

## DIM, Calcium D-Glucarate, Women's Health Herbs Are Effective "Natural Estrogen Blockers." *False Intel!*

Breast Canswer:

The theory of blocking the body's estrogen receptors to prevent our body's estrogens from binding is illogical. More absurd is blocking the receptor with another estrogen! If the body's estrogen was the problem, the body would cease to manufacture or reduce levels. Our body's estrogen is not the problem. Women have excess estrogen due to the overexposure of environmental estrogens bombarding the system. This overexposure creates an imbalance in the hormone levels which confuses the pituitary leading to numerous health issues. Don't block high levels of estrogen with another estrogen, it never works it still stimulates that estrogen receptor, you have to balance high estrogen levels by raising progesterone and testosterone.

I always find amusing is the number of women who are on "natural estrogen blockers" and are also using estrogen supplementation, flax or bioidentical estrogen. Ladies, take a moment and think that one through. You are taking an estrogen *and* using an estrogen blocker. Does that even make sense?

This supplement is especially harmful to breast cancer survivors. They put their hope in trusted medical professionals and they are not only endangering their treatment of reducing excess estrogen, as you can see with thermogram from breast cancer survivors, but also possibly risking their probability of recurrence.

DIM, calcium D-glucarate, women's health supplements and a specific Chinese herbal treatment (cannot name due to legalities) claim to be "estrogen blockers" or "weak estrogen," that block the estrogen receptors. But as our thermograms indicate, this does not seem to be true.

DIM is produced from plant hormones of cabbage, broccoli, Brussels sprouts and cauliflower and claims to reduce estrogen within the body.

Calcium D-glucarate is the calcium salt of D-glucaric acid that is found in apples, broccoli, cabbage, bean sprouts and brussels' sprouts. It can supposedly promote detoxification and hormone balance. However, calcium D-glucarate is not an essential nutrient, and therefore, no deficiency state can exist in the body.

I was truly excited to have a product that could decrease estrogen and vascularity in the breasts "naturally." In fact, I even conducted a test pilot study with the highest grade of calcium D-glucarate I could find.

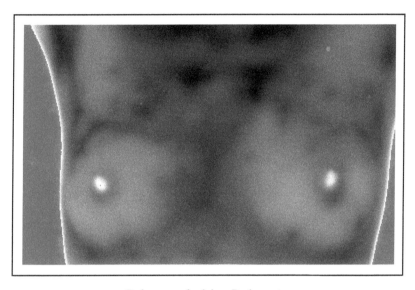

Before use of calcium D glucarate.

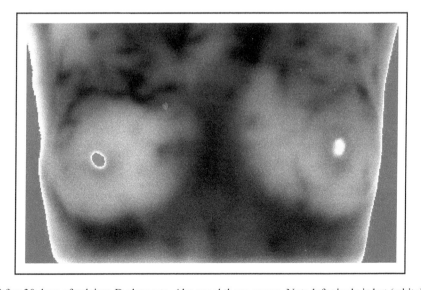

After 30 days of calcium D glucarate. Abnormal thermogram. Note left nipple is hot (white)

*Pilot Study (Refer to color pages for complete set of images from pilot study.)*

A six-month study to demonstrate that calcium D-glucarate is a "healthy" supplement for the breasts, by reducing risk by decreasing vascularity or neoangiogenesis in the breasts. Thermographic monitoring was to be performed for six months, every thirty days. Patient consumed manufacturers' daily suggested amount of two pills daily. After four weeks, patient reported that she had gained six pounds, and experienced mood swings, breast pain (which she had never had before), abdominal bloating and cramps. First thermogram showed an increase in the left nipplar delta T to outside normal limits. Due to increased health symptoms and breast health risk, patient discontinued study after thirty days.

With this study participant, the nipplar delta T (temperature difference) between the breasts, a thermographic measuring tool, increased and was now outside of normal limits, when the supplement was supposed to be reducing the stimulation. Of course, this rise in vascularity increased potential risks. In addition, the participant gained six pounds and her breasts were sore for three weeks straight. I was stunned and disappointed, as I never thought that calcium D-glucarate would actually increase vascularity as well as symptomology. I cannot be sure if it was the product's preservatives that were toxic or the active ingredients of the product itself that were estrogenic. Avoid these gimmicks, as we will discuss in the chapter on supplementation, as most supplements have too many toxic side effects.

I highly suggest avoiding all "natural" estrogen blockers, especially if you have breast cancer and are trying "alternative" treatments. As you can see in the visual examples provided, DIM, the specific Chinese herbal treatment, and calcium D-glucarate can increase vascularity and thermal activity, or not affect vascularity at all. This is a potential risk factor for breast cancer. We highly advise you not to experiment if breast cancer is present!

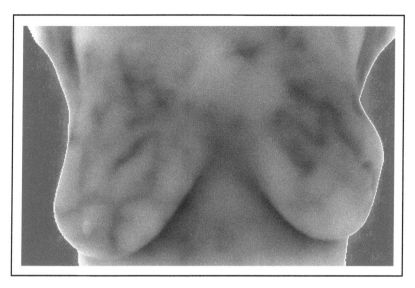

Breast cancer patient using DIM, calcium D-glucarate and popular Chinese herbal treatment containing xiang fu for several months prescribed by her doctor to block estrogen. Does it look like this supplement is blocking estrogen by decreasing vascularity? Note unusual hypervascular pattern. Lumpectomy performed in left breast.

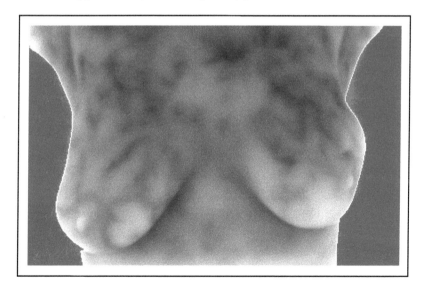

Repeat thermogram one year later. Breasts should be non-vascular, or "blocking estrogen" as supplement claims. Note increased vascularity in left breast. This patient was shocked that these supplements didn't provide the treatment for her cancer, blocking estrogen, which they claim to do. Doctors are recommending this as an alternative cancer treatment!

259

War Story:

One example is a lady who has recurrent breast cancer. A lumpec-tomy was performed in September 2011 and by February 2012, she was diagnosed with recurrent breast cancer, which was estrogen receptor positive. Her new doctor believed that the surgeon could have spread the cancer, but that can't be proven. However, when reviewing supple-mental history with the patient, she mentioned she had been using DIM and calcium D-glucarate after surgery until the recurrence. Again, this can't be confirmed and we are *not* saying that these products caused recurrence, but don't be a lab rat and take risks when treating cancer. After observing the effects of these products with thermograms for a few years, we know it definitely did not aid her into recovery. We believe that with Tamoxifen, her chances of recurrence, even with a "botched" surgery, would have been drastically reduced.

The Chinese herbal supplement we have referred to above contains three herbs: *yu jin* (turmeric root), *xiang fu* (cyperus rhizome) and *huang qi* (astagalus root). This product claims to block "bad" estrogen with "healthy" estrogen, but what escapes their intent is that *xiang fu* is a phytoestrogen. As we have shown throughout the book, phytoestrogens (like soy, flax, black cohosh, and bioidentical estrogen) are not "weak" or "healthy," but rather act as "strong" or "unhealthy" estrogens. And what have we learned that such estrogens do to our breasts? They stimulate our breasts cells!

In Chinese medicine, the effects of herbs and herbal formulas have been continually studied for thousands of years. This has *not* been done with Western herbs, and as we see in the supplemental chapter, this has created many issues. Although this is a simple formula, there is no historical mention or study on this particular formula, particularly with regard to breast health. It is important to understand that, in Chinese medicine, each formula is chosen or created for *each* patient, with the historical or traditional formulas being used as a guideline. Also, each formula may have herbal properties that are contraindicated in some patients, meaning not just anyone can use any formula. Herbs are medi-cine and are meant to be used in conjunction with the appropriate diag-nosis of each individual patient. Do not receive Chinese herbal advice from a doctor who isn't a Chinese medical practitioner, as they do not understand the intricacies of herbal medicine. This is not a practice one learns during a weekend seminar.

There are many products being sold as "hormone balancing" or promoting "women's health." Avoid all of these products, as they typically use estrogenic ingredients, causing increased risk and hormone imbalance. Don't block your body from doing its job correctly. First get a thermogram to determine hormone levels. If a hormone is low, then treat by balancing with the low hormone, which is usually progesterone.

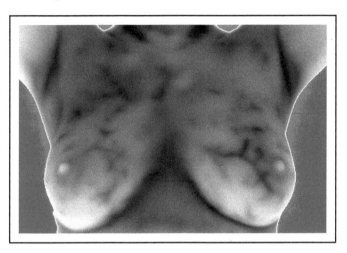

Using DIM. Does it look like this supplement is decreasing vascularity? Note unusual hypervascular pattern. Progesterone deficiency imbalance.

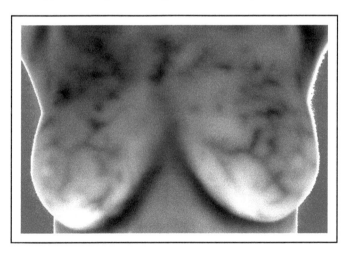

Repeat thermogram one year later. Breasts should be non-vascular, or "blocking estrogen" as supplement claims. Note unusual hypervascular pattern. Progesterone deficiency imbalance. "At risk" thermogram.

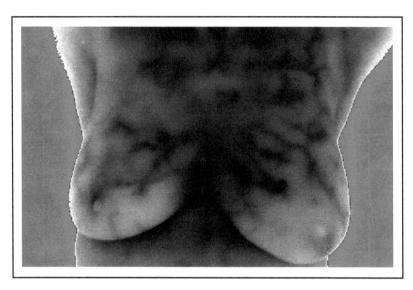

Breast cancer patient using DIM and calcium D-glucarate prescribed by her doctor to block estrogen. Does it look like this supplement is blocking estrogen by decreasing vascularity? Right breast has cancer and is abnormal.

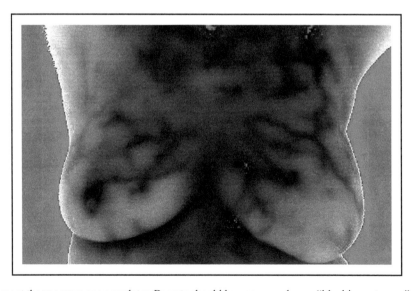

Repeat thermogram one year later. Breasts should be non-vascular, or "blocking estrogen" as supplement claims. Note increase in vascular patterns, which be evidence of neoangiogenesis. Right breast remains abnormal.

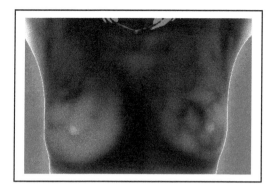

Using popular Chinese herbal formula containing xiang fu to block estrogen. Note unusual hypervascular pattern. Progesterone deficiency imbalance.

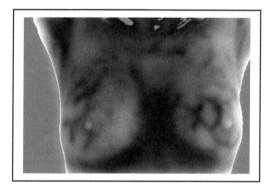

Repeat thermogram one year later. Still using "natural estrogen blocker." Breasts should be non-vascular, or "blocking estrogen" as supplement claims. Note increased vascularity. Progesterone deficiency imbalance. "At risk" thermogram.

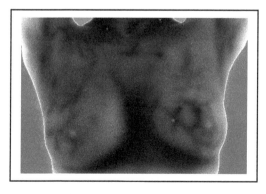

Repeat thermogram one year later. Still using Chinese herbal formula. Do breasts look healthy? Is this product "blocking estrogen?" Note unusual hypervascular pattern. Progesterone deficiency imbalance. "At risk" thermogram.

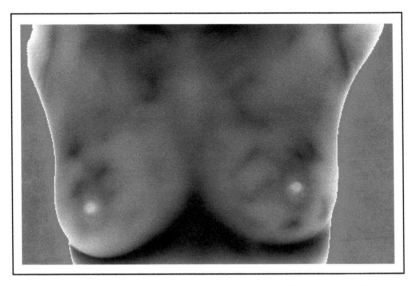

Using popular Chinese herbal formula containing xiang fu to block estrogen. Note unusual hypervascular pattern. Progesterone deficiency imbalance.

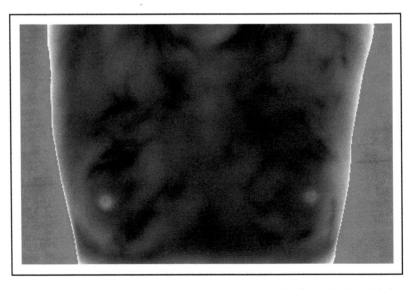

Repeat thermogram one year later. Still using Chinese herbal formula, plus added a supplement that claims to stop angiogenesis. Breasts should be non-vascular, or "blocking estrogen" and stopping angiogenesis, as supplements claim. Note increased vascularity. Right breast abnormal.

# Tamoxifen: Do or Don't

Breast Canswer:

Tamoxifen is an estrogen blocker and it does its job well. Many women do not want to use Tamoxifen because of its side effects, but if the cancer is estrogen receptor positive, it can be a valuable weapon in blocking the estrogen from "feeding" the cancer. It is in emergency medicine where Western medical approaches have the ability to be extremely beneficial. Yes, there are side effects from Tamoxifen, but once the cancer has developed to the stage that it is detectable, many of these side effects become a lesser evil, especially when death is a possibility.

Dr. Hobbins never radiated the breast or used chemotherapy, in fact, he used Tamoxifen quite differently than how all other doctors use it, he uses it as a treatment before surgery and quite successfully on cancers that are localized, usually stage one or stage two. It enables the tumors to shrink to the point that many patients do not require a lumpectomy or mastectomy. Dr. Hobbins describes Tamoxifen as having the ability to "melt" the cancer away and is able to observe the treatment process with thermograms and MRIs.

However, most other doctors do just the opposite. They first perform the lumpectomy or mastectomy and then administer Tamoxifen as aftercare. It is important to realize that doctors are not entirely at fault for such invasive decisions. Their choices are often based on insurance company policy, malpractice insurance coverage, and the licensing board as they find it difficult to risk their livelihood justifying a treatment protocol not dictated to them from third party interests.

Part of the reason Dr. Hobbins was comfortable with his medical approaches is that he is a surgeon, thermologist, and expert interpreter of mammography, MRI, and ultrasound (see Dr. Hobbins' role in mammographic research in the '60s, in the introduction). This means that all these modalities were made available and conducted by the same practitioner without the cumbersome process of communicating among several doctors. As an example, if a cancer didn't shrink within a certain time with the implementation of Tamoxifen therapy, the decision to perform a lumpectomy or mastectomy could then be evaluated. Every woman is unique and responds differently to treatment, which is why close monitoring of the patient with many modalities is important.

I read for a large alternative cancer treatment center and see breast cancer all day long. I regularly recommend Tamoxifen to patients with estrogen receptor positive cancer. If the neoangiogenesis is minimal or localized then alternative treatments might work. However, some cancers are invasive and past the point of alternative therapy. If a few months on Tamoxifen decreased the chance of mastectomy, it might be an alternative to consider. Or if an invasive case of breast cancer is no longer manageable with alternative or holistic forms of treatment (Tamoxifen might be a wise choice). If a thermogram indicates a minimal vascular pattern, then alternative or holistic therapies may be attempted with close monitoring by thermogram and MRI.

Side effects are always a complaint, but unfortunately, Tamoxifen is the most reliable estrogen blockers, which works to decrease the availability of estrogen to the cancer. If the cancer develops to the point that there is a need for pharmaceutical intervention, then there has been a neglect of breast health. The suggested usage length of Tamoxifen is five years, but patients rarely continue administration for that long due to its side effects, hot flashes and night sweats. Dr. Hobbins often treats these side effects with testosterone, decreases the side effects of Tamoxifen.

If women choose to quit Tamoxifen, I suggest to first confirm neoangiogenesis and/or vascularity has been reduced dramatically in the breasts or graded a thermographic score of nonvascular. Once the breasts are nonvascular, follow the antiestrogenic tips in this book. Monitoring of the breasts should be done with all imaging modalities, and if vascularity increases, then return to a treatment with Tamoxifen. Obviously, this is all done in close communication with a medical doctor.

I continue to be amazed at how many women who currently have or have had breast cancer remain on bioidentical estrogen. If these are estrogen receptor positive cancers, then they are most likely "feeding" the cancer or increasing their risk of recurrence!

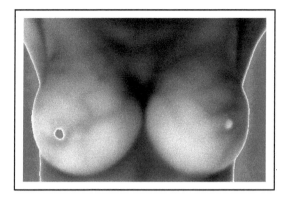

Invasive breast cancer stage II of left breast. Note neoangiogenesis in left breast.

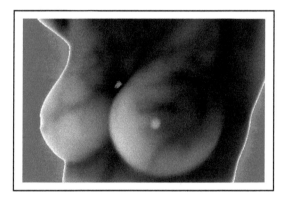

Invasive breast cancer stage II of left breast. Dr. Hobbins put this woman on Tamoxifen because he said it would reduce the size of her tumor so mastectomy wouldn't have to be performed, just a lumpectomy.

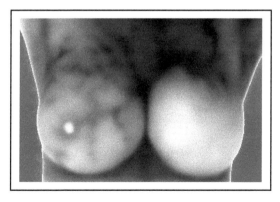

Invasive breast cancer stage II. This woman was only 36 with two children and after a month of Tamoxifen and conferring with her surgeon decided to proceed with a mastectomy.

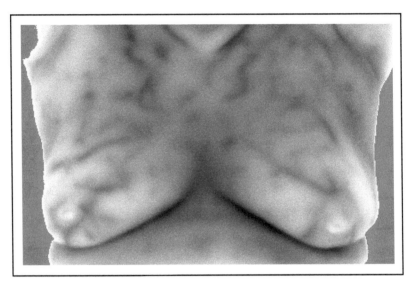

Unusual vascular pattern. Severe progesterone deficiency imbalance. "At risk" thermogram.

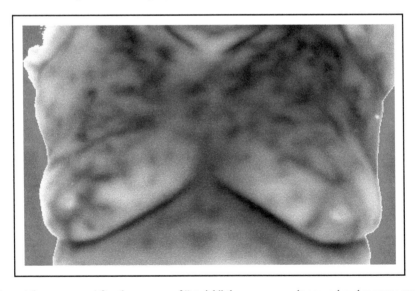

Repeat thermogram. After three years of "at risk" thermograms ultrasound and mammogram report finding in left breast. Abnormal thermogram confirmed neoangiogenesis in left breast. Tamoxifen is recommended to "cut off" estrogen supply.

# Japanese Women Eat Lots of Soy, That's Why Their Breast Cancer Rate Is Lower. *False Intel!*

Breast Canswer:

There is a misconception that breast cancer is lower in Japan due to their consumption of soy. This is a breast cancer myth. In fact, breast cancer rates are rising in Japan. The average Japanese woman's caloric intake of soy is only 1.5 percent, as stated in *The Whole Soy Story*. Japanese women eat very little, if any, soy cheese, soy dogs, soy ice cream, and soy milk. All of these are highly processed when compared to edamame and tofu. You have all heard that when Japanese women move to the U.S., the breast cancer statistics for this demographic shifts to 1 in 8 which is strongly due to our poor diet. In fact, many health experts believe the increase in breast cancer incidences in Japan is due to the influence of our "western" diet.

The Japanese diet is rich in omegas from the large amount of fish they eat, antioxidants and crucifers consumed from raw vegetable, and most importantly, iodine from all the seaweed. Iodine is a great advisory in the prevention of cancer (see "Nutrition—Eat Your Medicine" chapter). American women eat more processed foods, are high in carbohydrates (becoming sugar), refined sugar, and chemicals. Most people in America don't think that they eat a lot of soy, but it is in virtually every processed food, resulting in our high rate of breast cancer. Check the ingredients of everything in a bag, box, can or wrapper. Look for soy or soya emulsifier.

The key to being healthy is eating a balanced diet of real foods. Japanese women exemplify this and that is the reason breast cancer is low, however this is changing.

Don't buy into the Japanese women breast cancer myth, it will only increase your risk. Get educated, get the facts. Read *The Whole Soy Story: The Dark Side of America's Favorite Health Food* before you continue to spread this misinformation.

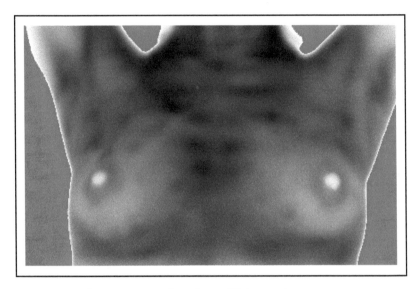

Japanese woman from Japan. Slight vascular pattern.

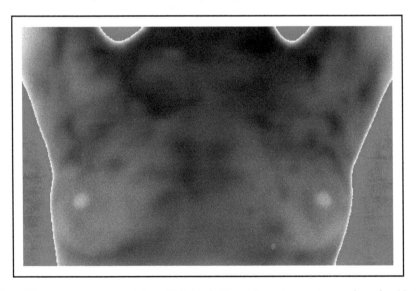

Repeat thermogram one year later, still living in Japan. Reports no estrogen therapies. Note increased vascularity. "At risk" thermogram.

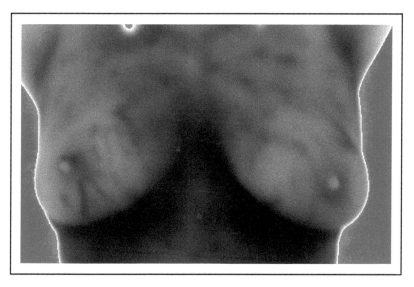

Soy diet. Note unusual hypervascular pattern. Progesterone deficiency.

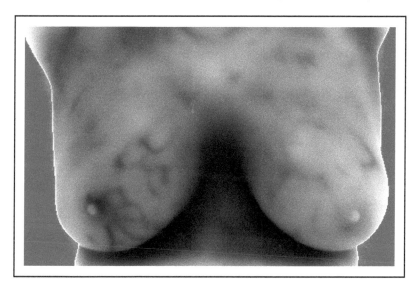

Repeat thermogram one year later. Soy diet. Note increased vascularity.
Right breast abnormal.

# Progesterone Is the Same as Progestin.
## *False Intel!*

Breast Canswer:

I am constantly amazed by the amount of MDs who believe progesterone is the same as progestin. Progesterone is produced by the corpus leutum at the end of our cycle. Progestin is a synthetic, manmade pharmaceutical. It was scientifically created to be similar to our progesterone, but is not an exact copy. Progestin is patented so the company that holds the patent can sell it.

Progestin causes many side effects. This list is from the *Physicians' Desk Reference*:

*Warning:*
- There is an increased risk of minor birth effects in children whose mothers take this drug during the first four months of pregnancy.
- The physician should be alerted to the earliest manifestation of thrombotic disorders.
- Discontinue this drug if there is sudden, partial or complete loss of vision.
- Detectable amounts of progestin have been identified in the milk of mothers receiving the drug. The effect of this on the nursing neonate and infant has not been determined.

Contraindications:
- Thrombophlebitis, thromboembolic disorders, cerebral apoplexy; liver dysfunction or disease; known or suspected malignancy of breast or genital organs; undiagnosed vaginal bleeding; missed abortion; known or suspected pregnancy.

Precautions:
- Because progestin may cause some degree of fluid retention, conditions which might be influenced by this factor, such as epilepsy, migraine, asthma, cardiac, or renal dysfunction, require careful observation.
- May cause breakthrough bleeding or menstrual irregularities.
- May cause or contribute to depression.

- The effect of prolonged use of this drug on pituitary, ovarian, adrenal, hepatic, or uterine function is unknown.
- May decrease glucose tolerance; diabetic patients must be carefully monitored.
- May increase the thrombotic disorders associated with estrogens.

Adverse Reactions:
- Breast tenderness and galactorrhea
- Sensitivity reaction such as urticaria, pruritus, edema or rash
- Acne, alopecia and hirsutism (excess hair growth)
- Weight changes
- Cervical erosions and changes in cervical secretions
- Cholestatic jaundice
- Mental depression, pyrexia, nausea, insomnia, or somnolence
- Anaphylactoid reaction and anaphylaxis
- Thrombophlebitis and pulmonary embolism
- Breakthrough bleeding, spotting, amenorrhea, or changes in menses
- Fatigue, backache, itching, dizziness, nervousness, loss of scalp hair

Progestin information by Dr. John Lee from his book, *What Your Doctor May Not Tell You About Menopause.*

## Progesterone Causes Cancer. *False intel!*

Breast Canswer:
Another misunderstanding we encounter all the time is that doctors regularly tell their patients that progesterone causes cancer. This is completely false. When a woman is tested for breast cancer, one of the tests they run is a receptor test called immunohistochemistry. They test to see if the beast cancer is affected by hormones:

1. Estrogen receptor positive.
2. Progesterone receptor positive.
3. Hormone negative (meaning that the cancer has no hormone receptors).

Around 80 percent of breast cancers are estrogen receptor positive. Twenty to around forty percent of breast cancers that are estrogen receptor positive are *also* progesterone receptor positive.

Now here is the misunderstanding. Estrogen receptor positive cancers *may* be progesterone receptor positive, 20-40 percent of the time. There is no breast cancer that is estrogen receptor negative with a progesterone receptor positive result. Dr. Hobbins has *never* seen or heard of this. What this means is that, if a cancer is progesterone receptor positive, it is also estrogen receptor positive, and therefore, progesterone by itself cannot cause cancer, this only occurs in conjunction with estrogen.

## Cleanses Are Healthy for the Breasts.
### *False Intel!*

Breast Canswer:

Liver, colon, and kidney cleanses do not decrease vascularity in the breasts or balance hormones. Our thermography research has never been able to prove this medical theory. We've had several doctors and patients try to decrease vascularity in the breasts with cleansing and they were never able to prove it.

There is a belief that detoxifying the liver, colon, and kidney will optimize body function. First, most toxins are stored in the fat cells, cleanses that are specialized for the above organs will not decrease this specific accumulation. Second, the toxins that are most concerning and potentially dangerous to the body are commercial grade petrochemicals from daily household products and foods that will take *years* to dispel from the body—supplements are too basic to remove them. Third, most cleanses are supplements that have preservatives, and may be contaminants, that are toxic to the body. Fourth, people who are deficient should never detox as this is too draining to the body. These people need to be nourished or strengthened to allow the body to function properly to naturally dispel toxins.

If you still feel the need to cleanse, just eat fruit, veggies, or broth for a couple days. Some people may choose to fast. However, avoid carbohydrates, as they will bind the intestines and break down to sugar.

Also, avoid juice as this is just sugar—instead, blend or make smoothies with "whole" foods.

Some people may choose to fast. Fasting for a short period has been proven to be beneficial and may be a great option.

To improve the efficiency of the liver, consume dandelion greens with your salads as a nutritional treatment for a short period of time. This is a Chinese herb that targets the liver and cools heat, resolves toxicity, and drains. This medicinal was historically used for breast abscesses. Only use this medicinal for a short time treatment, as this herb is cold and could cause side effects.

To improve the efficiency of the kidney, consume salt with iodine, as salt is the raw material of the kidneys and iodine will help prevent breast cancer.

If you want healthy organs, eat them. Organ meat is considered a super food. Why do you think grandma and grandpa were so healthy? We no longer consume organ meat and it is affecting our health. In most cultures, you eat like for like. If you have digestive issues you eat menudo, intestine. If you have weak tendons, consume Pho. Starting to get the picture? If you want a strong, healthy liver, heart, kidney, then consume it. The best is wild; if you know a hunter ask him or her to bring back the organs you want. The next best option would be to find grass-fed organic beef or contact a bison/buffalo farm. Instead of cooking liver I suggest cutting it up into small pieces about the size of a quarter, freeze the excess, and I consume one small piece a day. I also purchase pâté. If you don't like the flavor I found spreading a fig preserve or any flavor you prefer makes it more enjoyable.

Stop buying gimmicks. If you want to dispel toxins from the body the only known medical practice that achieves this purpose, other than through urination, is through sweating, either from a workout or a sauna.

## Liver Detoxifies and Metabolizes Estrogen.
### *False Intel!*

Breast Canswer:

Another medical assumption is that the liver detoxifies and metabo-lizes estrogen. These are false claims that we will walk you through so you'll stop wasting money on supplements that have no effect on the liver and breasts. The liver undoubtedly plays a role in filtering the blood and storing it, but the term "detoxification" is incorrect as it implies that it removes toxic substances.

If liver is detoxified why would it expel right back into the digestive tract just to be reabsorbed? If the liver is detoxified, it would exit the body like the kidneys. This is key, if the liver detoxified it would have to rid the body of these toxins by dispelling them directly, not to be reabsorbed. Hormones, especially supplements, are filtered out through the kidneys and flushed out with urine.

If the liver detoxified estrogen, then why are there high levels of estrogen, from birth control pills and hormone replacement, therapy in our water systems? It is well documented, so much that is becoming an epidemic that medical waste including synthetic estrogen is in our city water system, and rivers and oceans, affecting us and the wildlife. The liver does *not* successfully metabolize estrogen supplements.

If the liver detoxified then bile couldn't be produced in that organ, it would be broken down, as well.

Why is eating considered liver healthy? Because the animal's liver doesn't detoxify and is not toxic.

In fact, toxins are stored in the fat cells. Sweating is beneficial and helps to remove toxins from our system, therefore keeping your body weight down and less fat cells for toxins to be stored in,

Let's look at how our hormones, namely estrogen, are metabolized in the body. As you will see this does *not* include estrogen supplements like flax or birth control pills. As you just read, our body isn't capable of metabolizing all or the entire form of estrogen supplements. Our body will use and get rid of *our* hormones that it makes efficiently. The body knows how to take care of itself, supplements are throwing a curve ball at the body and it is not always able to metabolize them effectively.

If there is no fertilization, progesterone decreases as the corpus luteum degenerates, while estrogen also decreases, or being oxidized another word is metabolized and this results in the uterus shedding its lining. The unfertilized egg degenerates and exits out of the body with the menstrual blood. The egg is shed directly out of the body. This begins day one of the menstrual cycle. The body produces exactly the

276

amount of hormones needed, then naturally sheds the remaining out with the menstrual blood and through the digestive tract to the kidneys and out with the urine.

If you wanted to test if the liver metabolized estrogen you could measure estrogen blood levels going into portal vein and leaving during follicular phase as compared to luteal at is the only way.

The liver is the largest organ and we can't survive without it. It produces bile, which breaks up fat into smaller pieces for the small intestine and that is why the liver exits into the digestive tract. The liver has always been a store house for energy. The kidney has to decide what is dispelled or not dispelled in the body along with the right colon, which is the exit for impurities and absorption of what is good or waste.

The liver along with the digestive tract does *not* directly metabolize or detoxify estrogen, balance hormones or reduce risk of breast cancer; however, having a healthy liver strengthens our underlying constitution, similarly as having great digestion.

## Gum Disease Causes Breast Cancer.
### *False Intel!*

Breast Canswer

Gum disease does not cause breast cancer. Something you need to be aware of: Due to false claims made by amateur thermologists, the medical community is not accepting the incredible screening applications of breast thermography. As consumer advocates for breast thermography we want to explain these false claims to help set your minds at ease, so you can move forward in a more productive manner, decreasing breast cancer.

An unnamed thermography academy and certification center, overseen by an MD, posted this picture with caption, *"Some dentists have long claimed a relationship between oral bacteria and breast cancer. This picture to the left exemplify [sic] how the bacteria spread through the lymphatic (immune) system and can enter the breast. For any doctors interested in incorporating Thermography into their practice visit our website...."*

277

There is no evidence that breast cancer is caused by bacteria. For 15 years Dr. Hobbins interpreted thermograms for a clinic in Texas determined to prove this theory. They were never able to. If these claims were valid I would have included this vital information in our first groundbreaking book. In order to discuss a disease we must understand the mechanism behind it. Let's go back to school, shall we?

Bacteria 101. We are made of bacteria, lots of 'em; in fact, we can't exist without them. There are, believe it or not, *good* bacteria. Did you know that? It all starts in the beginning. The womb is a sterile environment. We are first exposed to our mother's bacteria in the vaginal canal; in fact if a mother has a cesarean section and the baby isn't exposed to her bacteria, it could possibly be fatal for the infant. There is a widening trend in delivery and operating rooms to wipe the c-section baby down with fluids from the mother's vaginal tract immediately after birth, just to restore these necessary bacteria. In the beginning infants are so sterile their poop has no smell and is sweet. Bacteria are so vital to our existence that without it we can't even digest our food.

Bacteria doesn't travel in one direction, it is all over our body and travels everywhere, in all directions. If you have a boil on your finger you can draw blood and prove bacteria is located there, but there is no directional flow of the bacteria.

We all know there are also bad bacteria, and the body is fighting it all the time. It is what strengthens our immunity and why you don't want to over expose yourself to antibiotics, especially anti-bacterial hand sanitizers and household products. You become too sterile and weak, like the infant.

This is just one part of the story; now we need to explain lymphatics in order to give you the entire picture.

Lymphatics 101. The lymphatics begin in the appendages – feet and fingers – and travel up (*not* down, as amateur thermography clinics and dentists claim) to the left side into the jugular and subclavian junction under the left clavicle. There are no shortcuts. One more time, the flow of lymph is from feet *up*, is a separate closed system all on its own, it has its own channels, just like the circulatory system. If you get an infection in your fingers and get a red streak, that's not the venous system, it's the lymph system and the way the body rids itself of infection.

Some of you may be thinking, "What about the heart?" Great question! With a root abscess that bacteria can possibly travel down the venous system, not lymphatic, into the heart, and if that valve has an injury or is weak that bacteria can cause an infection. But, an endocardial infection on the valve can be blamed on flow of bacteria from anywhere, not just the mouth.

From the face the lymphatic does travel down the side of the neck to the jugular, this is true; however, from the breast it goes up to the axillas or underarm, not down from the face to the breast. That we know, and we are accepting evidence from lymphatic specialists that there is no direct connection from face to breast.

Dr. Hobbins, who is a surgeon, says surgeons used to perform radical mastectomies, which are a complete removal of the breasts and chest muscles, the pectorals, and he never saw proof of the lymphatics system connection that these amateur thermologists and dentists are suggesting.

This thermogram is claiming proof of lymphatic connection from the face to breast. What amateur thermologists don't understand is that a thermogram can only measure the skin temperature. The breasts are actually a part of the integumentary system or skin and we can monitor the blood vessels within them or the circulation of the breasts. Thermography cannot measure the tissue of the breast, which is the function of the breast, just the skin which contains the vascular structures of the breast. The lymphatics are simply too deep to be seen. What you are seeing in the thermogram is stimulation of the vascular structures or blood vessels, not the lymphatics.

Let's rule out further arguments:

Lymphedema - is accumulation of the lymph fluid after damage to the lymphatic system, causing swelling, which is seen on a thermogram as cold.

Cellulitis - is a bacterial infection in the skin and the fluid is the same temperature as the surrounding tissue, which would be uniform, seen as hot in a thermogram. Again, the skin would also be hot due to increased circulation and the two couldn't be isolated in a thermogram.

The vascular patterns seen in this thermogram are coincidence, which is not the same as correlation. It is possible to have a root abscess and a breast abscess simultaneously without one causing the other. We do recognize that a person's immunity might be lowered, allowing for simultaneous infections. That vascular pattern is unrelated to teeth because it is anatomically impossible. That possible abscess in the breast is moving up and would drain in the upper quadrant.

A patient sent me a study saying she had proof gum disease causes breast cancer. This is what the researcher stated, "95 percent of breast cancer patients have root canals, therefore root canals cause breast cancer." Really? That I need to explain this fallacy is frustrating, but here it is. If 95 percent of people who have a broken leg have root canals, it wouldn't mean that root canals cause broken legs. Coincidence does not mean correlation.

Next, I will put to rest the holistic explanation, as I am a Chinese medical physician. Dentists and amateur thermologists claim the teeth are connected to the breast meridians. First, there is no such thing as a breast meridian. There are actually several meridians that run through the breast. I assume what these physicians are trying to say is that the stomach meridian runs directly from the mouth down to the breasts – but it doesn't stop there, it actually ends in the feet. This is correct, but as I explained from a biomedical perspective, bacteria are everywhere. I assume what they are trying to state is there is an energetic component. In fact, many Chinese medical doctors believe that the liver has more influence on the breasts than the stomach. Chinese medicine teaches that emotions can influence the organs, and issues with the organs can cause emotional imbalances. The liver is the most arrogant of the organs; in other words, the liver is a bully and overacts on other organs, which may cause stagnation to the breasts and may possibly cause an additional emotional imbalance as well.

While a root canal may be harmful to the body, it should not be used to scare the patient into spending thousands and subject themselves to evasive extractions to heal the breasts. Amateur thermologists and dentists telling women to extract their root canals to reduce risk to the breast is unfounded, is fear mongering, and creates unnecessary concern while not addressing the true issue. Eighty percent of breast cancers are fueled by estrogen; excess estrogen or progesterone deficiency should be addressed, not bacteria, which is an integral mechanism to our survival. That leaves only 20 percent of breast cancers caused by unknown factors.

Chew on this, gum disease doesn't cause breast cancer.

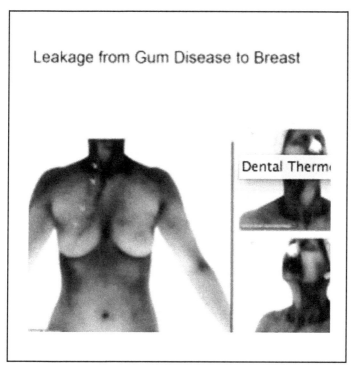

An unnamed thermography academy and certification center, overseen by an M.D., posted this picture with caption, *"Some dentists have long claimed a relationship between oral bacteria and breast cancer. This picture to the left exemplify [sic] how the bacteria spread through the lymphatic (immune) system and can enter the breast. For any doctors interested in incorporating Thermography into their practice visit our website…."* This is NOT proof. Thermography can ONLY measure the skin temperature, it cannot monitor the lymphatic, which are too deep and what this M.D. is claiming. This is a blood vessel from the subclavian to the breast.

## Estrogen Is Found in Milk. *False Intel!*

Breast Canswer:

A patient told me she went to a breast cancer seminar and the nurse practitioner told attendees to only drink nonfat cow's milk due to estrogen levels. She believed that estrogen was stored in the cow's fat cells and would affect the consumer, so only nonfat was safe.

There are a ton of misconceptions about dairy and I'm excited to clear them up. Milk and dairy have been consumed for thousands of years with little to no problems until recently and is a beneficial healthy fat and cholesterol if you are able to digest it properly.

When a human mother or cow is nursing, their body produces hormones differently, so that during the nursing state, the breast milk and cow's milk does not have estrogen. Yes, estrogen is stored in the fat cells, but milking cows are in constant nursing state and there is little to no estrogen in the fat cells. When cows or mothers are nursing exclusively, the body has stopped producing eggs so pregnancy is rare. It is the synthetic commercial-grade estrogen (hormones) given to the cows that causes fibroids and masses in the breasts and uterus.

The nurse also said to only drink nonfat because estrogen is stored in the fat cells. Milking cows are in constant nursing state, and there is little to no estrogen in the fat cells. However, many skim milks, even organic, have powdered milk added to them. Powdered milk is processed with high heat. This heat changes and oxidizes the healthy cholesterol in the milk. This bad cholesterol can cause plaque formation in the arteries that healthy cholesterol does not. An Australian study found that rabbits fed oxidized cholesterol had 64 percent increase of cholesterol in the arteries versus rabbits that were fed healthy cholesterol.

Another important fact is that both homogenized and pasteurized milk are toxic to the body because the milk is processed with heat. This heat reduces the size of the milk molecule to one-tenth of a micron. This reduced milk molecule is now small enough to escape through small holes in our intestines, allowing this acidic element to freely travel in the bloodstream and into the organs, causing unforeseen health issues.

Now this is where it gets interesting, that now acidic particle can escape the digestive tract and travel anywhere in the body. Many of these acidic particle end up in the blood vessels, which causes plaque and heart issues. When Dr. Hobbins was in med school in the 1940s arteriosclerosis did not exist! In med school, they would have to perform one to two autopsies a night, which was usually the homeless who have sold their bodies, meaning they did not have a good diet, and they did not present with arteriosclerosis. Another interesting fact is when the government decided to monopolize the dairy industry and homogenize milk, which before was delivered straight from the cow, did these issues increase, hardening of the arteries? The answer is no.

Organic raw milk, which is unpasteurized and non-homogenized is a healthy form of fat. Avoid non-organic milk due to synthetic estrogens, which may be given to some cows.

## Coffee Causes Breast Cancer and Fibroids.
### *False intel!*

Breast Canswer:

Can't survive without your morning cup? Me neither, you're going to love me after reading this! Organic coffee does not *cause* cancer.

First, coffee is a stimulant that increases circulation. Circulation is beneficial. Fibroids are due to stagnation. Now you know what causes 80 percent of breast cancers, yes, estrogen. Coffee is a plant estrogen, but a very, weak one, weaker than green tea, so one cup in a relatively healthy person should not significantly increase your risk of hormonal disorders or breast cancer. However, coffee is the one of the most highly sprayed crops and the pesticides are not only toxic, but contain commercial-grade estrogens, which may cause health issues over a long period of time. The pesticides used on the coffee may be causing the issue, *not* the coffee bean itself. Splurge, spend more on the organic and drink up.

Many uncertified thermography clinics are telling women to not drink coffee because it causes hormonal disorders, fibroids and cancer. They also tell women not to drink tea before a thermogram. They clearly don't understand thermography or breast cancer. Coffee increases circulation *inside* the blood vessels. Thermography is monitoring the blood vessels of the breasts looking for specific vascular patterns that disease form, neoangiogenesis and vascularity. Vascularity is stimulation of the existing blood vessels, usually due to estrogen. Vascularity and circulation are different. Breast thermography can only monitor the outside of the blood vessels, it cannot see deep inside. I challenge thermography clinics to prove me wrong all the time. Take a thermogram, have the woman drink –two to four cups and then take another thermogram looking for increased vascularity. Trust me, you won't see it, I've already tried. Coffee doesn't increase vascularity in the breasts, thus increasing risk of breast cancer. Fifty years of breast thermography and we can't prove that theory.

Now, I'm going to share with you how healthy coffee is – vindication ladies!

Studies have shown that coffee is one of the largest source of antioxidants, outranking both vegetables and fruits combined. Wow! You learn something amazing every day! There is more. Studies examined the effect of caffeine on the brain and showed that it improved mood, reaction time, memory vigilance, and general cognitive function, with a lower risk for Alzheimer's and dementia.

Due to the stimulation effect of caffeine on the central nervous system, it raises metabolism and mobilizes fatty acid from the fat tissue, decreasing weight! Yes, you read that correctly – coffee makes you skinny, enjoy.

## Vaginal Estrogen Creams Keep the Vagina Moist. *False Intel!*

Breast Canswer:
Since most women are estrogen dominant; vaginal atrophy is not due to a decline in estrogen or an estrogen deficiency issue. This medical fallacy will be explained further in this section.

The vagina is quite possibly one of the most misunderstood parts of a woman's body. The vagina is a smooth muscle with two glands (which are also smooth muscle) that when stimulated secrete vaginal fluids. The medical community believes location means correlation, in other words, those in the medical community will tell women that the vagina is controlled by the endocrine system or hormones, specifically, estrogen. This is absolutely false! Trust in physiology, not medical rumors.

As you have learned, estrogen deficiency is rare. In fact, moisture increases in the vagina at ovulation, which corresponds to increased levels of progesterone. The eventual drying of the vagina is *not* an indicator of a decrease in estrogen; in fact, the majority of women who complain about vaginal dryness have excess estrogen! I want to repeat that since I have to deprogram most of you: Almost all of my patients who complain about vaginal dryness have too much estrogen; therefore, lack of estrogen is not the problem.

But then you have to ask: What is the problem?

Eyes, ears, nose, mouth, and vagina. These are examples of the orifices of the body, openings to which the environment has contact. As we age, *all* the orifices will naturally dry out, but using an estrogen cream to keep the vagina moist is simply not the correct treatment. Moisture increases in the vagina at ovulation, which corresponds to increased levels of progesterone. Estrogen deficiency is extremely rare— the eventual drying of the vagina is not an indicator. More importantly, estrogen vaginal creams increase breast risk.

Important safety information:

Possible side effects of vaginal cream:
- Breast cancer
- Cancer of the uterus
- Stroke
- Heart attack
- Blood clots
- Dementia
- Gallbladder disease
- Ovarian cancer
- High blood pressure
- Liver problems
- High blood sugar
- Enlargement of benign tumors"

It may be true that the cream itself may be keeping your vagina moist, but this has nothing to do with estrogen. As soon as you place something into the vagina you are stimulating it, causing – guess what? – increased moisture. Ever think it is just the moisturizing properties of the ingredients that keep the vagina moist? Try using an over-the-counter cream without estrogen to keep the vagina moist. I suggest an organic coconut oil as an overnight cream or lubricant. Keep it in the refrigerator, use a small spoon to make a ball and insert with finger or applicator nightly or as needed. My patients respond quite well with this application. I don't condone the application of petrochemicals into the vagina as the skin is very thin and porous like your mouth, which makes it absorb more.

All smooth muscle, including the vagina, is influenced by the sympathetic nervous system. If you want to improve vaginal health, treat the sympathetic nervous system. How do you do that, you ask? Chinese medicine. Acupuncture works on the sympathetic nervous system. I recommend seeing an acupuncturist and a Chinese medical herbalist (they may be different). An acupuncturist can strengthen the sympathetic nervous system directly without any side effects, as well as address other issues you may present with. It's holistic medicine.

The herbalist will make a customized herbal prescription just for you (avoid an herbalist who wants to sell you pills and who uses phytoestrogen herbs). There are herbs that create moisture in what is called the lower jiao, where the vagina is located. The drying of the vagina might be an indicator of something else which your herbalist may also address with just one herbal formula; this is holistic medicine, treatment of the entire body all in just one formula (bottle).

In western society, people don't go to the doctor until they are sick, which is why we have doctors who can only treat illnesses. Treating an illness or condition is so much more difficult than preventing it in the first place! This is why I am always strongly recommending Chinese medical doctors for prevention or anti-aging. They can see an imbalance before the disease. To be a healthy society we must be proactive, not reactive. Start treating for vaginal dryness before you have it, because once you do it is harder to reverse.

A good way to bring moisture to the skin and muscles is to eat foods that will do this for us and slow down the signs of aging. As we age blood is shunted to the organs for survival, that leads drying of the skin, causing wrinkles, hair turning gray and fingernails becoming brittle. In Chinese medicine and many other cultures, you eat like for like, if you have weak digestion you eat Menudo, a spicy soup made from tripe. For weak tendons eat Pho, a meat and noodle soup. You get the picture. If you want healthy skin, nails, hair and muscles (the vagina) eat meat or drink bone broth. Water hydrates, but it is the blood that moisturizes.

Want to know what else can help moisturize the vagina? Play time. Yes, that's right, stimulate the area. Stimulation to the clitoris causes the glands at the opening of the vagina to secrete fluids. You can do this by yourself, with a toy, or include your partner - although if you're having painful intercourse due to dryness, you may want to warn your partner ahead of time that this is "therapy" and not necessarily foreplay. (But involving your partner in your treatment may bring you closer and may lead to other healthy fun alternatives, you never know.)

Additional tips for vagina health and cleaning:

On the pH scale the vagina is considered acidic, and you want to keep that balance in order to reduce bacterial growth and infections. Douching with vinegar is simple and effective. Some people suggest apple cider, but white vinegar works just as well, too. I happen to prefer organic as the vagina is porous and absorbs everything.

For maintenance, use half vinegar, half warm water. Regular maintenance douching, once a week, or as needed, keeps the vagina at a healthy acidic balance, reducing risk of infections and abnormal discharge. For more severe, cases like a yeast infection or severe discharge you can use all vinegar and daily.

If you suffer from chronic yeast and bladder infections, you might want to get rid of your panties for a healthier lifestyle. Wearing panties, especially a thong, traps heat and dampness, which allows bacteria to grow and could increase yeast and bladder infections that tend to grow in warm moist climates. This tip is especially important during workouts. I'm shocked by the number of women who wear panties at the gym, especially with yoga pants. Trapped heat and sweat increases risk of infection or dampness.

Many women wear synthetic, tight panties or wear control-top hose, these can cause constriction, which may lead to stagnation in the lymphatic system. There is a major chain of lymph in the groin area which you don't want to obstruct. No panties allow for air circulation, which will keep the area dryer. Don't wear panties with pants or shorts, but be appropriate: If you're wearing a dress or skirt, be sure to put the panties back on.

Some critics say not wearing panties increases your risk of rashes, lice, and infections. I've personally been panty-free since 2001 and I've never had a rash or a case of lice. Along with simple nutritional changes and proper cleansing ditching my panties has dramatically reduced chronic infections. I encourage all my patients to be brave, be panty-free. Many will testify to the same results, reduction of chronic infections and constrictions for a comfortable, healthier lifestyle.

If you are worried about discharge, let's get some facts straight. A small amount around ovulation is normal and essential for fertility, a nice way to "check in" to see if your body is healthy. However, if you have more than this, and/or it has a smell, this is *not* normal and is a health issue. A smell is usually a tell-tale sign of an infection, and that can usually cleared up with antibiotics. Nowadays many women are choosing a more natural approach. Abnormal discharge, including smell, can easily and quickly be cleared up with a customized herbal formula from a Chinese medical or Ayurvedic physician. You'll want find one of these two holistic physicians who specialize in herbs and will make a customized herbal formula (make sure it is a customized formula and not in a pill form). Gynecological issues, including dampness, can be treated quite easily with herbs tailored specifically for you with no side effects caused by antibiotics and hormones.

Next, clean the outside daily with organic soap. Synthetic soap, antibacterial soap and even natural soaps have hormones, pesticides and petrochemicals. You know that clean, squeaky feel you get with these soaps? That is not good. These soaps strip your skin of its natural acid mantle. Yes, the body knows how to protect itself; it has been doing so for thousands of years. The skin is also acidic and when you remove this protective film it causes dryness and is prone to bacterial infection. Organic soap properly cleans the skin without damaging it like these horrible soaps.

The vagina is smooth muscle and is porous, similar to your mouth. Anything placed in the mouth or vagina is readily absorbed, more so than on the skin. Tampons contain bleach, sawdust and petrochemical that are quickly absorbed into our system. It is vital to invest in your health and only use organic tampons. For play time you'll also want to invest in saving the vagina by buying BPA free and petrochemical free condoms and vibrators.

# Vaginal Estrogen Creams, Estrogen Rings and IUD With Hormones Are not Systemic and Won't Affect the Breasts. *False Intel!*

Breast Canswer:

This was taken from the website of a popular name brand vaginal cream. Please refer to the "Collateral Damage" Appendix chapter for all others forms of estrogen and their side effects.

> Using estrogen alone may increase your chances of getting strokes or blood clots... dementia. Serious, but less common side effects include breast cancer, cancer of the uterus, stroke, heart attack, blood clots, dementia, gallbladder disease, ovarian cancer, high blood pressure, liver problems, high blood sugar, enlargement of benign tumors.

Many doctors *still* believe that if you apply something such as estrogen to one area of the body, it will not affect another. But if they were to go back to childhood and recall the song... "The hip bone's connected to the thigh bone, the thigh bone's connected to the...," they might remember that the body is one system, and therefore, completely interconnected. Estrogen applied to the abdomen, wrist, thigh, or vagina with pills, pellets, or patches will travel to the specific receptor sites in the body, such as the uterus and the breasts, increasing the risk for breast and uterine cancer. Nearly everything that we ingest or place on the skin ends up, in some portion, in the circulatory system. By the suggestion or implications of these physicians, a nicotine patch would only have effect at the site of direct contact. But we know this to not be true.

Even though you are putting the estrogen cream in your vagina, it still creates estrogen stimulation or vascularity in the breasts. When estrogen is applied to any part of the body, it naturally seeks out estrogen receptors, even those in the breasts. That is the same application method and theory of how bioidentical estrogen cream works. Once a patient removes the vaginal estrogen cream, estrogen, or IUD, their vascularity or stimulation decreases, and this can be seen in thermograms.

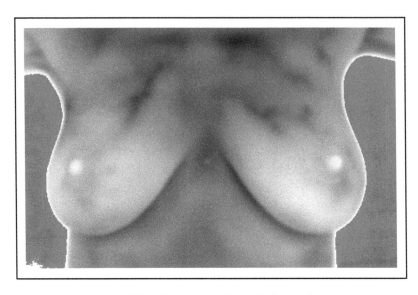

Before use of IUD with hormones. Note slight vascular pattern.

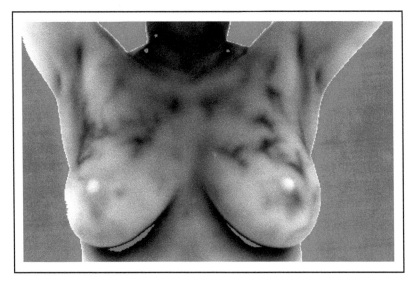

With IUD containing hormones. Note increased vascularity. Abnormal thermogram.

# Estrogen Helps with Prolapsed Uterus or Vagina.
## *False Intel!*

Breast Canswer:

The majority of women are estrogen dominant; therefore, prolapse of the uterus and vagina is not due to estrogen deficiency. I had a doctor tell me he will never stop medicating his patients with estrogen for prolapse of the vagina, even after most of his patients' thermograms were abnormal. It is my opinion that, if he is not the reason for their breast conditions, then at the very least, he is aggravating their conditions with all his estrogen prescriptions. He claims he has read all the latest studies from Europe and that he is at the forefront of study-based knowledge.

Ladies, the vagina is a muscle and the uterus is supported by ligaments—they have nothing to do with estrogen! Think of the uterus like a gourd with the round part at the top held in place by ligaments and the neck of the gourd at the bottom above the vaginal canal. With childbirth, these muscles get stretched and for some women, so relaxed the uterus will fall into the vaginal canal.

Supplementing with hormones will not help with a prolapsed uterus or vagina as these muscles are not influenced by the endocrine system. Ask yourself this: Does a pulled muscle or tendon injury benefit from hormonal therapy? No? Then why would the vagina, a smooth muscle, benefit from hormonal therapy? Location does not mean correlation.

If one has issues with prolapsed organs, it is advised to see a Chinese herbalist, as this can be treated with herbs if addressed in the early stages. The key is the early stages.

Many ladies are choosing to treat a prolapsed uterus with a pessary. Pessaries are used as a nonsurgical approach to the treatment of mild pelvic organ prolapse. Pessaries may also be used to treat uterine prolapse during pregnancy. The pessary holds the uterus in the correct position before it enlarges and becomes trapped in the vaginal canal. Pessaries do not cure pelvic organ prolapse, but help manage and slow the progression of prolapse. They add support to the vagina and increase tightness of the tissues and muscles of the pelvis. Symptoms improve in many women who use a pessary and for some women, symptoms go away. Pessaries are fitted specially for each woman.

If these preventive practices don't work, then surgery is an option.

The uterus and breasts are healthy when there is a balance between estrogen and progesterone. When estrogen becomes excessive, then risk of uterine and breast cancer increases. Synthetic estrogens and progestin (a synthetic form of progesterone) do not protect your uterus or your breasts as they are bioidentical and not an exact copy of your body's hormones.

## Painful Sex Is Due to Lack of Estrogen.
### *False Intel!*

Breast Canswer:

Painful intercourse is not due to estrogen. Pain during sex is due to three issues, infection, prolapse or tightening of the vagina. Estrogen does not affect the tissues of the vagina because it is a muscle, which means it will not assist with painful sex. However, lubricating this muscle may assist, as discussed in detail in the next section.

Pain during sex can be due to an infection and trust me – you'll know when you have an infection. The smooth muscle of the vagina can become inflamed and sore. Clear up the infection and the pain will diminish.

When you are pregnant the uterus and the ligaments holding, the uterus is stretched. Think of them like a rubber band, if you stretch it for nine months it will become lax. Pain after childbirth is caused by a suctioning action, from the penis in the vaginal canal. When you first start having sex, there is no pain, but once the pressure builds from continuous thrusting of the penis, the now relaxed ligaments allow the uterus to be pulled through a small opening into the vaginal canal causing pain. When the penis is removed, the pressure is released and the pain subsides. If pain continues during sex a *pessary*, a medical device similar to the outer ring of a diaphragm, can be used during sex to hold the uterus in place.

Now some of you are thinking, "Dang, childbirth ruins me!" Don't stress, the pendulum swings the other way. You know the saying "use it or lose it?" Well, with the vagina it is true. As we age the vagina muscle will tighten, literally. For women who have not stretched out their vagina from giving birth if they don't have sex as they age the vagina will tighten and the penis will no longer fit. To keep the vagina from tightening regular sex or stretching either with a partner or by yourself will keep it pliable.

## Get the Facts!

If you want to fight a disease, breast cancer, or fix a disorder, hormone imbalance, it is imperative to understand how the body works, physiology, and that is why this chapter is critical to your health. The medical community is misinforming us about hormones and that is why there is an increase in breast cancer, estrogen dominance, Low T and early puberty. I walk you through physiology to explain medical assumptions and rumors so that you can have the knowledge to fix yourself!

# 8. Supplements: The Enemy You Thought Was Your Ally

## Breast Fact: Supplementation Increases Breast Cancer Risk

There is little to no money in creating a healthy society, while there are billions to be made perpetuating sickness.

A five-year study in Sweden involving 30,000 women taking a multivitamin increased their risk for breast cancer by 19 percent. Many studies show that vitamins and supplements have virtually no effect and/or are increasing disease including cancers. The American Cancer Society lists vitamins and supplements under risk, "Factors with uncertain, controversial or unproven effect on breast cancer risk," stating "So far, no study has shown that taking vitamins reduces breast cancer risk."

Wendy Sellens, DACM, LAc

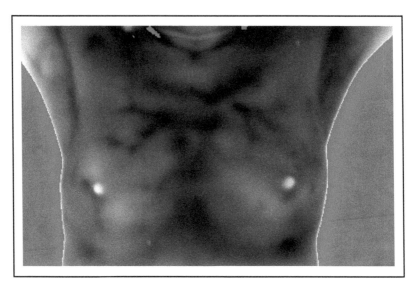

Woman reports no recent history of estrogen therapies. Reports "lots" of vitamins. Note unusual vascular pattern. Progesterone deficiency imbalance. "At risk" thermogram.

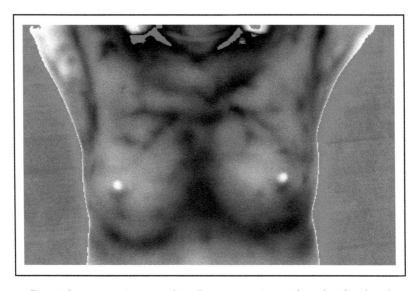

Repeat thermogram two years later. Reports no estrogen therapies. Continued supplement and vitamin use. Note same unusual vascular pattern.

Most of the public truly believes supplementation and vitamins are nutrition, when, supplements are the equivalent of fast food. Supplements were intended to "supplement" people's poor diet choices, not become a foundation for health. The ingredients are cheap chemicals that increase the risk of contaminants and toxins entering the body in high daily dosages. This includes "whole food" or plant food supplements and the new "medical foods"; the preservatives that give them a shelf life are toxic to the body.

Recently an FDA investigation uncovered that companies were selling fraudulent and potentially dangerous supplements. They discovered that four out of the five products did not contain any of the herbs listed on their labels. Testing of the supplements labeled "medicinal herbs" often contained cheap fillers like powdered rice and household plants, and more surprisingly substances that could be harmful to people with allergies. Popular with the cancer industry, medicinal mushrooms were found to be high in heavy metals.

Now, if you are sick then it is understandable to be using supplements and/or pharmaceuticals, but if you are healthy you shouldn't have to supplement. Do you know who has the lowest incidence of cancer in in the U.S.? The Amish. They grow their own food, work outside, don't smoke or drink and don't use supplements or pharmaceuticals.

In 2015, supplements were a reported $37 billion industry. With supplement sales sky rocketing, why aren't Americans healthier? Why do most cancer rates, not just breast cancer, continue to rise in America? Why is America not leading the world in healthy individuals? If supplements really were healthy, then thermograms, a marker of breast health, would reflect their claims – but they never do. Recently, editors of two highly prestigious medical journals revealed to the public that as many as half of medical studies are at best unreliable, and at worst simply false. Maybe we should consider why companies are having studies manipulated. To sell products?

For years, Dr. Hobbins and I have told women to get off all their supplements. This is the most difficult pill for them to swallow, even more so than estrogen, because we have been programmed to believe a pill can make you better. As one of the founding members of the American Holistic Medical Society, Dr. Hobbins has educated his patients for years about the ineffectiveness of supplementation. He explains, "Some supplements are acid and some are alkali; some are oil-based and some are aqueous (water soluble). This means that they do not mix well when they are purified and then added back together. Multiple vitamins inactivate each other, making salts of each other and blocking absorption." Many supplements don't consist of just the vitamin or mineral; many other chemicals are added. Chemicals that create the lubrication so they don't stick together, synthetic ingredients of the gel or capsule and preservative for shelf life which are all contained within a plastic bottle. Supplementation is simply not as beneficial as we have been conditioned to believe.

It is a rare account that a patient reports to me that they do not take any supplements. So many people are caught up in the belief that pills are nutrition. When women come to me with a list of supplements, my first question is, "How do you feel?" With all their supplementing, many women only feel marginally better. Spending thousands of dollars attempting to fix every problem separately with a specific pill wouldn't make many feel good either. Our body strives for perfection if you allow it to maintain balance, which is achieved through proper diet and water, physical and mental health, and a stable, clean environment.

We can exemplify supplementation through baby formula. It would be hard to find someone who does not believe that breast milk is a superior choice to formula. People innately understand that if it comes from the mother, it is what's best for the child. Breast milk is the epitome of "organic." This source of natural nutrients is not only from the person most genetically familiar to the child, it also provides the baby with its immune system, as the infant has not yet developed. Formula is a processed form of food with nutrients added, but due to this process, it may not be bioavailable to the baby. Many formulas have preservatives and stabilizers so they can sit on your shelf for *years*! It's the same with supplements—they are processed and filled with preservatives and stabilizers that may be poisonous to the body. Have you ever wondered why infants who are fed formula have difficulty returning to breast milk? Infant formula is high in sugars. In addition, the lining of the formula can is made from petrochemicals that contain ecoestrogens, and therefore, women are feeding their infants hormones or estrogen with each meal!

We also encourage women to avoid plant-based or "whole food" supplements and medical foods, as the label is really just a marketing ploy. Plant-based supplements have grown more popular as consumers learn the side effects of synthetics. However, plant-based supplements still require a preservative, which is poisonous to the body. I asked one patient with an abnormal thermogram if she was taking supplements. She replied "No." Later she informed me she was taking "whole food" supplements. Whole food in a pill form? What? If it is a pill, powder or liquid, and it's "in addition to" regular food intake, then that is a supplement! Whole foods are actually real foods, like an apple. They cannot be called "whole foods" when they are not in their original whole form! Ladies, again, be careful with propaganda and deceptive methods in an attempt to sell you stuff.

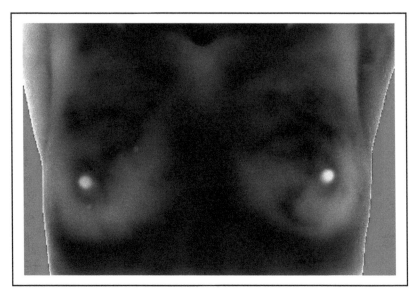

Woman reports no recent history of estrogen therapies. Reports using 16 medical grade, mostly "whole food" and "organic" supplements daily. Note unusual vascular pattern. Progesterone deficiency imbalance. "At risk" thermogram.

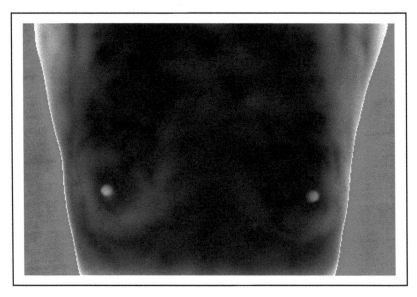

Repeat thermogram two years later. Reports no estrogen therapies. Continued supplement and vitamin use. Note increased vascularity. "At risk thermogram.

Whole foods are fresh, not ground down and dried up to be administered into powder or liquid form. Whole foods contain enzymes and nutrients when eaten fresh. When dried and processed to form a supplement, the enzymes are destroyed. As a natural living food source, whole foods will eventually rot or degrade. This process can be extended with preservatives, but the food is no longer in its natural state and now contains toxins. Whole food supplements, unless specified, require a preservative to sit on a self. When a supplement is processed, you take a chance of containments polluting the supplement. This happens all the time; it is only when someone dies that the supplement is pulled from the shelf. Most importantly, if the whole food supplement is not organic, you are consuming large amounts of pesticides.

Food has to have vitality. For example, look at organic fresh peaches versus canned peaches. Which do you think has life or vitality still in it? The fresh peach has the nutrients your body needs while the canned peaches are literally dead. When fruit or veggies are cut, they are exposed to the air and begin to oxidize or break down. Once this occurs, the enzymes degenerate and become inactive in just a few hours. The enzymes of the peach help break down the sugar within and make the nutrients bioavailable to our body. This concept is the same for supplements. They have no vitality and are cheap, deficient, alternate versions of the "real" thing. They are fast food in a pill. How healthy is eating fast food every day?

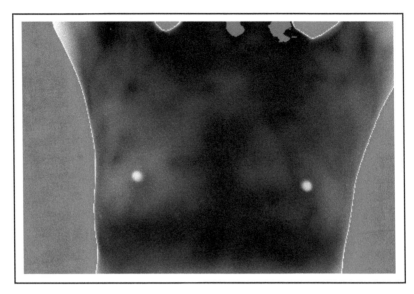

Woman reports no recent history of estrogen therapies. Reports 34 medical grade vitamins/
supplements daily prescribed by integrative doctor. Note unusual vascular pattern.
Progesterone deficiency imbalance. "At risk" thermogram.

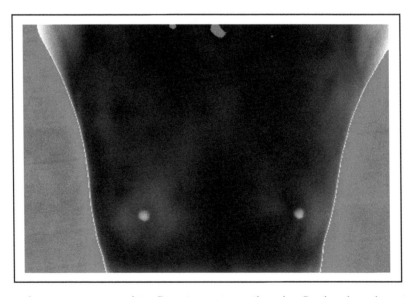

Repeat thermogram two years later. Reports no estrogen therapies. Continued supplement and
vitamin use. Note same unusual vascular pattern.

The next argument that I hear is, "My friend cured his cancer with X (insert name) supplementation, so I am going to do the same." First, a person with cancer is very sick, and their supplements are being used as a treatment. People who are ill or sick need to supplement, as they must outweigh the risk, toxicity, versus the benefits. They may have acquired a disease because their body was so deficient or toxic it couldn't fight off the disease. This person needs to nourish and build up their body and immune system to fight the disease. The body is always striving for balance and requires a continuous balance of nutrients. Do you think health really comes from cramming ten thousand mushrooms into a single pill? Isn't that the same as saying, "Go eat half a cow, because the body needs protein?" Is bigger better?

Secondly, remember the person who acquired this disease may have been overstressed, consumed a poor diet, overtaxed their body with work, and performed either excessive or insufficient exercise, allowing the body to become weak and susceptible to disease. Now that they have a disease, they are not just eating a certain supplement, but probably eating better, getting enough sleep, reducing stress, and possibly engaging in mild exercise. There are always other factors to consider in someone's story. But we do admit there are miracles, too

How are we supposed to know what works when we take a handful of pills morning, day, and night. Seriously, which of your supplements are working? Start with one, if there is no change for thirty to sixty days, try another.

Make it simple for your body. For example, minerals work together like a lock and key. What if you use a calcium supplement? Well, this increases your calcium, but now you may be out of balance with your magnesium, sodium, and potassium. With a comparative deficiency, the body may react in a new way and the problem has either transformed, shifted, or become compiled. My suggestion is that before supplementing with pill formed "food," try and eat a healthy diet of meats, seeds, vegetables, fruits, and dairy. Essentially, what most of the arguments for supplementing come down to is laziness.

Supplements confuse the pituitary, the "general," which monitors our body's functions. All supplements are going to have a different effect on the pituitary. Studies will eventually show this. Each supplement has several ingredients—multiply these by the number of supplements a person takes and it adds up quickly. People think they are only taking a couple, but it is the amount in each pill that adds up to *many*! You can't take hundreds of supplements and not affect the control center of the body.

"You tell me not to supplement, but then you tell me to use progesterone cream?" Again, only supplement when you are sick. Almost all women are progesterone deficient; they have to balance their estrogen levels with progesterone. Most women will have to do this for the rest of their lives due to the strong effects of environmental estrogen. We start many women out with a high percentage of progesterone cream, but once they are balanced and able to combat the environmental estrogens, they can switch to a lower percentage. Every woman is different; one might use a higher percentage while another uses a lower. Some may need to use progesterone cream daily, while others require only a couple times a week. Treatment is individually based and monitored with thermography, along with patient/physician dialogue. Never use progesterone pills due to synthetic formulas, toxic ingredients, preservatives and risk or contamination.

Keep in mind if you take something for your fingernail, it will be absorbed somewhere else as well. Our body is interrelated. You may be polluting your body by trying to fix a single part. This is why it is important to see a holistic physician, Chinese medical, Ayurvedic, or homeopathic. They will nourish or strengthen the whole body while targeting a weaker area. Supplementation is micromedicine, not holistic or macromedicine. Chinese medicine is the oldest medicine in the world; it has stood the test of time, five thousand years. Schools would research specific herbs for hundreds of years. Each formula and each herb has a list of contraindications which are applied to each person individually. Western herbs and supplements simply do not have this incredible amount of experience and clinical study; they are lacking.

Supplementation is *not* medicine. As a traditional Chinese medical physician, the holistic or natural medicine so many of us look for is not within supplementation. Supplementation chases symptoms, often based on lab results, and is the laziness of health practices. When a lab result indicates that vitamin D levels are low in a patient, what does the typical physician do nowadays? Instead of telling the patient that they are most likely not getting a sufficient amount of sunlight exposure, their advice is to take a pill. Don't chase symptoms by taking a pill for each one, as it eventfully causes further imbalances. Instead, fix the cause or the root of the problem.

When a physician assesses the patient, it should be done as a whole, or holistically. This is not to say that Western medicine does not have its strong points, it does; particularly emergency medicine. Yet from the position of preventative medicine, and in the case of health education, a mammoth absence exists. When the human body is seen as an intricate operating unit, the ability to maintain a healthy, functional body is not determined based upon microscopic analysis and derived conclusions. Rather, one must step back and see the forest beyond the trees. It may seem like a new age cliché, but balance is the key to health.

Optimization should be achieved in all aspects of health, not just in what is identified at that moment. How the body presents at that moment may dictate treatment, but the body as a whole requires much more attention and balance if it is to remain or become healthy. Proper circulation of fluids and energy, intake of nutritious food, and water, and emotional stability is how the body maintains health and prevents disease. This is how we stay young. Not by taking tests, chasing symptoms or injecting ourselves with who knows what.

In traditional Chinese medicine, the physician reads the patient's pulse and looks at their tongue (the only muscle of the body you can see), skin, fingernails, and eyes, and even assesses their odors. Subtle changes in the body act as indicators of imbalances and potential pathologies, helping to predict disease before it becomes serious or more advanced. Many will read this and think that I am just promoting a biased opinion of which medicine is the best, namely my chosen field of traditional Chinese medicine. However, my opinion is both subjective and objective, and I have found that the holistic medicines, such as Oriental medicine, homeopathic and Ayurvedic medicine, are the forms of medicine that address the body as a whole and attempt primarily to maintain health, not just treat symptoms. All medicine has its areas; knowing your expertise and limitations in medicine is fundamental for ethical treatment of patients.

Healthy people should get their vitamins and nutrients from foods. If you choose to take vitamins, make sure they are a single vitamin taken without any other vitamins or supplements. As discussed above, multivitamins or several vitamins taken together have incompatible ingredients that are poisonous to the body. Start with one vitamin or supplement and see how it "feels" for you. Then add another. Make sure your vitamins or supplements are yielding results.

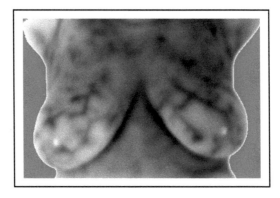

Woman reports "lots of supplements and vitamins." No estrogen therapies reported. Note unusual hypervascular pattern. Severely progesterone deficiency imbalance. Abnormal thermogram.

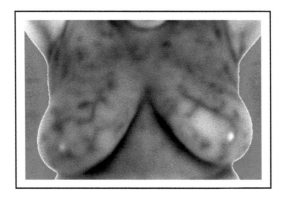

Repeat thermogram six months later. Continued use of supplements and vitamins. Abnormal thermogram.

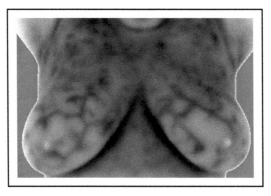

Repeat thermogram six months after removal of supplements and vitamins. Vascular pattern within normal limits. "At risk" thermogram.

Strategic Operation: Supplementation Usage
(Refer to color pages for complete set of images, color and black hot).

For two years, I observed a patient who was emotionally tied to the numerous vitamins and supplements she ingested. She believed health was found in a bottle. After a year of abnormal reports (for six months, report of a right nipplar delta T, then six months later switch to a left nipplar delta T), I suggested removing all supplements and vitamins from her routine, with the exception of krill oil. We observed her every three months; in six months, her breasts had equilibrated and were deemed "vascular uniform." However, her vascularity did not decrease. She still has a severe progesterone deficiency, but her nipplar delta T stabilized, which is important, as 83 percent of cancers have a nipplar delta T. This demonstrates stimulation may be caused by some vitamins and supplements.

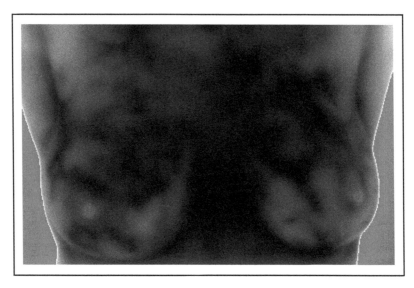

Woman reports no recent history of estrogen therapies. Reports using several medical grade supplements and vitamins. Note unusual hypervascular pattern. Severe progesterone deficiency imbalance. "At risk" thermogram.

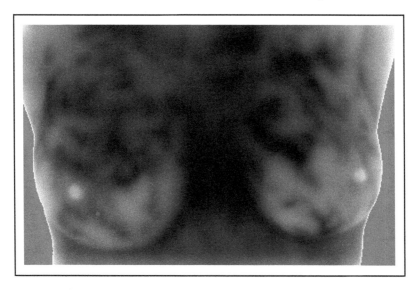

Repeat thermogram two years later. Reports no estrogen therapies. Continued supplement and vitamin use. Note same unusual hypervascular pattern.

It may be apparent by now that I try to get all my patients off supplements, that is, unless they are severely ill. Supplementation is not a healthy practice; it is the equivalent of fast food. It is understandable that people are so busy and caught up in the fast-paced life which most of us live, but we must take the time to nourish ourselves. Just like the over supplementation of estrogen creates dangerous imbalances, supplementing with vitamins, minerals, etc., is a similar thing. Eat your medicine daily in the form of healthy organic foods, and stop being pill poppers. True health comes from daily practices of good health and not from magical pills in the elusive quest for the fountain of youth.

# 9. Progesterone

As we've learned from previous sections of this book, progesterone is a hormone, derived from cholesterol that is only made by the corpus luteum when an egg is expelled. Progesterone is an important counterbalance to excess estrogen, the major contributor to the rise in breast cancer. It may be argued that, when women are deficient in progesterone, they increase their chances for other cancers as well. In this section, we will shed much more light on the hormone progesterone and the myths and misinformation that surround it.

During ovulation, a woman makes 10–20 mg of progesterone a day, while a pregnant woman makes 300 mg a day by the end of her term. This is because progesterone is needed to maintain the pregnancy, as too much estrogen in a women's system will either not allow for the implantation of the fertilized egg or causes the inability to sustain the pregnancy. This is exemplified when a woman wishes to abort a pregnancy the physician may utilize the option to inject the patient with estrogen to discontinue the pregnancy.

Even if a pregnancy persists when there is an excessive amount of estrogen, often after a woman gives birth, she experiences what is known as post-partum depression. This is actually a severe hormonal imbalance between excess estrogen and deficient progesterone. The last remaining progesterone a pregnant woman can regain is in her placenta. Anyone who grew up on a farm or similar environment will notice that, after giving birth, the mother animal will consume the placenta. That is why, in ancient civilizations, women would make a medicinal tea out of the placenta. Interesting that past cultures from primitive times figured out hormone balance yet we still struggle with this concept today.

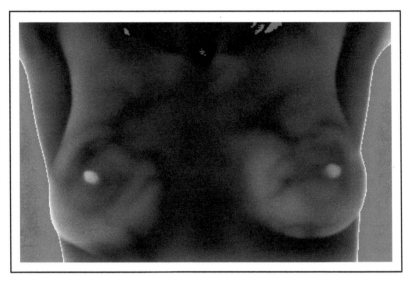

No hormones. Note hypervascular pattern and abnormal thermogram of left breast.

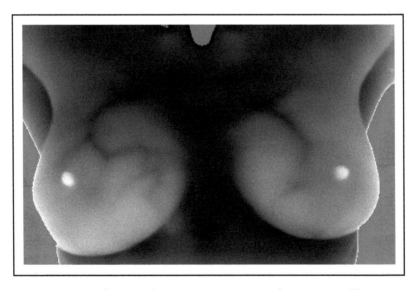

Repeat thermogram four years later. Woman reports use of progesterone. Thermogram demonstrates decrease in vascularity by removing estrogenic foods/products and applying progesterone cream to the breasts. Normal thermogram.

Before tackling the dilemma of menopause, let's look into the reason we go through all of this—procreation. Our bodies are set up to drive us to procreate, a.k.a. make babies. Hormones truly control us. Progesterone increases and decreases throughout the cycle, ranging from 2–3 mg a day to 30 mg at its peak. The increase in progesterone at ovulation results in an increase in basal body temperature that prepares the body for fertilization; this is how women can measure ovulation time. This increase in progesterone also causes the sex drive a woman feels at this time, as well as the desire for children.

When the body stops producing eggs, the result is no more progesterone and estrogen, and women become menopausal. Women who are overweight might have higher estrogen levels, and therefore, more severe symptoms of menopause due to estrogen storage in the fat cells. Weight is also a nationally accepted factor that increases risk for breast cancer.

However, most women experience signs and symptoms of menopause. This is due to exposure from environmental and synthetic estrogens, HRTs, and BCPs, phytoestrogens, flax, soy, bioidentical estrogens, and ecoestrogens in petrochemical products, *not* because of their body's estrogen. Symptoms of menopause, night sweats, irritability are from excess estrogen (or progesterone deficiency) and low testosterone *not* from an estrogen deficiency. It is these environmental estrogens that bombard us on a daily basis that create women's hormone imbalances. During menopause, most women have excess estrogen and are low in progesterone. Now if this is true, why in the heck is estrogen given to menopausal women? Does this make any sense at all?

Many women are now anovulatory in their twenties and thirties, meaning they have periods, but don't always produce an egg. This becomes quite a problem because progesterone is not produced due to the lack of an egg, which leads to a cascade of other effects, including the absence of a period (amenorrhea), infertility and an increase in the risk of breast and uterine cancer. Let's face it, due to the amount of environmental estrogens in our present day lifestyle, we are basically all on the pill. As statistics clearly show, this is a dangerous situation. Thermograms can monitor hormone levels and treatment with holistic medicine can alleviate many of these medical issues, including amenorrhea and infertility.

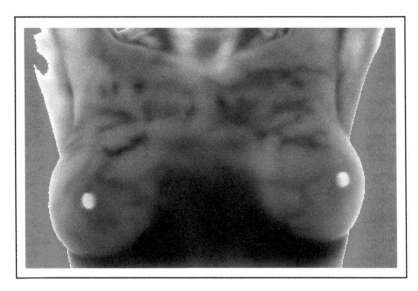

Before starting progestogen cream. Note unusual vascular pattern.

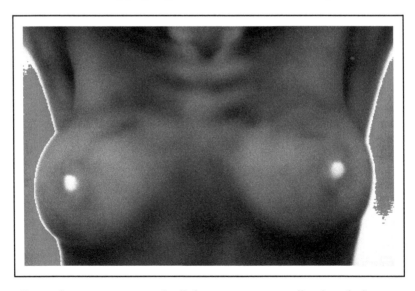

Repeat thermogram one year. Applied progesterone cream directly to the breasts.
Note decrease in vascularity. Normal thermogram.

In the late '70s and '80s, Dr. Hobbins studied with the original bioidentical hormone researchers in France. They examined the effects of different forms of estrogen, progesterone and testosterone on the body.

Dr. Hobbins' desire was to increase the circulation of progesterone into the skin by using niacin as a stimulant in his study, "Double Blind Study of Effectiveness Transcutaneous Progesterone in Fibrocystic Brest Conditions Monitored by Thermography," William Hobbins, MD (1986). However, he discovered that progesterone coupled with niacin dissipated too quickly. A fat-soluble progesterone used alone was required as it accumulated in the skin.

These doctors also found that progesterone in pill form does not decrease stimulation or vascularity to the breasts, due to the fact that most of its properties get destroyed in the digestive system. With regard to progesterone cream being applied to the wrist, thigh, and abdomen, they found that it does not reduce stimulation or vascularity in the breasts because it is not local and dissipates in the bloodstream. The same results were found with progesterone suppositories applied rectally, as well as with sublingual or under the tongue application. Sublingual dissipates in the circulatory system and pills get digested in the digestive system. So don't believe the hype concerning these forms of progesterone. Some PMS and symptoms of menopause might decrease minimally with the above applications, but the concern is breast cancer. Due to the vascularity and neoangiogenesis caused by excess estrogen stimulating breast cells, the only way to reduce risk and stimulation is to apply progesterone cream directly to the breasts.

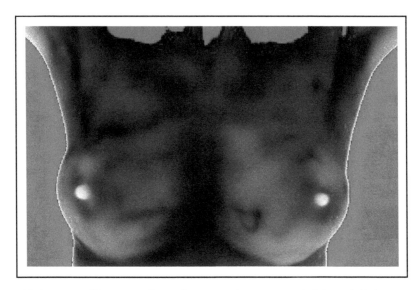

No hormones. Note unusual vascular pattern. Progesterone deficiency imbalance. "At risk" thermogram.

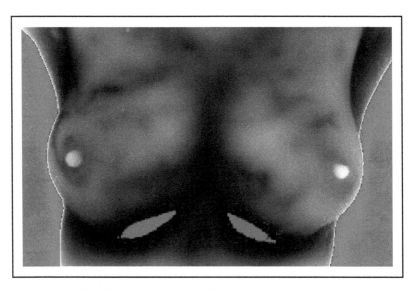

Woman reports using sublingual progesterone for two years. Note no change in the unusual vascular pattern. Sublingual progesterone dissipates before it reaches the receptors in the breasts. Progesterone deficiency imbalance. "At risk" thermogram.

Here is a list of which approaches should be made in regards to our breast health **with progesterone cream.**

- Don't begin application until the breasts have fully matured (typically at the age of twenty-five).

- Try to consult with an educated physician who utilizes breast thermography to measure hormone balance, as blood tests are unreliable which results in inaccurate hormone results.

- Use compounded or USP progesterone cream. Avoid wild yam or "natural" progesterone they may have estrogenic properties.

- Only use progesterone by itself, *do not* have it combined with other hormones, herbs, essential oils, or supplements.

- Progesterone cream must *only be applied to the breasts.*

The following are falsehoods of progesterone cream:
1. Progesterone cream must be applied to the arms, thighs and abdomen—*false*
2. Progesterone cream doesn't work because it is fat soluble—*false*
3. Progesterone pills and sublingual (under tongue) drops work—*false*
4. Blood and saliva tests are accurate for estrogen and progesterone—*sometimes false5*
5. Progesterone causes cancer—*false*
6. Progesterone and progestin are the same—*false*

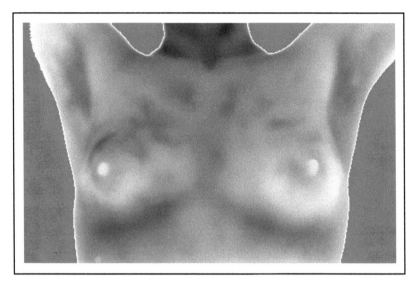

Woman reports using progesterone pills. Note unusual vascular pattern in right breast. Progesterone pills can get destroyed in the GI tract. Abnormal thermogram.

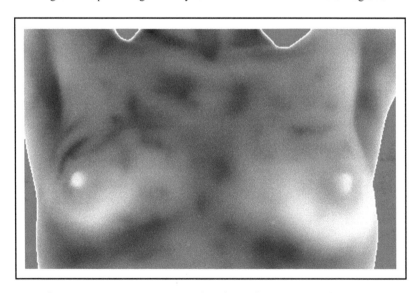

Repeat thermogram. Woman reports continued use of progesterone pills. Note unusual vascular pattern in right breast. *If* vascularity is due to estrogen stimulation progesterone pills are unable to balance. Abnormal thermogram.

## Fat-Soluble Compounded Progesterone
## Cream Applied to the Breasts

As stated above, progesterone cream must be applied directly to the breast daily in order to balance out the estrogen. This is because the progesterone receptors are located in the breasts. Regardless of this medical fact, some doctors continue to state that progesterone cream is not to be applied on the breasts. No explanation is given. Why? If you have a cut on your finger, you don't apply Neosporin to your elbow, do you?

What seems to be another form of misinformation is the notion that, because progesterone cream is fat soluble, it is ineffective. But it is the fact that progesterone cream *is* fat soluble that creates the key to its success. Fat soluble means it is stored in the body. The skin acts as a reservoir for progesterone cream so that it may accumulate in the breasts. Over time, it builds up and counters the overstimulation of estrogen, resulting in the balancing of these hormones. It is this balance that decreases infertility, breast tenderness, cramps, heavy periods, fibroids and signs of menopause, night sweats, weight gain, etc.

Many doctors tell women to only apply progesterone during the last fourteen days of their cycle, the leuteal phase. This is incorrect, as most women are severely progesterone deficient. It is vital to find a physician who is educated in thermography so they can work with you to determine the appropriate dosage and length of use by monitoring levels with thermography.

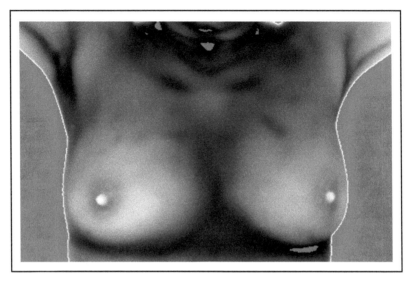

Woman reports using progesterone cream daily for ten years applied to the breasts. Normal thermogram.

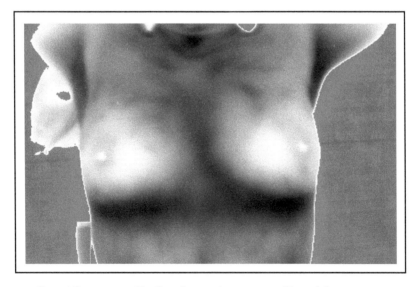

Repeat thermogram. Continued progesterone cream. Normal thermogram.

## Compounded Progesterone Cream

It is important that the progesterone cream used is a compounded progesterone cream. Some MDs, chiropractors and naturopaths make their own creams, and although their thought process is correct, unfortunately, the other ingredients they include in the creams have estrogenic effects that counter progesterone and often increase vascularity and neoangiogenesis in the breasts.

Wild yam is the most popular source of progesterone for these creams. However, estrogen is derived from this source as well, so women should be cautious. This is why it is important to use a compounded pharmacy, as they correctly develop the progesterone without any estrogenic properties.

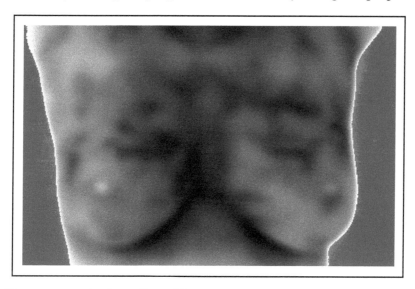

Woman reports using "natural" or wild yam progesterone cream. Note unusual vascular pattern that could be from estrogenic properties found in cream. Progesterone deficiency imbalance. "At risk" thermogram.

Avoid buying and taking suggestions from health food stores as their employees are most likely educated by propaganda. Many times, I suggest a compounded progesterone cream and the patient goes to her local health food market to buy it. The employee there excitedly tells her instead about an over-the-counter, wild yam progesterone cream that is wonderful at treating women's health issues! False! This form of progesterone cream usually contains estrogen, and the patient's repeat thermogram shows an increase in vascularity or neoangiogenesis every time. Again, progesterone must be extracted correctly, usually by compounding pharmacies.

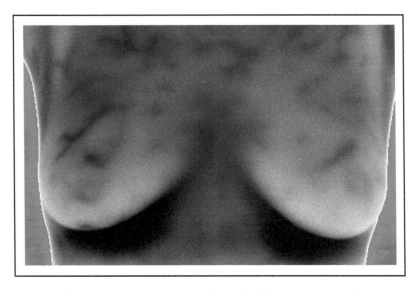

No hormones. Note unusual vascular pattern. After initial thermogram showed a progesterone deficiency imbalance she started using a progesterone cream recommended by another doctor.

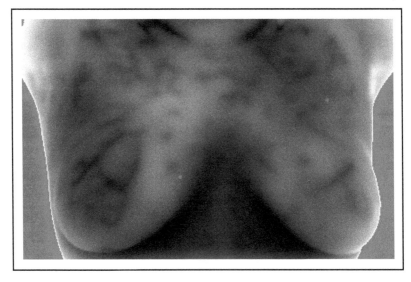

Repeat thermogram three years later. Used a progesterone cream that contained phytoestrogens, or tainted progesterone. Note increase in vascularity. Right breast abnormal.

We see this time and time again in our patients' repeat thermograms. Every patient is convinced that their doctor is "fabulous" with hormones. The patients are advised to get a compounded progesterone cream that requires a prescription, so they ask their doctor for one. Often times, the doctor instead tells patients that they are deficient in other areas, and therefore, creates a cocktail cream with additional elements. This may appear beneficial—after all, why not address everything at once? But that is the flaw; if other factors are put into the treatment, it becomes difficult to isolate and differentiate the responses. And this is exactly what we see; something has interfered with the original intent of the cream and we get contradictory results with nothing to draw definitive conclusions from.

Start with just a progesterone cream for thirty to ninety days, and then reevaluate. So many doctors send their patients out the door with hundreds of dollars of various pills, believing they are doing the correct treatment. How do they know *what* is working? Keep it simple, start with a compounded progesterone cream, and then add one form of treatment at a time. Your body will tell you what is working, as tests are not always reliable, which brings us to our next topic.

What we have found to be quite a dilemma is the heavy reliance on blood and saliva tests. Many of our patients who receive a progesterone deficiency grade score from us are later told by their medical provider that they are estrogen deficient. What is becoming increasingly apparent is that blood and saliva tests are not accurate. Based on thermographic findings, they do not have the ability to test for exogenous estrogens but only natural occurring estrogens. This might be accurate if we were isolated from the environmental influences, but that is not reality. These women would not present with an array of excess estrogen symptoms and thermographic findings of vascularity if they were truly estrogen deficient. Labs have their strong points but they are not the end all, be all of diagnostic tools. Rather, there should be an evaluation of the patient as a whole. Listening to the patient is extremely important. At the same time, breast thermography is not a diagnostic but rather a screening process. If the breasts were hormonally balanced, there would be no vascularity. Our breasts don't lie.

Quite often, I hear from women that they have tested really high for progesterone. If this were true, their thermography would reveal breasts with "nonvascular" results. I have never seen this, and again, blood and saliva tests are not accurate.

Here's a tip, look at the doctor who gives you hormone advice. How do they look? They should appear healthy; not overweight or prematurely aged. I have imaged many doctors who advise women on hormone treatments, and yet not one of them has a hormonally balanced thermographic image.

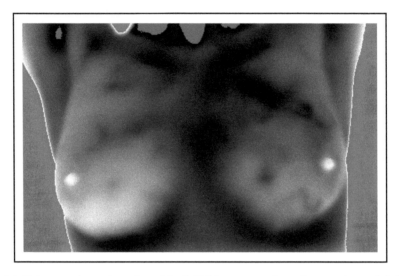

Soy diet. Note unusual vascular pattern. After initial thermogram showed a progesterone deficiency imbalance decided to use progesterone pills because research claimed they were more effective.

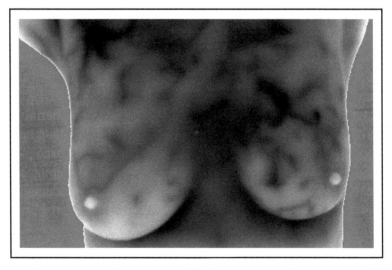

Repeat thermogram. Used progesterone pills for one year. Note increase in vascularity. Progesterone gets destroyed in the digestion before it reaches the receptors in the breasts. Left breast abnormal.

How does a thermogram enable the detection of hormone or endocrine imbalance, you might ask? Let's first look into the fact that estrogen stimulates the breast cells, which we covered in our breast anatomy section. To quickly review, once we reach puberty, our body begins producing estrogen in order to develop sexually. This leads to the development of our breasts and the reproductive maturity of our body. While in the follicular phase of our cycle, our breasts are tender and growing. During the luteal phase, progesterone surges, countering the estrogen, and our breasts cease to develop. This goes on month after month during puberty, and the breasts continue to mature until about age twenty-five. While this may be in the distant past for many of us women, try to recall what happened to our breasts when we started taking The Pill. They got bigger, right? This is because of the estrogen. You also probably gained weight, again due to the estrogen.

As we've stated, estrogen stimulates the breasts, stimulation causes an increase in activity, and this increase in activity causes heat. In addition to providing a delivery system for the body's countless activities, blood flow also provides the warmth. When a thermogram is performed, it picks up heat. The room is cooled and a cold stress challenge is applied, which initiates a systemic vasoconstriction (closing of the blood vessels); therefore, the areas that are not of natural nerve innervations (cancer can create its own blood supply to "feed" off) are not responsive to this temperature differentiation. This will detect the areas of the breast, generally referred to as "hot spots," which are overstimulated and at a higher risk for breast cancer. This is usually seen in the breast that is suspicious for cancer, while the other breast remains cool.

When a woman has an endocrine or hormone imbalance, both breasts are stimulated when placed in a cool room and will have "hot spots." Referred to as "vascularity," this indicates a progesterone deficiency, or excess estrogen. Ultimately, vascularity is stimulation. If we are balanced, in regards to estrogen and progesterone, the thermogram would not indicate any vascularity because there is no stimulation. No stimulation = no heat and no vascularity. It is a wonderful test for a patient to observe, as the results are easy to understand and distinguish with their own eyes. When a woman experiences pain, tenderness, soreness, irregular menses, infertility, dense, fibroids or cystic breasts, symptoms of menopause, this is all likely due to the overstimulation of estrogen.

Many of our patients are relieved, yet frustrated, to find that years of various symptoms and discomfort are due to excess estrogen, which can usually be addressed through dietary changes and perhaps the use of progesterone cream. These women grow even more excited when they are finally able to shed those five to ten pounds of excess weight that they were unable to lose prior, no matter how hard they tried. Why is this? Estrogen is a fat-storing molecule, and women tend to store this additional weight in the abdomen, hips, and thighs. Again, think about the side effects of birth control pills: weight gain and larger breasts. Estrogen, estrogen, estrogen. Also, why do we always hear how "there are all these hormones in our beef and it's making our children fat." What hormone do they give these cows? That's right, estrogen. This is also why it is imperative to avoid flax and soy, especially with developing children.

Let's review a little bit here. Thermography can measure exogenous estrogen based on breast stimulation, whereas saliva and blood tests seem to be ineffective in regards to this vital contributing factor. Therefore, these tests are going to report false hormone levels, and as doctors generally base their treatment plans on such tests, they are blind to the damage that is inflicted on the health of the female population. This cannot be an excuse for these practitioners, as so many of them refuse to listen to their patients' complaints or do objective research on the treatment strategies most commonly provided by pharmaceutical companies.

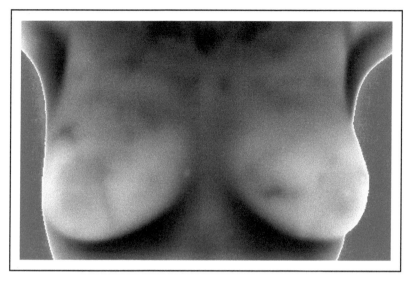

Woman reports using progesterone cream for several years. Normal thermogram.

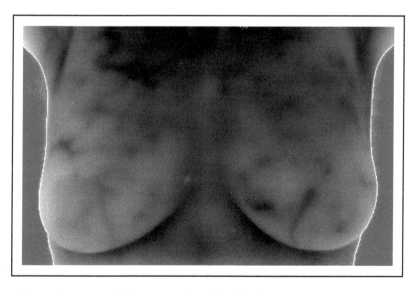

Repeat thermogram. This woman changed application and applied progesterone cream to wrists. Note increase vascularity. Progesterone receptors are in the breasts, not the wrists, arms, abdomen, or legs.

"I had my first thermography done in San Diego. It was confusing with the "results" they gave me. I did some research before having another one done, and came across Pink Image. Reading the other reviews greatly impressed me. I am 67 turning 68 in a week, and I WISH I had known about the information Dr. Wendy Sellens shared with me now back when I was having 2 weeks on and 2 weeks off of flooding periods as I neared menopause! Her natural recommendations would have cleared all of that up I am sure! After the thermography test this time, Dr. Sellens took the time to tell me how to create better breast health. I got the progesterone cream she recommended, and applied it to the breasts as she recommended and WOW!!! what a difference!!! I feel calm, more energy, like someone I used to like and know-ME AGAIN!!! There are a lot of progesterone creams out there-you want to use only what she says to use-one with NO Estrogen or phyto estrogens that will only make your problem WORSE. To feel like I do now (and I have only used the cream for about 7 days) was worth the cost of the thermography 10 times over, because what price health?! We have been on a fixed income since 1998 as my husband had a PTSD breakdown from combat and no longer could work. I had tried a progesterone cream years ago that had wild yam (a phytoestrogen!) added to it, and I felt weepy, sad, bloated, and weak. It actually made me feel worse!

*The fact is ladies, we are all estrogen dominate when in peri and actual menopause, and we don't need any more estrogen, as that is the problem.*

I was using "healthy" things like flax, and soy that were ruining my health. The soy ruined my thyroid! Flax just feeds estrogen, along with some other things that turned out not to be healthy either. The fact is, what Dr. Wendy recommended WORKS and she doesn't sell it, she just tells you what it is and you buy it at Sprouts, Amazon or even online from Walmart! Thank you, Dr. Wendy, I feel like a new woman!"

Linda

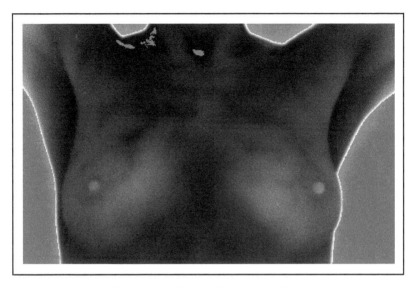

No hormones. Note mild vascular pattern.

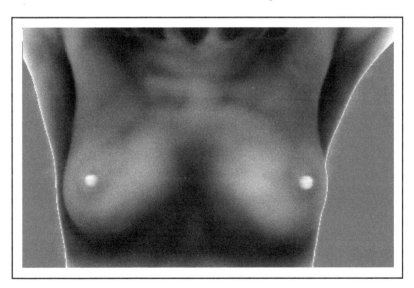

Repeat thermogram three years later. Woman reports use of progesterone. Thermogram demonstrates decrease in vascularity with use of progesterone cream. Normal thermogram.

# Progesterone Does Not Cause Breast Cancer

Another misunderstanding we encounter all the time is that progesterone causes cancer. This is completely false. When women are tested for breast cancer, one of the tests they conduct is a receptor test, called immunohistochemistry. This test establishes if the breast cancer is affected by hormones, to determine if its estrogen receptor positive, progesterone receptor positive or hormone negative (meaning that the cancer has no hormone receptors). Eighty percent of breast cancers are estrogen receptor positive while 20-40 percent of estrogen receptor breast cancers are progesterone receptor positive. Here lies the misunderstanding: estrogen receptor positive cancers *may* be progesterone receptor positive, but there has never been a breast cancer that was estrogen receptor negative *with* a progesterone receptor positive result. What this means is that if a cancer is progesterone receptor positive, it is also estrogen receptor positive, and therefore, progesterone by itself cannot cause cancer.

Another reason for the belief that progesterone causes cancer is a study conducted where six hundred women were studied for the effectiveness of Tamoxifen, a drug given to women with breast cancer. Tamoxifen blocks estrogen from stimulating the breast cells. This is very important in estrogen receptor positive breast cancers, as estrogen promotes cancer growth in these types of cancer. In the study, three hundred of the six hundred women with breast cancer were given Tamoxifen and the other three hundred were given a placebo. Of the three hundred women who were not given Tamoxifen (placebo patients), three got uterine cancer, and interestingly, of the three hundred women who were given Tamoxifen, three of those also got uterine cancer.

So the incorrect conclusion that was derived from the results of this study was that because estrogen was not present, progesterone must have caused the cases of uterine cancer. Yes, from this study, uterine cancer had the similar frequency in breast cancer patients regardless of treatment by Tamoxifen. In no way does this conclude that progesterone *caused* these incidents of uterine cancer. The theory that progesterone caused cancer was an assumption, which is not evidence! Don't let dangerous assumptions affect your health.

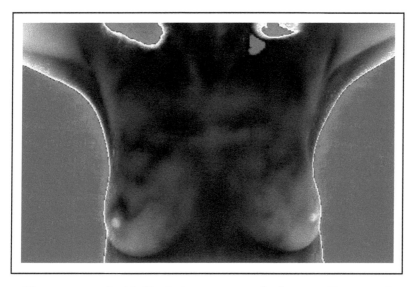

Woman reports using bio-identical estrogen cream for five years. Note unusual hypervascular pattern. Right breast abnormal.

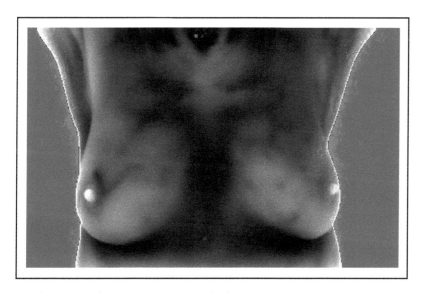

Repeat thermogram five months later. Started using progesterone cream and stopped using bio-identical estrogen cream. Note decrease in vascularity in the top halves of the breasts. Thermogram within normal limits in five months!

# Common Mistakes

It is extremely important to thoroughly inspect the foods in your household. We must make sure that the main phytoestrogen additives, particularly soy and flax, are not in the food that we consume on a daily basis.

War Story:

One patient returned for her follow-up thermography, and her breasts were more vascular than before, even after supposedly eliminating estrogen and phytoestrogens from her diet. She was very frustrated! We had done everything correctly, but her breast thermography and symptomology hadn't subsided. I kept telling her that she has to solve this mysterious source of phytoestrogen—she was ready to strangle me. Finally, a couple of weeks later, she reported back to me that her "juice-man" was putting one-fourth cup of flax into her afternoon juice. That is a huge amount of phytoestrogens! Following the removal of her juicing habit, her breasts decreased in vascularity and her complaints disappeared.

As mentioned above, many times I send women out to get compounded progesterone cream and their doctor, based on labs, will add elements to the cream. Many of these special cocktail creams now have phytoestrogens in them, and therefore, eliminate the purpose of having a progesterone cream. These women will return, and lo and behold, their breasts are worse. They tell me "I got the progesterone cream from my doctor like you told me." But when I look at the bottle, it has all these extra ingredients added. Ladies, stick with compounded pharmacies *only* and compounded progesterone cream *only*, with no other added ingredients. If this is not effective within one to three months, then there needs to be a reassessment of the condition and a new approach or treatment established.

With my patients, I constantly use the "keep it simple" motto. If a woman presents with an endocrine imbalance, we begin the first thirty to ninety days with hormone balancing. When a follow-up thermogram is done and it shows that she is thermographically balanced, yet she still has insomnia, weight gain, etc., I then treat her with nutrition and Chinese herbal medicine. The diet is typically the first change that I suggest for nearly all of my patients, so hopefully, by the time they return for another thermogram, they have implemented this. I'm not a fan of clinics that test women, find that all levels are low, and prescribe sacks full of supplements. The woman walks out the door with a few hundred dollars in supplements and no knowledge of what is actually going on. If, by chance, they do happen to get better, what is working? Are they sentenced to a life of continuous supplementation? I should hope not!

If a patient is really stubborn and wants to supplement, I have them remove all supplements for three months and only use progesterone and testosterone. When they have a nonvascular thermogram, we add supplements. The addition of one supplement at a time allows the patient to observe how her body is responding. Then we perform another thermogram sixty days later. If there is vascularity or stimulation, we know which particular supplement is causing it. We keep doing this for all supplements to see which ones work. From my clinical experience, many supplements create vascularity.

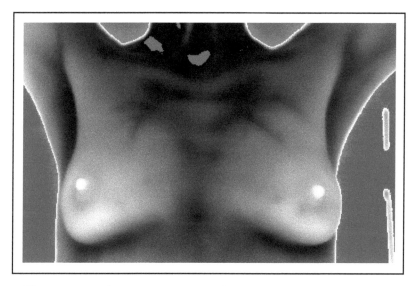

Woman reports using progesterone cream for eight years. Normal thermogram.

Remember, keep it simple. Start with progesterone and maybe testosterone. Start slow and see how you feel. You are in charge of your body; your doctor is there to make educated suggestions, hence the extensive education. But ultimately, *you* have the final word and only *you* know how *you* feel. This is *your* health.

# 10. Breast Cancer

"At Johns Hopkins Hospital in 1898, Dr. Halstead reported his five year survival rate of 48 percent with radical carcinoma of the breast. The survival rate, as now judged some fifty years later at the same institution with all the new modalities… have not provided the female any increased safety in being cured from this malady."

William Hobbins, MD, "To Mammogram or Not," 1969

## How Cancer Cells Grow

How cancer is created is still a relative mystery. At present, the most popular theory is from the works of Dr. Nicholas J. Gonzalez in his book, *The Trophoblast and the Origin of Cancer: One Solution to the Medical Enigma of our Time.* He believes that the inception of cancer is probably caused by an initial stem cell or a trophophite cell in the body. Trophophite cells are not stem cells, but similar in characteristics, as they can change into any other cell. One trophophite cell may enter any cell in our body and transform it into a normal cell or into one with the terrible characteristics of a cancer cell.

These cells cannot be found in blood tests or organ histology, but it is known that they exist. It is not certain how trophophites achieve this transformation (infection, chemical irritant, X-ray) or when this catalyst occurs, but these cells come out of nowhere and create cancer. Two people can have an infection, and one gets cancer and the other doesn't. There is no proven theory as to why this occurs. Cells will not invade other cells of the same organism, which is why cancer isn't contagious. It is the trophophite cell that invades or changes a normal cell into a cancer cell.

Cancer starts as an abnormal cell that has mutated from its original healthy state. Every time a cell divides, there is a chance for mutation. The body has a couple of amazing processes that minimizes copying of abnormal or unhealthy cells. One way to actually minimize "poor reproductions" is with enzymes called repair endonucleases. They can fix the cell *before* division or replication. However, if a cell is damaged beyond viable replication, there is another process called apoptosis that will destroy the unhealthy cell. This is like a self-termination program that further prevents abnormal cellular growth.

There are many causes for mutations including radiation, electricity, toxins, pollutions, etc. Some people believe that cancers come from a virus, which may very well damage a cell and thereby cause a weakness.

If a cell mutates to become a cancer cell, every 90 days it has the ability to replicate or double this flawed genetic material. Because these cells replicate at an exponential rate, the cancer grows the most at the later levels of development. If the cancer is the size of a grape (which takes around six to ten years to become that large), then in ninety days, it doubles to the size of an avocado pit.

The genetic material of a cell is organized into chromosomes that have cap-like ends called telomeres. These "caps" degrade with every cell division until the genetic material is no longer protected, at which time the cell is triggered to self-terminate. The enzyme telomerase has the ability to replace these caps, creating a cell that never dies, and therefore, perpetually replicating into what we find as a cancerous mass. The genetically mutated cancer cells create this telomerase, and therefore, cancer.

This mass of tissue is called a tumor. These cancer cells grow and push other cells out of the way, taking or occupying their space. Tumors are divided into two types: benign and malignant. Benign means that the mass *is not* cancerous, and is therefore unable to spread to other parts of the body. Malignant refers to a mass that *is* cancerous, with the potential to spread and invade other regions of the body.

A tumor is interesting because it has a protective protein barrier around it that is not recognized by macrophages (immunological cells). When you get sick or hurt yourself, the body sends out a cleanup crew of macrophages that detect foreign invaders, destroy, and consume them. The protein barrier protects the tumor by blending in, like camouflage, so the body doesn't recognize it as a foreign invader.

Metastasis is when the cancer cells break free and travels to another area in the body. It is not certain what causes this, though one theory explains it as follows: cells are held together tightly by an extracellular matrix, and the cancer cell may have an enzyme with the ability to destroy this bonding product, allowing cells to leave and invade other regions of the body.

People don't actually die from cancer itself, but rather from its waste product (excrement).

"I knew something wasn't right a few years back and I was urged to get a thermogram. Unfortunately, I hadn't done my research and settled on a clinic that was not FDA approved. I was misinformed and for quite some time had false confidence. Almost 6 months ago, at age 36 I was diagnosed with stage 2 breast cancer. This is when I realized I needed to do my homework, my own research, and be my own advocate. I was on a mission to decode my own pathology report. Not an easy task I might add. I've learned cancer is a mystery. Whose research and recommendations do you believe? After a lot of research, I decided to have an FDA-approved thermogram at Pink Image in Solana Beach, CA. There, I met board certified thermologist, Wendy Sellens, L.Ac. She informed me that I had options. She quickly sent my screening results and pathology report to her advisor, creator and founder of the certified breast thermology model, William Hobbins, MD. Dr. Hobbins had me contact him right away and gave me a short lesson on the very specific type of breast cancer I had and shared an alternative path that I should consider. He gave me words of truth, hope, and courage. Dr. Hobbins asked if he could pray with me and instantly, I realized the power of my faith would have to play the primary role in my recovery.

"It is vital that when getting a thermogram, it is an FDA-approved thermography camera. I want to thank Wendy Sellens at Pink Image, for her professionalism, compassion, and true discernment. She was a critical member of a team that literally helped save my life."

Sarah

# Types of Breast Cancer

*Noninvasive (in situ) Breast Cancer*

In this scenario, the cancer cells remain in their place of origin, the lining and ducts, and have not spread. This is stage 0 cancer or DCIS. Dr. Hobbins does *not* consider this to be cancer because only 5 percent of DCIS ever becomes cancer. Yes, that means 95 percent of DCIS are not cancerous. DCIS actually looks different than cancer. DCIS is an adenoma that has for some unknown reason gone "crazy."

Due to the nature of DCIS, nowadays many women choose to live with or treat it alternatively and not use traditional modalities like lumpectomies and radiation. This is where breast thermography works so well! It monitors the breasts for activities concerning changes in DCIS and observes neoangiogenesis caused by stimulation. If there is an increase, treatment can be advised immediately.

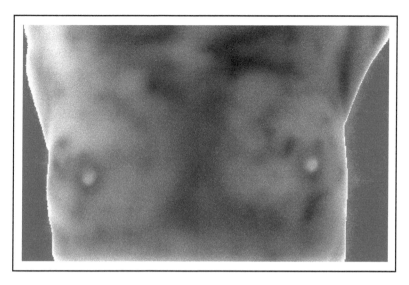

DCIS in right upper breast. Good prognosis for alternative treatment.

## Invasive Breast Cancer

Invasive or infiltrating, breast cancers spread beyond the lining into the ducts or lobules and eventually to other parts of the body like the lymph nodes. A breast cancer in stage I, II, III, or IV means it is invasive with stages determined by how different cancer cells look from normal cells.

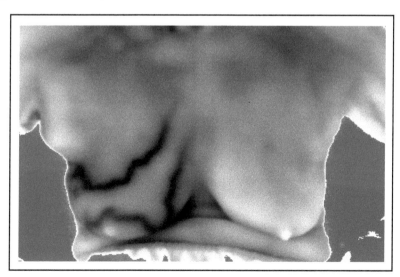

Invasive Stage IV lymph node breast cancer.

## *Invasive Ductal Carcinoma (IDC)*

As the name indicates, this cancer is in the lining of the milk ducts, which carry breast milk from the lobules to the nipple. This is the most common type of breast cancer, with subtypes determined by the appearances of the cancer cells. Subtypes of IDC are tubular, mucinous, medullary, and papillary.

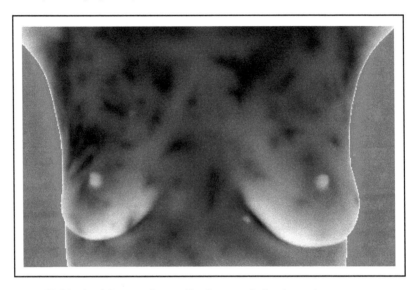

IDC in the right upper breast. Good prognosis for alternative treatment

## *Invasive Lobular Cancer*

This makes up a small portion of breast cancer, and as the name suggests, it is found in the lobules, where breast milk is produced. This cancer doesn't typically form a lump but rather a thickening of the tissue in an area of the breast. This cancer has a higher possibility of being bilateral, or spreading to both breasts, and is highly recurrent, meaning you can get it again.

## *Inflammatory Breast Cancer*

This is the most aggressive of all cancers. It develops and spreads very rapidly and can occur at any age. It is also the rarest of breast cancers; only 6 percent of breast cancers are inflammatory. Inflammatory breast cancer is many times mistaken for a breast infection called mastitis, which is often effectively treated with antibiotics. Since breast cancer is not common in young women it is often mistreated, and because younger women have a higher metabolic rate, this form of cancer is very dangerous. In addition, it typically does not form a lump.

Signs and symptoms of inflammatory breast cancer are the following:

- Rapid change in the appearance of the breast over the course of a few days or weeks
- Thickness, heaviness, or visible enlargement of one breast
- Discoloration that gives the breast a red, purple, pink, or bruised appearance
- Itching
- Unusual warmth of one breast
- Dimpling or ridges on the skin of one breast, similar to an orange peel
- Tenderness, pain, or aching
- Enlarged lymph nodes under the arm, above or below the collar bone
- Flattening or turning inward (inversion) of the nipple

## Paget's Disease of the Nipple

Paget's carcinoma involves the nipple and/or areola and is rare. Characteristics are usually a pimple, or red, ulcerated or crusted area that does not heal. The malignant cells are a telltale sign and are called Paget cells. Paget's disease will also accompany a tumor or tumors in the underlying tissue.

## Sarcoma Breast Cancer

This cancer is very rare and occurs in the connective tissue that is made up of muscles, fat, and blood vessels. Sarcomas that occur in the breast are phyllodes, tumors, and angiosarcoma.

## Triple-Negative Cancer

A cancer with negative testing for all three hormone tests is called a triple-negative cancer. What this means is that the growth of the cancer is not fed by estrogen, progesterone, nor by the presence of HER2. Because of this, the cancer will not respond to hormone therapy like Tamoxifen. Triple negative cancer makes up about 10–20 percent of cancers.

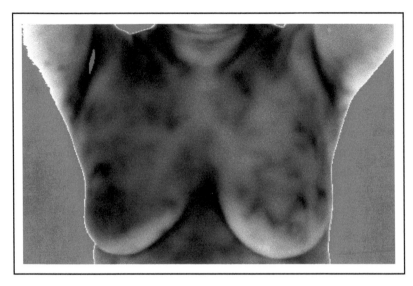

Triple negative cancer in right breast. Patient continues to use a bioidentical estrogen patch. Note unusual vascular patterns in left breast.

## *Bilateral (Both) Breast Cancer*

Only 5 percent of breast cancers are bilateral (both breasts).

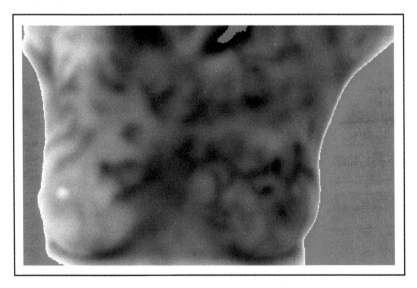

Positive mammogram for right breast. However, left breast is abnormal. Suspected carcinoma in left breast also. Look at the images. Which breast looks more vascular?

# Recurrence of Breast Cancer with Mastectomy

It is still possible to get breast cancer even though a woman has had a mastectomy. A mastectomy will not stop breast cancer; it reduces the percentage of recurrence. Fifteen percent of breast cancers are located in the Tail of Spence, which is not removed with a mastectomy. Cancer can also occur in the chest wall, which is not removed. Many women have come in extremely upset with recurrence after a double mastectomy. They believed they could not get breast cancer again, but this is simply not true. Be aware that, with a double mastectomy, you are only reducing your percentages, not eliminating the possibility of breast cancer.

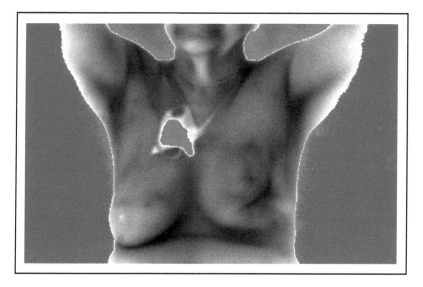

Recent mastectomy of left breast.

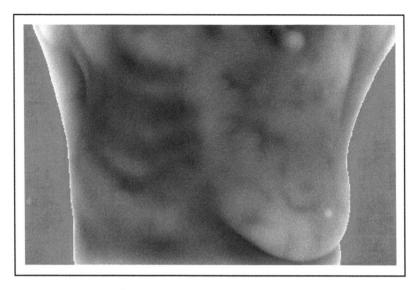

Recent mastectomy of the right breast.

## Hormone Status of Breast Cancer

Around 80 percent of breast cancers are fueled by our own hormones, which is why receptor tests are given once it is determined that breast cancer is present which is called immunohistochemistry. ER+ or estrogen receptor positive, means estrogen causes the breast cancer to grow while PR+ or progesterone receptor positive, means progesterone *may* cause the breast cancer to grow. This is not entirely true, and it is therefore very important to once again cover this topic, as doctors will tell you progesterone causes cancer.

Here are the facts. Around 80 percent of breast cancers are estrogen receptor positive. Twenty to forty percent of that 80 percent are progesterone receptor positive. Read that again to understand completely. Estrogen receptor positive cancer may be progesterone receptor positive, but there has never been a breast cancer that was estrogen receptor negative (meaning not affected by estrogen), while being progesterone receptor positive.

What this tells us is that a cancer positive for progesterone receptors must be positive for estrogen receptors, and therefore, progesterone by itself *cannot* cause cancer.

More importantly, if you are estrogen receptor positive, you are given Tamoxifen, which blocks the effect of estrogen to the cancer and the breast. It does not block the effect of progesterone.

HR- hormone receptor negative means the cancer is not affected by your hormones.

# Genetics

*HER2 gene* or epidermal growth factor receptor is a genetic alteration that tells the cell not just to double, but to make multiple copies. Medications are available that shut off the HER-2 gene, thus reducing the ability for the cancer to multiply at this accelerated rate.

*BRCA1 and BRCA2* (Breast cancer susceptibility gene 1 and 2) are genes that belong to a class of genes called tumor suppressors. In healthy normal cells, BRCA1 and BRCA2 prevent mutation of the DNA. Mutations of BRCA1 and BRCA2 are linked to hereditary risks of breast and ovarian cancer.

> Women (and occasionally men) at high risk of breast cancer (due to family history, BRCA genes, prior breast cancer history, etc.) should consider using certified breast thermography yearly or even several times a year to monitor breast health and screen for changes in the breast tissue and vascularity (screen more often for high risk or image changes over time).
>
> When I say certified breast thermography, I mean high resolution, black & white thermography cameras that reveal vascularization patterns in the breasts, NOT the low resolution color thermography cameras that merely image surface temperature differences.
>
> Naturally, I choose Pink Image for thermography because of the high quality of the cameras they use, the training of their image readers, and their vast experience

in the thermography field. I've lost count how many years I have been going to Pink Image for thermography. Wendy Sellens, the Pink Image founder and owner, was trained by the medical doctor who pioneered the use of high resolution thermography cameras to monitor breast health.

I discovered thermography after my gynecologist noted certain areas of concern in my breasts during office visit exams. Two years in a row, I was sent for diagnostic level mammograms (higher radiation exposure) and ultrasounds, yet each time mammography and U/S could not detect anything unusual, because there was no tumor (yet). I have dense breast tissue, which mammography does not distinguish well from cancerous tissue.

However, high resolution thermography did reveal increased vascularity in the same areas of concern noted by my doctor during annual office exams. Increased frequency of thermographic imaging was recommended to monitor for further changes.

The following two years I scheduled my routine annual screening mammography to be performed in the afternoon the same day as thermography, after the thermography screening was performed in the morning - to be a scientific as possible (my husband is a research scientist) I wanted the condition in my breast tissue to be as similar as possible for each screening method. Further changes have not been detected with thermography, so I have scaled back my mammography screening frequency to about every 4-5 years to avoid reduce my exposure to radiation, while continuing with annual thermography monitoring.

Other than the cold room necessary for the thermography imaging (the skin needs to be very cool) and the need to hold the arms up high for a few minutes to cool the skin before and while the images are taken, there is no physical contact with technician or machinery at all (or painful breast compression as with mammograms).

Thermography is 100 percent radiation-free, unlike mammography.

Unlike mammography, thermography can be used by women of any age at any stage of their lives, by women with breast implants, and by breastfeeding women.

I'm not anti-mammography "screening" nor do I refuse all mammography (I'm just using it less often as a routine screening tool as long as my scheduled thermography images are not indicating worrisome changes). Mammography is, of course, necessary for diagnosis if/when an actual lump or tumor is detected or if thermography reveals risky vascularity increases in the breasts or evidence of an unusually high vascular area of the breast.

Certified high resolution thermography is an excellent screening tool all women and men can safely trust to monitor their breast health. I trust Pink Image with my thermography imaging."

Anna

## Risks for Breast Cancer

All of these risks are supported by studies and recognized by the American Cancer Society and National Cancer Society. Eliminating some of these risk factors could decrease the probability of breast cancer.

1. Age. The older we get, the longer our breasts are exposed to carcinogens (things that cause cancer) such as petrochemicals, estrogens, pollution, and radiation.
2. Age of menarche (first period). The earlier a girl begins puberty and starts developing breasts, the longer her breasts were exposed to factors that may increase her risk of cancer.
3. Hysterectomy and oopharectomy. This is the removal of the uterus and of the ovaries, respectively.
4. Weight, excess estrogen stored in fat cells.
5. Age of first pregnancy. The earlier the age of first pregnancy, the less risk of breast cancer. Conversely, the later the age of the first

pregnancy, the higher the risk. Lack of childbearing increases the risk even more.

6. Breastfeeding. The number of children you breast feed decreases the risk of breast cancer, which is attributed to the increased circulation created by nursing.
7. Birth control pills and hormone replacement therapy. Exposure to synthetic estrogen increases your risk of breast cancer (see "Chemical Warfare").
8. Family history. Genetics may increase risk.
9. Race. Jewish and African descents are considered more vulnerable.

We have added the following to this list:

10. Phytoestrogens, soy, flax, black cohosh, red clover, etc.
11. Bioidentical estrogen, cream, patches and pellets.
12. Ecoestrogens, BPA, parabens, etc.

"I am only in my late 30s and already have had several friends my age diagnosed with breast cancer, one who passed away at the age of 37. Why are the rates going up? Why are women getting cancer at an earlier age? What can we do to decrease risk and prevent Breast Cancer? The answers are in this book. This is an amazing resource for all women. We can make lifestyle choices to decrease our risk! I have used the information in this book, as well as thermographic imaging, to take action to decrease my risk factors. I am a health care provider, and use this book as a resource in my private practice to educate my patients, and in my faculty teaching position as well."

Erica

# 11. Certified Breast Thermography Survival Guide

Thermography was shown as the highest risk factor marker (for breast cancer). It was found to be a 10 times higher risk marker than family history.

William Hobbins, MD, "Thermography-Highest Risk Marker," 1977

Breast imaging in the United States is a billion-dollar-per-year industry!

All imaging should be performed in conjunction with other screening modalities, as no single imaging modality is 100 percent accurate. If we are truly going to wage war on this disease, we must think of the various medical imaging modalities as our arsenal. Each technique does not need to be performed every year, but when a suspicious abnormality exists, women should utilize as much of the breast imaging arsenal as possible. Just as one weapon is used in a certain situation, others may be used in another. When there is a concern, we should double-check those findings with other imaging techniques, such as ultrasound, mammogram, and MRIs. We need to protect our breasts, and the only way to do so is if we have a clear image of what is happening within them!

*Quick Cancer Cells Lesson*

Every time a cell divides, there is a possibility of mutation. This is important because substances such as toxins and free radicals can mutate the cell by interfering with DNA replication. This can be very dangerous because cell division replicates these mutations and may eventually create cancer.

Every ninety days, a cell doubles in your body through mitosis (cell division). Unfortunately, this includes cancer cells.

- 90 days = 2 cells
- 1 year = 16 cells
- 2 years = 256 cells
- 3 years = 4,096 cells
- 4 years = 65,536 cells
- 5 years = 1,048,576 cells

(Breast cancer isn't usually detectable by mammogram till around year six)

- 6 years = 16,777,216 cells
- 7 years = 268,453,456 cells
- 8 years = 4,294,967,296 cells

Depending on the age and density of the breasts, a mammogram cannot detect cancer until it has been growing for almost six to eight years. For the mass to be large enough for detection, it usually must grow to the size of a small pea. Unfortunately, after this many years, it becomes much more difficult to treat, especially with alternative medicine. A thermogram can detect an abnormality during the first few years, at which stage it may not necessarily be a cancer and therefore has the best chance for treatment through habit and lifestyle changes.

> Thermography is, as the word suggests, a graphic recording of temperature. The invention of the thermometer was observed by medical scientists as a major breakthrough in disease diagnosis and management. As early as the recorded paper of Hippocrates, the area of the breast where wet mud dried first was the most significant area for surgical consideration. Early in this century, "evapograms," using alcohol and lamp black films, were used to take a thermal surface temperature of the breast.
>
> William Hobbins, MD, "Breast Thermography—A Vital Screening Tool for the 1983 Woman"

# How Thermography Works

Thermography is a superficial screening procedure that monitors small changes or abnormalities in the skin by analyzing the blood vessels. Healthy breasts should be symmetrical or the same on both sides. Symmetrical vascular patterns, same on both sides, are created by blood vessels with the same temperature. A thermogram that is asymmetrical or has a difference (vascular pattern or heat) from one breast compared to the other is considered a potential risk or abnormal.

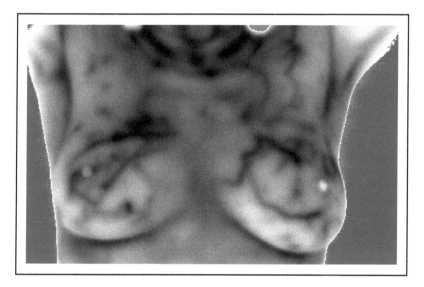

Thermography monitors the blood vessels in the breasts.

Think of thermography as similar to a thermometer. When a child has a fever, the mother takes the child's temperature for early detection of an illness. While it may not yet be clear which illness the child has, a common cold or something worse like meningitis, the fever is a warning signal to start treatment. Thermography should be utilized similarly to the thermometer—when a fever in the breasts is detected, the cause may still be unknown, but treatment should begin.

Since commencing his mammographic research in 1965, Dr. Hobbins has searched for a measurement tool for early detection. At first, he thought it would be mammography, but in 1971, he realized it was thermography. Its sensitivity makes it ideal for breast cancer screening, and more importantly, breast health treatment, as it can detect minute changes in the breast in a short amount of time, usually just a couple months. This is vital for women monitoring breast health, DCIS, breast cancer, or suspicious abnormalities.

> "Prevention is the "cure"! This book clearly shows (using advanced medical thermal imaging) how the effects of many commonly used products, along with exposure to a multitude of chemicals are increasing our risk for breast cancer. I love this book and highly recommend it to any woman who wants to be proactive and help to prevent breast cancer instead of our current model of mammography "screening" starting at age 40. By the time you see something on a mammogram you are already sick, meaning the tumor is already formed. Using thermography as the first screening tool (recommended to start in our 20's), gives women the power to take control of their breast health. Women with genetic risk factors now have a way to monitor their breast health without constantly worrying or having a radical double mastectomy, which only lowers your risk (as described in this book). Finally, a book that gives current information on all forms of estrogen (bio-idential, flax, soy, etc.)! Thank you to both Dr. Hobbins and Wendy for this visual description of what's going on in our breasts. This book is bound to be controversial, but as the book states...the thermographic pictures don't lie. This truly is a revolutionary finding!"

K. Porter

# Thermography Versus Mammogram, Ultrasound and MRI

> Thermography screening of the breast does not find breast cancer. Thermography screening does identify a female population which is at higher risk than the population at large. Thermography screening is biologically safe. Thermography screening increases the opportunity to intensify educational emphasis.
>
> William Hobbins, MD, "Mass Breast Cancer Screening with Thermography, 25,000 Cases," 1975

Thermograms are not superior to mammograms and *do not* replace them. A mammogram is an effective imaging tool when used appropriately and usually after the age of fifty. Dr. Hobbins created the breast thermography interpretation model as an early screening procedure for breast cancer, with the intention that breasts considered thermographically high risk would be sent for further testing with a mammogram. This way, not *all* women are given mammograms. Especially since a mammogram is only 48 percent accurate for women under fifty and 68 percent for women over fifty. In November 2009, the US Preventative Services Task Force (USPSTF) updated it recommendations for an annual mammogram from forty years of age to fifty. In 2016 the American Cancer Society changed its recommendations for an annual mammogram from 50 to 45 and even more surprising, that women 55 and over scale back their mammograms to every other year. Performing a thermogram before a mammogram reduces unnecessary mammograms for relatively "healthy" women, while decreasing exposure to radiation.

Saying one imaging is superior to another is like saying airplanes are superior to cars, they are equally important, as needed. While it may be a wise choice to fly from Los Angeles to New York, would it be a better choice to fly from Los Angles to Long Beach, California? In this instance a car may seem the appropriate choice.

Thermography analyzes the blood vessels looking for vascularity, stimulation of the existing blood vessels or neoangiogenesis, new blood vessels, within the breast and can only measure the skin temperate, therefore, it cannot "see" deep into the tissue to "detect." However, since benign and malignant breast disorders and/or diseases are fed by the blood vessels monitoring them may find a disorder or disease before other imaging. That is why thermography is not a replacement for a mammogram, but an adjunctive screening procedure.

Mammogram are an x-ray monitoring for calcifications or anatomical anomalies. Mammograms tend to have an issue with dense breasts and many women get recalled due to inconclusive reports, which increases access to radiation. Also, women with implants have a risk of rupture due to compression. Mammograms have too many false negatives, meaning they have a high percentage of missed cancers. This is one of the reasons why the national age for an annual mammogram was increased from forty to fifty years old.

Sensitivity is the ability to detect. Thermography is 90 percent sensitive at monitoring abnormal vascular structures. Accuracy is the issue detected was what you wanted to find. Accuracy with mammography changes with age due to denseness of the breasts. Mammograms have high false negatives – missing issues, especially at younger ages due to dense breasts. Thermograms have high false positives – finding too many issues, due to high sensitivity; however, this is what makes it beneficial.

Ultrasounds are sonography or sound waves, which records the echoes as the sound waves bounce back to determine the size, shape, and consistency of soft tissues, usually fibroids and tumors in the breasts. Ultrasound has too many false positives; meaning they have a high percentage of detecting too much.

For the breasts an MRI with gadolinium contrast is required. This dye is radioactive. Thermograms are monitoring for neoangiogenesis. MRI can confirm neoangiogenesis because the dye will leak out of the new blood vessels, thus increasing suspicion of breast cancer. Biopsy is detection and actually confirms cancer.

Together, all four imaging modalities give a better, more complete picture of the breast. Thermography can begin at around age 22 every three years, if normal, in the 30s every two years and at age 40 annually *with* an ultrasound, if normal. Abnormal reports *always* require further imaging, in the order below. Use other imaging "as needed" not annually.

Breast Screening should proceed in this order:

1. Thermography
2. Ultrasound
3. Mammogram
4. MRI with contrast
5. Biopsy

> "After my OBGYN refused to provide me with an Ultrasound and insisted on yet another mammogram (which always comes back inconclusive due to my dense breast tissue), I went to get a thermogram at Pink Image.
>
> Wendy provided me with a full write up on what was happening and then debriefed over the phone with life changing recommendations on what to do to rebalance my hormones and lower the estrogen levels in my body. I cannot be more grateful to Wendy and the whole process and cannot recommend her enough! Please go see her - it may save your life."
>
> Masha

Ultrasounds have too many false positives, meaning that a particular condition or attribute is present or too many biopsies are done due to positive ultrasounds. If women were to get their thermogram before an ultrasound the thermogram could indicate a possible area of concern then the ultrasound could confirm with a positive or negative report, this may reduce the number of false positives. In a perfect world after the age of 35, I believe, every woman should have an annual thermogram and ultrasound, both are biologically safe and through imaging corroboration ensure a breast health issue wasn't unnoticed.

Many women these days do not want yearly exposure to radiation from mammograms. Thermography is a safe, painless, noncontact, and nonradiation screening that detects breasts that are a potential risk or have an abnormality. Thermography monitors the blood vessels therefore it is recommended to begin around the age of 25 or for women with dense breasts for preventative breast screening. High risk thermograms are sent onward to ultrasound, mammogram, or MRI with contrast. If one of these tests is positive, then the patient is most likely beyond the preventative stage and more aggressive medical approaches may be required. If negative, then the patient can be treated with less aggressive medical modalities and make the lifestyle changes included in this book.

> "I was fortunate enough to have Pink Image as my first breast thermography experience. I have a family history of breast cancer, so it has always been a concern. Being in my mid-thirties, mammography seems premature, yet, no screening seems negligent. A physician of mine explained the difference between the two screening technologies and recommended that I seek out Wendy Sellens for breast thermography. The technician was kind and informative and I could see, for myself, the vascularity issues that were of a concern. I shortly thereafter received an explanation of findings from Wendy, a wealth of knowledge, and I am now on a path of prevention thanks to her and this great imaging technology.
>
> Additionally, the book, Breast Cancer Boot Camp (link below), is an incredible eye opener. It's a must read. Chapter after chapter is packed with amazing information. The material presented in this book is well organized, easy to understand and accompanied with visual confirmations (thermograms). Shocking discoveries about everyday things women are doing and physicians are recommending that may be contributing to higher risks of breast cancer. We must educate ourselves as women and take charge of our health. Don't let this information go unnoticed and unrecognized. I highly recommend this book."
>
> Michelle

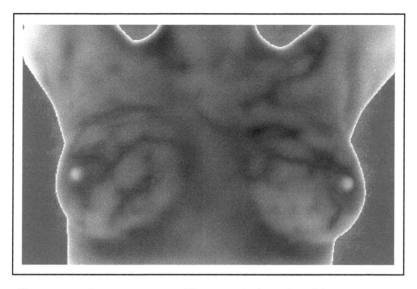

Thermogram of a pregnant woman. Thermography is a safe, painless, noncontact, nonradiation screening. It is safe for women who are pregnant or nursing and have a breast health concern.

Thermograms should begin at age twenty-two, when the breasts are fully developed. This will set a baseline, so that any abnormalities are spotted quickly. Dr. Hobbins reports, "In our screening program in Eau Claire, Wisconsin, 42 percent of the cancers found were in women forty-nine years of age or under." This is also when breast cancer is more aggressive. For ages forty and under, thermograms are suggested every two to three years depending on risk, and annually after forty.

# Breast Thermography Imaging

Breast thermography looks at the entire breast in contrast to mammography, which only looks at the compressed area. This is important because thermographic images include the axilla, or the armpit, where the lymph nodes are located. Thermograms also include the Tail of Spence, where approximately 15 percent of breast cancers can develop. Not only is this important for initial evaluations, but it is also vital for women who have received single or double mastectomies, as a mammogram cannot detect the above mentioned areas where cancer can still develop. Even after mastectomy, breast cancer recurrence is still possible in the chest wall and Tail of Spence. Mastectomy does not eliminate breast cancer, it just reduces possibility of recurrence.

In thermogaphy, there are several image-viewing angles: Anterior view (straight on), left and right oblique (sides of the breasts), and inferior (underneath the breasts). For ladies with larger breasts, it is recommended to put your hands on your head and try to touch your elbow together behind your head while arching backwards. This forces your breasts up during screenings. It is important to never touch the breasts during the imaging session, not even with a tissue, as this will corrupt the image because the hands are three degrees cooler.

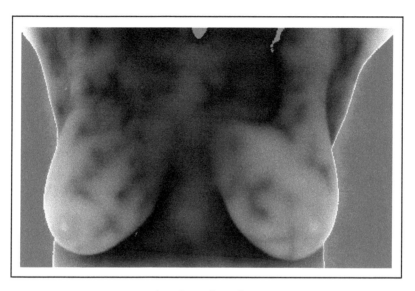

Anterior or front view.

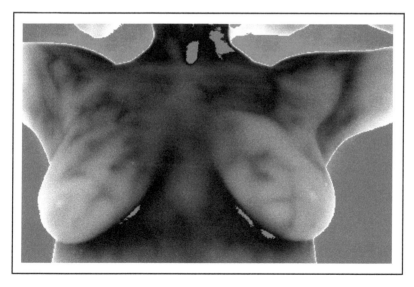

Under view.

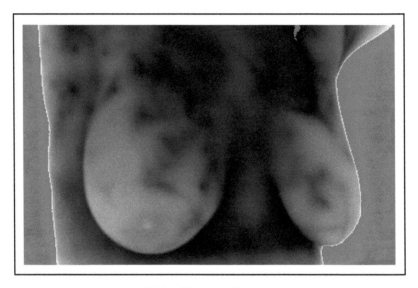

Right oblique or side view.

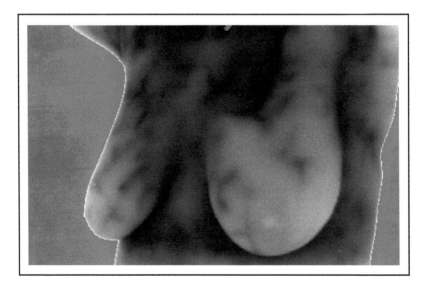

Left oblique or side view.

## Why Certified Breast Thermography

Thermography is not a standardized practice; meaning, anyone can open a breast thermogaphy clinic and read as they please. The majority of breast thermography clinics and academies are *not* meeting the minimum standard requirements for breast thermography. This is one of the major reasons I wrote this book to explain the purpose for requirements in breast cancer screening and to list them! Below are the minimum requirements created by Dr. Hobbins and a group of medical doctors in the early '70s. It is important that breast thermography clinics and academies meet these minimum requirements at the very least, so that the best possible images and interpretation can be performed on the breasts. Keep in mind that these requirements are just for breast thermography.

Thermography on other body parts, such as the knees, neck, back etc., are much easier to diagnose, and therefore, requirements are not as strict. Thermography is usually used in pain clinics as an alternative test for chronic pain or injury of a specific area; it is not used on the entire body.

Be wary of clinics conducting full body scans. Thermography cannot see lungs, kidneys, or the cervix directly; remember this technology is limited to superficial skin temperatures and it can't "see" past the skin into the tissue, muscle or organs! Avoid this gimmick, as it is usually in conjunction with the sale of supplements.

Organs have referral patterns, so abnormalities of the organs can be seen in thermography but not directly over the organ. (For example, Dr. Hobbins had a woman complain about pain in her palm. With the aid of thermography, he determined that the source of the pain was her lung. As a result, further testing was conducted and lung cancer was confirmed. Since he is a surgeon, Dr. Hobbins immediately removed the tumor. With early detection from thermography and Dr. Hobbins' expertise, the patient was fine. Thermography for the diagnosis of organ issues is very extensive and precise, and Dr. Hobbins is the only qualified doctor presently using this method.)

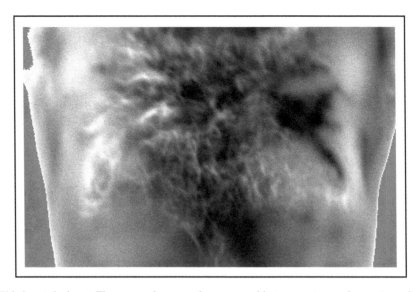

This is not the heart. Thermography can only measure skin temperature and cannot monitor past the skin into the tissue or organs. This claim was made by an M.D. and featured on another famous M.D.s show! These "specialist" don't understand thermography basics and are spreading misinformation.

"I do not live near Pink Image Breast Thermography, but I wish I did. I live in a different state. I have been using a local Thermography service to monitor my breast over the last 4 years. I have very dense breast tissue and in the past every time I would get a mammogram I would end up getting an ultrasound and had lots of scares. I was thrilled to find an alternative in Thermography. I picked up Wendy Sellens book last year "Breast Cancer Boot Camp". After reading it I started to question the Thermography reports I was issued. I consulted with Wendy and she reviewed the interpretations I received from the service I used. Wendy pointed out to me so many disturbing deficiencies in the interpretation of my exam. I see now that having Thermography services regulated would be a tremendous benefit to women. Thermography is a gift and an awesome tool, but put in the wrong, untrained hands it can be a detriment. I see firsthand the battle that Wendy faces as she tries to educate women and doctors. I know these practitioners mean well, but proper education and the right camera/tools/interpretation are key to making this a viable option for women moving forward. If you are using a Thermography service other than Pink Image Breast Thermography, please refer them to Wendy's website/ blog and her book. Wendy has started this Revolution. Let's rally around her."

Joy

## Gimmicks to Avoid in Thermography

Cancers are being missed with breast thermography and these are reasons why. Thermography is not regulated, and anyone can open up a clinic! Get the facts!

Avoid clinics that only interpret in color images. Thermography monitors the health of the breasts by monitoring the blood vessels, specifically looking for patterns, which are only seen in reverse gray imaging. Color is called secondary interpretation because the small changes in the blood vessels, the key to early detection, can't be monitored in color. However, women love color, its easy for them to see the thermal activity of the breasts.

Another reason to be aware of solely color images. Imagine a company who wants to sell a breast cream or a clinic that does a special breast treatment or massage, then performs another thermogram to show the change a few minutes later. Creams and oils applied to the breast are reflective and since an infrared camera detects heat, creams and powders change the measurements by blocking the heat. This is why you can't wear lotion or apply deodorant before a thermogram. The change in the color image before and after a treatment is due to the products properties interfering with the camera's measurements not the effect of the cream on the breast's underlying condition. Changes in the breast must be monitored by viewing the blood vessels, which is only seen in black hot.

Avoid clinics doing a three-month follow up. They claim, "a baseline cannot be established with one study because we have no way of knowing if this is your normal pattern...a three-month interval is used because this is the time it takes blood vessels to show change." Incorrect, changes in the blood vessels can been seen in a month, as demonstrated in this book. They are using the term "baseline" incorrectly. Your first thermogram is your baseline. It is used as a reference point to see an increase, decrease or no change in the blood vessel patterns. These clinics have to "double check" in three months because the camera they use is cheap, that is not strong enough for breast screening, has an optical line of 120 or 240. This is one reason why cancers are being missed. Breast thermography requires an optical line of 480 or higher.

The three-month follow-up is a "check-up" to double check they didn't miss anything. This is one of the reasons breast thermography clinics are missing cancer. One patient came in after performing breast thermography for six years and they missed stage four cancer. She had actually touted the benefits of thermography and felt betrayed. Again, thermography does not replace a mammogram, which discovered her cancer.

Most of these clinics do not discuss the blood vessels, give a TH score, thermographic score of each of the breasts, or give the delta T measurement, temperature differences between the beasts. Again, this is why they do a three month follow up, to reassess. What is even more distressing these reports are usually done by M.D.s.

Avoid full-body imaging; it is a gimmick. Many clinics do full-body images with false promises and charge more. Thermography can only measure *skin* temperature. It *cannot* measure and analyze temperatures of organs directly, they are too deep to be monitored. The breasts or mammary glands are unique organs, and their blood vessels can be monitored.

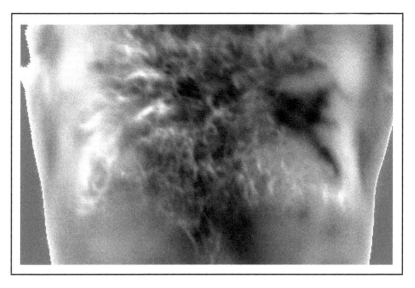

This is not the heart. Thermography can only measure skin temperature and cannot monitor past the skin into the tissue or organs. This is a breast issue in a male patient who was consuming large quantities of estrogenic sesame oil. Claims similar to this one, was made by a female M.D., who was interviewed by a famous doctor as an expert on breast thermography.

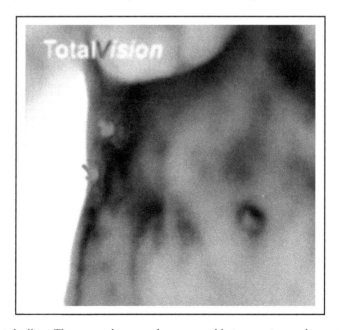

This is not the liver. Thermography can only measure skin temperature and cannot monitor past the skin into the tissue or organs. This claim was made by a M.D. who is an "expert" in thermography and has an educational program that certifies other M.D.s

Many women I imaged have their thermograms interpreted from a radiologist and one told me she is monitoring cancer of other organs, especially the uterus. No! Thermography cannot directly analyze risk of the uterus in the manner this radiologist was interpreting the screenings.

Many clinics use thermography to sell supplements. They tell women the red heat pattern, seen in color, under the breasts, is inflammation from digestive issues. No! This is what most women already know, heat from the breasts resting on the abdomen. It can't see the heat from your digestive tract directly over the actual organs.

Thermography is very effective in pain diagnostics. Avoid all other claims.

## Breast Thermography and Medical Insurance

Thermograms are a screening procedure; they do not diagnose breast cancer. The average cost is about $250-$300. At one time, thermography was covered by insurance, but due to a handful of doctors who committed insurance fraud, coverage ended in 1994. Presently, thermography is covered by a few supplemental insurance companies with the larger companies covering some women with histories of breast cancer. But for most women, breast thermography is not covered.

## Minimum Standard Requirements for Breast Thermography

To view all MSR examples for breast thermography, refer to color pages.

For breast thermography to be accepted by the medical community, all physicians, academies, and clinics should be meeting the minimum standard requirements which are based off thermographic evidence and studies.

Certified breast thermography should include the following:

1. Black hot or reveres gray scale analysis
2. TH score
3. Interpretation
4. Delta T and nipplar delta T
5. Major and minor signs
6. Cold stress test or sympathetic stress test
7. Personal breast cancer health risk (not required, suggested)
8. Monitoring breast health, hormones, and breast cancer (not required, suggested)
9. Camera optical line measurement

## 1. Black Hot or Reverse Gray Imaging

Certified breast thermography interpreters read images in both reverse grayscale and color, with reverse gray being more significant. Typically, when researching breast thermography, there are pages full of color images. What many clinics are missing is a vital key to determining the vascular pattern in the breast, as only grayscale and reverse grayscale enable the reader to see vascular patterns, which is actually vascularity and neoangiogenesis. Dr. Judah Folkman first hypothesized that tumors caused new blood vessel growth or angiogenesis. With thermography, vascularity can be observed, sometimes before there is a thermal or heat pattern. Since uncertified clinics only read in color, they are most likely missing vascularity, which is the true early screen marker.

Black hot or reverse gray scale is *vital* for all repeats. Breast thermograms are monitoring for any change in the blood vessels signaling an abnormality, vascularity, or neoagniogeneisis. Thermography clinics *must* do all repeats in black hot.

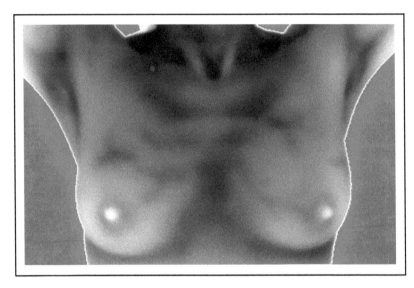

Initial thermogram. Note slight vascular pattern.

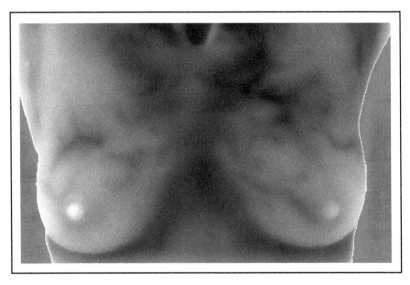

Repeat thermogram. Note increase in vascularity. Neoangiogenesis suspected in left upper breast. Abnormal thermogram.

"I was tired of getting my breast squashed and radiated each year and decided to look at other options. I heard of thermography some years ago but decided that this year I would take a closer look at it. After much research and let me stress much, I found Pink Image. I must say this experience has change the way my family live and eat. The thermography exam was quick and easy. No pain and no touching! It was determined that I was estrogen dominant and had patterns of hypervascularity in both breast. I was shocked at how my breast looked! Wendy suggested an ultrasound for follow up which I have scheduled for next week. I spoke to Wendy at length on how to improve my breast health which included going organic and omitting flax and soy from my diet amongst other things. I learned so much from this woman in such a short time. She is so knowledgeable and very easy to talk to. I feel blessed that I met her. And her book is Breast Cancer Bootcamp is must read. Go get it now!"

Monica

## 2. TH Score = Thermographic Score

Dr. Hobbins decided that the methodology behind thermography scoring should be modeled after the Pap smear. There are not just "normal" or "abnormal" reports, there are score levels. If a report has "normal" or "abnormal" without a score, this is not a proper report and is therefore not conducted by a certified clinic. Typically, only one breast can have a TH score of 3, 4, or 5. It is highly unusual for both breasts to have scores above TH2, as only 5 percent of breast cancers are bilateral.

*TH-1 = Normal or Nonvascular*—A healthy breast is nonvascular, which indicates a lack of neoangiogenesis (new blood vessels) and a negative cancer screen. Both breasts can receive a score of TH-1.

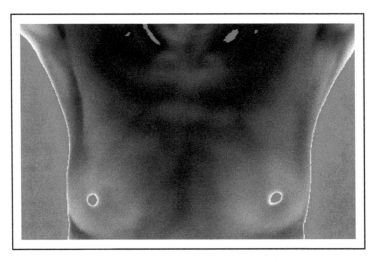

Bilateral TH- 1 nonvascular or normal.

*TH-2 = Vascular Uniform*—As thermograms compare one breast to the other, a vascular uniform score indicates that both sides exhibit vascularity or hypervascularity, which is more severe. Both breasts can receive a score of TH-2.

The exceptions to this presentation are breasts of pregnant, nursing, and still developing women. Vascularity during these times is considered *normal*, due to increased activity.

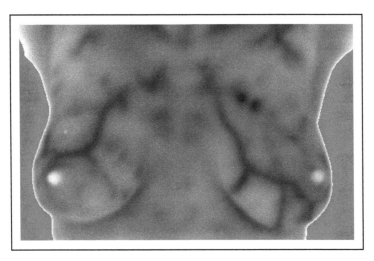

Bilateral TH-2 Normal vascular pattern for nursing mother.

Unfortunately, most women imaged nowadays fall into a score of TH-2, whereas twenty years ago, most women would be a TH-1. This is another reason why this book was written. Environmental estrogens are causing women's breasts to be at an unusually high risk for cancer.

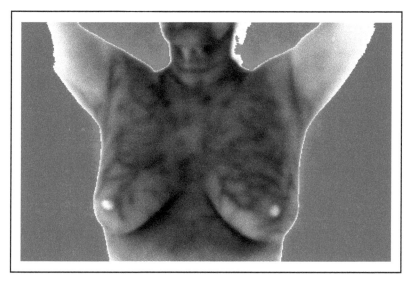

Bilateral TH-2 "At risk" thermogram. Not a normal vascular pattern for this woman.

A TH score of TH-3, TH -4, or TH-5 can only be assigned to *one* breast, because bilateral breast cancer is rare, comprising only 5 percent of breast cancers. This means both breasts are not high risk; usually only one can be. The other breast has to be a score of TH-2 or TH-1. I have seen several reports of bilateral TH-3, which is incorrect. Again, the breast can never have a bilateral score of TH 3. However, there is the rare occasion when both breasts are suspicious, but it is usually suspected neoangiogensis or carcinoma and the score would be TH-4 or TH-5 with a TH-3 on the breast that is of thermographic concern, never a bilateral score of TH-3.

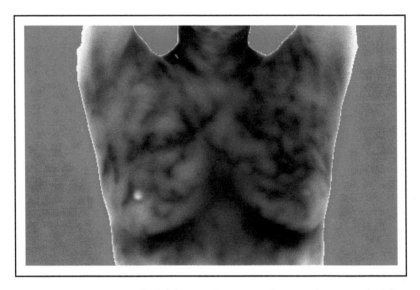

A score of TH-3 is given for left breast. Note concerning vascular pattern in right breast also, however, this is given a score of TH-2.

*TH-3 = Equivocal*—This score is given when there is a thermographic finding limited to *one* breast. In this case, the woman must proceed to other imaging modalities, such as ultrasound, mammogram, or MRI with contrast, to determine the issue. However, a portion of women with a score of TH-3 who return for imaging several months later are downgraded to a TH-2. This downgrade is possible if the questionable area stabilizes or decreases in vascularity or neoangiogenesis.

*TH-4 = Abnormal and TH-5 = Severely Abnormal*—In these cases, findings are considered significant, suspected neoangiogensis, and require further investigation such as ultrasound, mammogram or MRI with contrast.

Many uncertified clinics demand a three-month repeat to determine a baseline thermogram. As each woman has an individual thermal pattern, each case is determined independently. A woman who has a score of TH 1 or is nonvascular does not require an early recall. Some concerning TH 2 scores may require an early recall and some may not; it is a case by case basis. All TH 3 TH 4 and TH5 require an early recall.

Some of Dr. Hobbins' students changed the interpretation model that Dr. Hobbins taught them. Here is an example of one: Avoid a point scoring system or calculation system. There are several out there and one is called the CTA Breast Analytical System. They are based on a point system of 1—200. In the '70s, a large software company came up with an idea to have a computer diagnose thermography. To prove efficacy of this theory, studies *needed* to be conducted. This company initiated a million-dollar study for a statistical/scoring system for breast thermography, conducted by a radiologist at the University of Oklahoma. What this statistical/scoring system basically showed is that it created an average 28 percent error rate in breast thermography reports.

No other medical imaging modality utilizes a computer scoring system to interpret. For example, an MRI of the spine is read by a qualified radiologist, not a computer scoring system. The FDA approved breast thermography by physician interpretation, *not* a calculation system.

Another flaw in point scoring and the CTA Breast Analytical System and other computer-generated scoring systems is that thermography can be individualistic. Each interpreter follows basic guidelines to interpret, but every woman should be treated as an individual. Age, family history, age of first child, number of years on hormones and clinical findings, a lump or pain, are all factors that determine the TH scores and risk index included in a report. Scoring systems such as the ones mentioned above do not allow for individual variances. A computer cannot read neoangiogenesis.

Once the software company realized the flaw in this approach, they dropped the idea of a scoring system or using a computer to read breast thermography, even after several millions of dollars had been spent. Avoid interpreters trained by camera companies. These are point and click results and not true interpretation by observation of blood vessels or neoangiogenesis. Point scoring systems are untested, there are no clinical studies or data proving efficacy.

# 3. Interpretation

The reason for the subpar thermography clinics in the United States is that the interpreters are poor. The MDs who created breast thermography spent *years* of painstaking study and research. Dr. Hobbins toured the globe ten times educating physicians. Most qualified physicians were trained by him as there was no other doctors who educated large numbers of physicians. If you are in South America, Japan, or Korea, your doctor was probably trained by Dr. Hobbins. His class was a weekend course followed by readings of a hundred reviewed reports. Regretfully, that is all it took to become a qualified interpreter. The enormous error of this teaching technique is quite apparent now through the large number of mediocre interpreters, as seen in the example above, among many others. These interpreters were not properly trained and many changed breast thermography requirements without performing studies or statistical analysis.

On the other hand, my partner and I spent almost two years having Dr. Hobbins approve over 700 reports, as our goal was to become accomplished interpreters. A radiologist does not just take a weekend course to read mammograms—there should be integrity within the screening field of breast thermography as well. How can one justify screening a woman for breast cancer after a weekend course and a hundred reports? Would you trust your breast thermography interpretation to a physician with only a few hours under his/hers belt and no experience with breasts in a clinical setting? A patient seeking a cancer screening deserves to be seen by an experienced, knowledgeable practitioner. In my opinion, the reason that breast thermography requires a high standard is because it is individualistic, meaning each woman is unique and should therefore be treated as such. What may be considered normal for one patient is unacceptable for another; this is the difficulty in interpretation. Demand quality for your breast health. Ask who your interpreter is, where they were certified and who certified them. *Do not* be fooled by titles or academies—demand experience.

Currently, there are only two accredited thermography academies. There are other thermography academies, but they were started by camera companies and are for profit. The American Academy of Thermology was set up by MDs in the early 70s, which Dr. Hobbins is an honorary fellow. Dr. Hobbins assisted the chiropractors in creating the International Academy of Clinical Thermography and is a founding member and at one time vice president. Pain diagnostics, veterinarian, and commercial thermography are accredited in these academies. However, currently many of the physicians in these academies are no longer meeting the minimum standard requirements for the breasts.

Over the last thirty years, Dr. Hobbins has reached out and attempted to reeducate these physicians on the importance of following thermographic studies and clinical experience, but to no avail; they will not take his qualified advice. Surprisingly, many of these physicians are his students! As a result, we started the Women's Academy of Breast Thermography; we are the only academy currently meeting the minimum standard requirements for breast thermography. We founded this academy because women's health is the priority above all else!

"Dr. Hobbins scanned 100,000 women's breast for cancer during his career using thermography. His thermography images are excellent and far superior to any I have seen. I was surprised to learn that only 7 thermography centers in the USA scan and report correctly and that thermography results are utilized to assist women in lifestyle changes to prevent cancer. The outlook for breast cancer is bleak (it comes back in other body parts sooner or later). Mastectomies do NOT insure breast cancer will not reoccur. His knowledge regarding hormones and erroneous treatment is excellent.

Soy and flax are touted as great health foods, but contain an outrageous amount of estrogen. Small dosages of estrogen are in our drinking water. Elevated estrogen imbalance leads to breast cancer. Progesterone creams are often made from yams. It is necessary to remove the estrogen from the yams so progesterone creams treat not cause breast cancer.

What a wealth of information. Women and their physicians should read this book."

Rebecca

# 4. Delta T and Nipplar Delta T

Delta T is temperature difference between the breasts. Dr. Hobbins' studies in the '70s analyzed and determined temperature difference that could alert a possible disease. It is vital that the Delta T's determined by studies are being strictly followed in breast thermography. If a report is not listing delta T measurements or are either too high or lower than those listed for you in this book, then you are not receiving qualified thermography. Delta T's are what is called a threshold. If the threshold is set too low, then the interpreter is detecting variations that are no cause for concern, but obviously creates worry with the patient. If threshold is set too high, the interpreter is missing findings. Either way, make sure your report lists Delta Ts in the breast which is strictly following thermographic studies.

Delta T measurements outside of normal limits

1.0° C or higher at nipple
1.0° C or higher with finding
1.5° C or higher at periareolar
1.5° C or higher global heat
2.0° C or higher in isolated area (Major or Minor sign or vascular structure)
2.5° C or higher with finding in unilateral breast – mastectomy
3.0 ° C or higher in unilateral breast – mastectomy

The most important area to analyze in breast thermography is the temperature difference between the nipples (a.k.a. nipplar delta T). Eighty-three percent of cancers will have a hot nipple on the diagnosed breast. It is also important to note that patients using thermography as an adjunct viewing source of their breast cancer have a better prognosis if there is no nipplar delta T, meaning the cancer might be localized or in situ. Since thermography views blood flow in the skin that may "feed" the cancer, it may not actually see the cancer if it is deep or what is referred to as a shadowing lesion. When you are sick and feverish, heat finds a way to vent out of the body. In breast abnormalities, not just cancer, this heat escapes through the nipple. Think of it as a valve.

Because of this, if a nipple is a degree or more hotter than the other, this is a potential factor and the patient is sent for further testing.

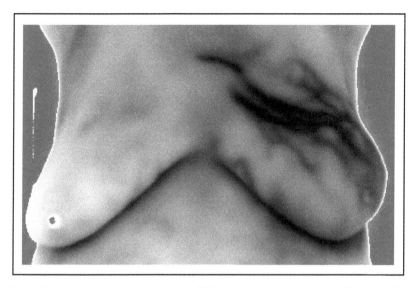

Cancer has a hot nipple, left, note color difference versus right nipple which is cooler.

## 5. Major and Minor Signs or Primary and Secondary Characteristics

Cancers tend to form certain patterns, and at one time, were categorized and classified by several studies and then catalogued into "thermograms' major and minor signs." Dr. Hobbins and a group of medical doctors included these patterns in the minimum standards. These patterns are taught to certified breast thermography interpreters so they can give women complete, detailed reports. These signs can determine the TH score or risk of each breast. That is why black hot or reverse gray is mandatory in thermogram imaging to view the blood vessels and the patterns generated in your breasts.

Once again, thermograms view blood flow in the breasts. As cancers tend to form specific patterns, having one or more of these major or minor signs with a temperature difference outside of normal can increase your TH score. Or as preventive screening, having one of these major or minor signs might be noted in your report, but because the temperature difference is still within normal limits, you are notified of this finding and then monitored with an early recall. It is then your choice whether or not to make lifestyle changes to reduce this sign, which is vascularity or neoangiogenesis.

Make sure the thermographic clinic includes your black hot or reverse grey images in your report. It is a wonderful visual for breast health and cancer screenings. You can see for yourself how healthy your breasts are!

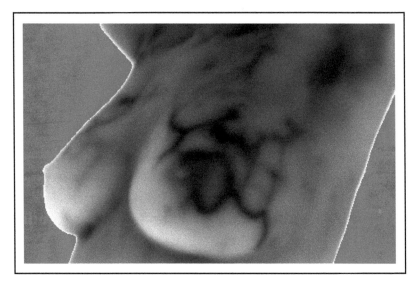

Major sign at 3 o'clock position adjacent to nipple.

# 6. Cold Stress Challenge

When a patient is cooled, the blood vessels constrict and a potential abnormality will not. The infrared camera detects heat that radiates from the unusual blood vessels. Most certified clinics use an air-conditioned room kept below 68°F. However, a cold stress challenge is always recommended and is actually mandatory with a TH score of 3, 4, or 5. A cold stress test includes ice packs applied to the forehead or back. Some clinics still use cold water. Water that is simply cool is ineffective. Do not apply ice water to the hands, as this requires the arms to be down. During a thermographic screening, the hands must be on the head while cooling down for ten to fifteen minutes. Having the arms up effectively raises the breasts, decreasing any reflective heat off the abdomen and cooling the lymph in the axilla (underarm). If hands are immersed in water, the breasts and axilla will not effectively cool.

"I am so grateful to have stumbled upon Wendy Sellens' Pink Image. I have been to another thermography center, which never seemed to get the room temperature where it needed to be, which can result in inaccurate images, and mislead the patient as to what is going on in their breasts. Wendy is deeply devoted to her patients and schedules a detailed consultation after her analysis of your images. Wendy also provides very constructive advice in regards to diet and other suggestions to improve the status of your breasts. I was having daily intermittent breast pain, and after following Wendy's advice, no more pain, and my 6 month follow-up showed vast improvement. Thank you so much Wendy!!!"

Liz

## 7. Personal Breast Cancer Health Risk

A personal breast cancer health risk is tallied for each individual. The health risk index is a nationally accepted risk for breast cancer, determined by a culmination of studies from The American Cancer Society, The National Cancer Institute and The American Radiology Society. These three organizations followed 250,000 women for five years as part of their research. Increased risk of breast cancer is determined by: age of individual, parity (age at time of first child), family history, weight, race, and exposure to synthetic hormone replacement therapies.

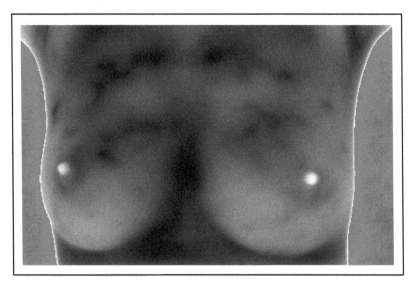

Low risk due to age, thirties, no family history of breast cancer, no history of BCPs or HRTs and nursed two children.

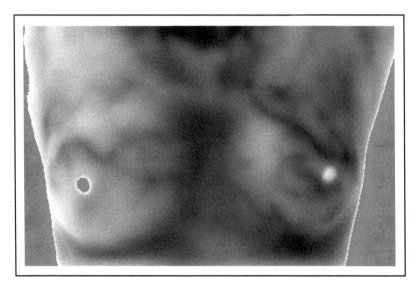

High risk due to age, forties, family history of breast cancer-mother, history of BCPs—twenty-five years, IUD with hormones—four years and no children.

# 8. Monitoring Breast Health, Hormones and Cancer: Not Approved by FDA

Breast health risk is determined by thermograms, which is the most important reason to implement them into a "healthy" lifestyle. Currently, only a couple certified thermography clinics know how to properly monitor breast health. By educating the consumer on the importance of breast thermography to determine breast health, consumers can then demand more certified clinics.

Hormone levels, estrogen and progesterone can be observed with breast thermography. Since thermography can monitor environmental estrogens, estrogen therapies, and the body's naturally occurring estrogen, it is an ideal tool for hormone and breast health treatments. Due to excess administration of estrogen therapies (bioidentical estrogen, soy, and flax) and environmental estrogens, most women have become progesterone imbalanced, which means progesterone deficient.

Breast health scales are therefore graded on a progesterone deficiency from mild to severe or 1–3 (relative). A score of TH-1 is normal, or nonvascular, and hormonally balanced. A progesterone deficiency score would not apply. Please note that hormone levels are just for breast health assessment and are not FDA approved for breast thermography.

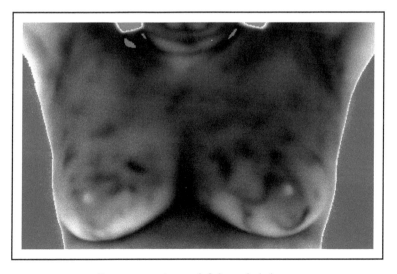

Severe progesterone deficiency imbalance.

Breast thermography can also monitor all traditional and alternative cancer treatments by analyzing vascularity or neoangiogenesis in the breasts. If a treatment is working, then vascularity or neoangiogenesis will be reduced. If it's not working or is causing an increase in the vascular pattern or neoangiogenesis, the patient can see the results with her own eyes.

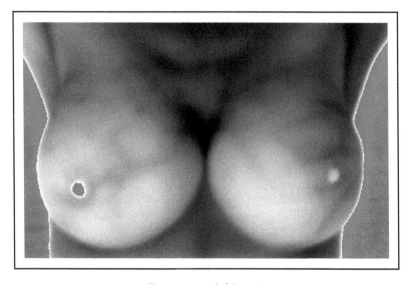

Breast cancer left breast.

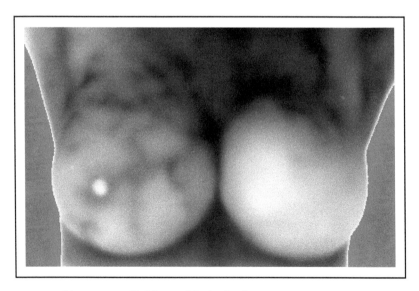

Mastectomy of left breast. Monitoring breast cancer treatments.

The Breast Thermography Revolution

Treatment can then be individualized for each woman and each cancer. Not all women and all cancers respond similarly to all treatments. When treating breast cancer, Dr. Hobbins wants to remind women that it took several years, six to ten, for cancer to be detected. So if cancer is not too aggressive, take time to try treatments before jumping into a mastectomy. Dr. Hobbins used nutrition to treat many cancers. With more aggressive cancers, he used Tamoxifen, a wonderful treatment that can strangle the cancer and actually reduce tumor size so that mastectomy or lumpectomy may not need to be performed. Tamoxifen cuts off cancer's food, estrogen. He also used testosterone to shrink many tumors.

By monitoring with thermography and other imaging modalities, Dr. Hobbins could observe treatments and adjust his protocols when necessary. Since he was a surgeon, if treatments weren't working, he could immediately perform a lumpectomy or mastectomy.

Dr. Hobbins also wants to remind women that breast cancer is a local problem if it hasn't metastasized. Why would you treat the whole body with harmful chemicals for a local problem? Many women are killed or their lives are shortened by traditional aggressive therapies. With many cancers, the implementation of breast thermography to monitor treatment can render these harsh therapies unnecessary. Breast cancer treatment has not changed in five decades; it is time to look for alternatives.

In 1956, Ray Lawson showed increased heat on the breast surface and venous blood of breast cancer. Gros and Guthrie of Strasberg, France, Pistolesi of Italy, and Atsumi of Japan correlated neoplasia (presence of new, abnormal growth of tissue) and thermal breast skin signal. Because of believing that heat was generated by the tumor, it was thought that the thermal signal would be directly related to the size of the tumor and therefore was not an early warning signal or good screening tool. Not until 1978, when Jean of Mellon-Carnegie University demonstrated an angiogenesis factor in breast cancer and breast tissue, were we able to find TO tumors. British surgeon, Lloyd Williams of Bath, England showed survival was directly related to the thermal expression better than any size, tumor marker or other method of calculating survival. This was done in the late 1960s and again in the mid-80s by the same surgeon.

In 1988, Judah Folkman from Harvard demonstrated that angiogenesis was necessary for neoplasia to move from in situ to invasive disease. He also demonstrated that an enzymatic stimulation of the vasculature took place from this angiogenesis factor. Presently, 300 or more drugs are being tested in stage 3 FDA trial to halt neoangiogenesis.

The 21st century paradigm is that when a normal breast thermal study changes, time for antiangiogenesis and expected thermal turn-off as demonstration of tumor regression will be the protocol. This will occur without identifying the tumor.

The thermal signal precedes clinical (including x-ray, ultrasound, diaphanscopy and MRI) by six to 12 months. Now early detection and acceptable nontoxic therapy is available and will be the protocol in the decades ahead for conquering this dreaded disease of women.

William Hobbins, MD, American Thermographic
Meeting, Orlando, FL, November 2002

# 9. Camera Optical Line

As is true with virtually all other imaging modalities, the quality of the breast thermography process begins with the imaging equipment used. Thermographic camera resolution is measured by optical lines; much like a digital camera resolution is measured in pixels. Therefore, the higher the number the better the resolution. Don't forget, these are our breasts, and we need the most detailed image possible.

The quality of thermographic cameras is based on two factors: resolution and sensitivity. Resolution is the amount of information that a camera is able to capture and is measured in optical lines. Sensitivity defines how accurately the camera is able to discern levels of thermal radiation (heat) and is measured in degrees C per level. It is desirable to have as high of a resolution and sensitivity as possible. Modern thermographic cameras have a resolution of 480 optical lines, with some cameras as high as 600 optical lines (more is better). The sensitivity of these cameras is at least .05 degrees C per level, with some achieving .025 degrees C per level (less is better). The minimum requirement for certified breast thermography should be a resolution of 480 optical lines and a sensitivity of .05 degrees C per level. Cameras with specifications inferior to these numbers may be used for imaging other areas of the body, but are not suitable to track the minute temperature variations required for breast thermography.

Most infrared cameras currently used for breast thermography have optical lines of 120 or 240. These cameras are only FDA approved for skin temperature variation and not for the breasts. Obviously, these cameras are cheaper and the images show the difference. Cameras with an optical line of 120 or 240 are appropriate for other areas of the body; they are not suggested for the breasts. Low optical line cameras yield poor images and little detail of the breasts, making them insufficient for breast analysis. It is imperative to have images from a high optical line camera to achieve the level of detail required to properly relate to breast thermography research. Superior technology is a key factor in certified breast thermography. After all, these are our breasts, and we must demand the best.

I use the Bales Tip camera, the first camera approved by the FDA for breast thermography. To this date, it is still the highest optical line (600) used in breast thermogaphy. This camera usually has a price tag in the six figures, but it is only when breast thermography is standardized or when women demand that their clinic use a higher optical line that money will be spent on the appropriate cameras. The minimum recommended optical line for breast thermography is 480.

When investigating breast thermography clinics, be sure to ask what camera they use and what its optical line is. Then search the camera's information to double-check they are correct!

## History of Thermal Technology

In 1979, Maurice Bales invented the first digital infrared camera. His MCT7000 camera was the first infrared camera approved for *breast* thermography (not skin) and is still the oldest listed on the FDA website. To date, no other medical infrared camera with an optical line resolution of 600 is FDA approved for BREAST (not skin) thermography. Maurice created the Bales TIP 600 optical line camera, along with other medical devices with his company, "Bales Scientific." The Bales TIP has dominated the medical community for four decades; he is truly a pioneer in thermographic technology. This section was contributed by Maurice Bales as a quick history in infrared technology, based on his experience.

The FDA approved Thermography as an adjunctive screening tool and issued a 510(K) to a company named Spectratherm. Their camera was all analog but had the best optical system in the world at that time. Spectratherm became an entity of General Electric, which placed the thermal imagers in medical facilities. In the 1970s, UTI purchased the rights to the Spectratherm camera from General Electric. UTI used the camera to image and record the quality of wire-bonding in the semiconductor industry.

A year later, UTI realized the drawbacks of their analog camera and asked Maurice Bales to have a look at their Spectratherm 900 camera and characterize it. It had a number of problems in the electronics, but the optics were the best in the world for that time. Along with Dave

Reinagal, Maurice Bales tested the imager and found it had a 6 bit resolution. Bales recommended that UTI completely redesign the electronics, while keeping the optics. They agreed and paid Bales and Reinagal to design it and supply two prototypes. It was to have a 200 degree C temperature range and be a 12-bit system. The first digital infrared imager was labeled UTI-9000. The design was a great success, being used mostly in the multilayer, printed circuit board testing. At this time, the military was the only one using more than two layers. The PCBs in the missiles were more than eight layers and the parts were soldered in with no sockets. Each board cost the manufacturer > $10,000 (in 1980 dollars!). So if the new board didn't work, it was very costly. Their new system had real-time image subtraction (also developed by Maurice as part of the redesigned electronics), which enabled them to take an image of a good board and then use that image as a reference to test the defective board.

UTI asked Bales to be the liaison in regards to all thermal imaging inquiries from various industries. One day in 1985, Maurice received a call from a doctor who wanted to discuss the specifications of the UTI 9000. The doctor had heard about the use of infrared imaging in medicine and was interested in purchasing a camera. After some discussion and demonstration, the doctor decided that he wanted to purchase a system with updated software. At that time, UTI decided they were not going to get involved with the FDA and declined the sale. However, since Maurice was manufacturing the electronics for the UTI 9000, an agreement was made that Maurice could sell medical systems and UTI could sell industrial systems. In 1987, Maurice attended his first American Academy of Thermology (AAT) meeting, where he met Dr. William Hobbins, and as they say, the rest is history.

Congrats, you just graduated from breast thermography basics.

# 12. Breast Cancer Boot Camp

## The Battle Plan

Welcome to Breast Cancer Boot Camp, ladies! The protocols provided are tested, tried, and true from fifty years of breast thermography evidence, clinical experience with patient results, and feedback. I have personally been in the trenches experimenting on myself as well as performing dedicated research to find the best possible treatments based on evidence and clinical experience. Breast Cancer Boot Camp will whip you into the strongest and healthiest version of you! Gear up and prepare for your mission… be diligent and patient… your hard work will pay off.

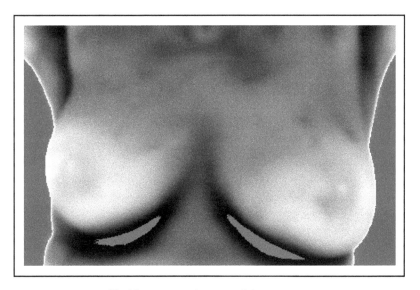

Healthy, nonvascular, normal thermogram.

Debriefing:

"After someone very close to me passed away from breast cancer at the young age of 42, I was determined to find a better alternative to annual mammograms. I did a lot of research and reading and found a recommendation for Pink Image and breast thermography. It made perfect sense to me, was completely safe, unlike mammograms, and could detect cancer up to 7 years earlier. When I met Wendy Sellens at Pink Image, it was clear that Wendy had a huge amount of knowledge, a passion for what she was doing and a true caring for helping others to avoid breast cancer. She has shared, and continues to share, so much knowledge as she herself is always striving to bring the best information to the forefront. I can't imagine why anyone would not take advantage of an opportunity to have a thermogram. They give you the information you need to avoid a situation that no one wants to be diagnosed with at a time when you can likely have a positive effect. Just as a side note, all centers performing thermograms are not the same. I have been to a few that use a very old method that is no where near as accurate."

Sherrie

## Self Care: Doctor's Orders-Have Fun

**First – YOU!**

How can you take care of others when you can't take care of yourself? Stress lowers the immunity, leading to many health disorders. The new trend is busy, busy, busy, give, give, give and face it, it is killing us.

Over the years with patients I have learned women put themselves last and that is one of the contributing factors to why so many are sick. Studies have shown happier people are healthier. Therefore, I have put self-care at the top of the list. To remind "us" what is important. When your needs are met and when you have found your balance, then you can care for others.

Doctor's orders – Be selfish!

Do *you*rself a favor – learn to say no. Most of you with kids can't even use the restroom without the lil' ones at your feet. It is imperative to find time for yourself. Get a massage, go have a champagne lunch with a girlfriend, or just read. Learn to be alone with yourself, it's addictive and will give you strength. Ladies, help each other out, take turns and schedule play dates if your husband is at work and you can't afford a babysitter. Don't allow others to judge you for taking some *me* time, it's saving your life. If they do, give them this book, save their life. Balance.

Have fun! First and foremost, life is meant to be enjoyed. We are to here love, laugh, and live. Fall in love with your partner, kids and even your job. Spend time with your family. Be with people who make you laugh and laugh often. Studies have shown women live longer healthier lives when they spend time with friends. Make a date with a friend. A joyful life is a balanced life. You work hard so play harder. Find out what makes you happy. Get a hobby, read, travel, ride horses, skydive…

Find your purpose. When you live with a purpose, it gives you something to strive for, which keeps your mind and emotions at a task. Bored people are stationary, and it also allows time to stress and worry. Keep busy with goals to avoid depression.

Finally, have cheat days. A restrictive lifestyle or diet binds the emotions, which increases disease. Freedom is healthy so, learn to cheat when you need it. Even if that means, pretending to take the garbage out to have a glass of wine.

There will be good days and days you feel blue. *Everyone* has bad days, you are not alone. My motto, celebrate your bad days. If it's going to be a bad day, make it the best bad day ever. Wallow, don't try to control others, cry, eat fatty foods, mope if you have to, but eventually put down the potato chips, get out of bed, wash your hair and get back to it. You have to experience the bad days to appreciate the good ones. Balance.

It is vital to find time for yourself and recover. When you are resting, because you are weak, it is not wasting a day doing nothing, you are allowing your body to recover. Self-care is a requirement for any healthcare regime.

# Breast Thermography

Your breasts are a window into your health. With a thermogram we first assess your breast health risk and create a regiment appropriate for your risk. Each woman is monitored throughout Boot Camp so she can visually "see" how treatments are affecting *her* breasts. Breast cancer patients can monitor their traditional western treatments and alternative treatments with breast thermography as well. A breast thermogram is simple evidence you can "see" with your own eyes, and determine for yourself how your treatments are progressing.

As you have learned by now, breast thermography is a painless, non contact, no radiation breast health risk screening procedure that monitors the blood circulation in the breasts for abnormalities. This makes monitoring safe to repeat, every 2–6 months if needed, based on an individual's risk. It is important to begin breast thermography early in life, around age twenty-five, to monitor every 2–3 years for changes in the blood vessels, especially if a woman chooses to use BCPs.

It is vital to only receive breast thermography from a qualified and trained thermography clinic. To find a qualified breast thermography clinic, please visit our website: womensacademyofbreastthermography. com The breast thermograms at these clinics are performed in black hot to assess breast health risk, interpreted by a highly trained thermologist and the physicians or practitioners are trained in helping women achieve their best health.

For women that have no qualified breast thermography clinics near them, you can still follow the Breast Cancer Boot Camp system on your own…that is why I have written this book. I have provided women with all the information and evidence they need to have an educated conversation with their gynecologist or nurse practitioner in order to obtain progesterone and/or testosterone. I have also emphasized the importance of finding a holistic doctor to use as your primary or secondary care physician. A holistic doctor can implement Breast Cancer Boot Camp easily into your customized treatment plan, just be sure they do not prescribe any phytoestrogens. The rest can easily be accomplished by you. I suggest you start your own revolution and form a Breast Cancer Boot Camp regiment. This way you can push and support each other.

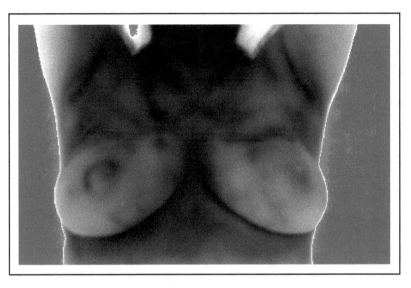

Initial thermogram Progesterone deficiency imbalance.
"At risk" thermogram.

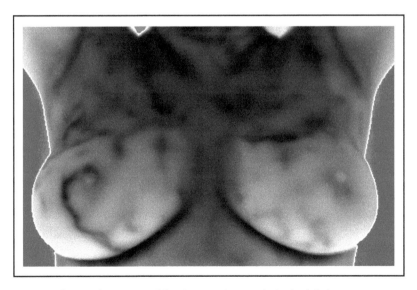

Repeat thermogram. Note increase in vascularity in right breast.
Abnormal thermogram.

Debriefing:

"Pink Image is truly the gold standard of breast thermography. I was sent to Pink Image when my health care practitioner saw something slightly suspicious on one or both of my breasts. After my results were mailed to me, I called Wendy Sellens and she explained my scores. I felt for the first time that I understood the basics of breast health. There is a TON of misinformation out there and it was so refreshing to get some clear information about how to care for "my girls." I now know what to do and what to stop doing.

"This test is safe for pregnant women, women who are nursing, and women with implants. This is the only test available for women from 25 to 39. The most reassuring fact is that thermography can detect cancer 6–10 years before a mass (or lump) can be felt. Do yourself a huge favor and go to their website, watch the informative videos, and read the articles. You will be amazed at what a great resource it is."

Carol

Debriefing:

"Ladies, this is a long story that began in 2000. It is a first hand account of my journey down the breast cancer road. Mammograms were routine with me up to that time. When I experienced an oozing from my right breast, I immediately went to the doctor. Upon examination, the doctor found no lumps and scheduled me for monthly visits that went on for one year. At the end of that time he scheduled me for a biopsy, which revealed an advanced and aggressive cancer. Mastectomy followed after which the radiologist took an ultrasound that showed the left breast was clear. About four months later I felt shooting pains in my left breast. By this time I had a new doctor because my insurance had changed. He immediately tested me. The diagnosis— aggressive cancer. A second mastectomy followed, then chemotherapy. The oncologist who followed me for 5 years declared in October 2006 that I was 'cancer free.'

"In December 2006 I found a lump on the chest wall. The oncologist was on vacation, (lucky for me I figured later on). My surgeon saw me, did a biopsy immediately, cancer had metastasized. This was followed by PET scan, bone scan, CT scan and other tests. I was turned over to the oncologist, who very glibly told me I had a year to live, but with chemotherapy, 2 years. A man who had never tested me properly, who said I was cancer free in October and now in January a death sentence! You guessed it, I walked right out and I am positive that God guided me down the road to alternative care. Like so many women who trust in our country's answer to cancer...barbaric cut, burn and poison treatments, I wised up and educated myself.

"It is 8 years and I am still here. Only God knows our death date, not man and specifically not an oncologist. All this to say that had I heard of thermography I would not have suffered so, (and continue to do), because of barbaric practices that scar your body and soul. In 2007 I was blessed to find information on thermography. Research led me and a friend of mine to Pink Image. We both had thermography in Murrieta, California, with Martin Bales of Pink Image, when our results were in, my friend, herself a cancer survivor, had a "hot spot" on her right breast which was cancer. Prior to this she had a left mastectomy with no evidence of a problem with the right breast even after months of follow ups. Early detection through thermography will save your body from invasive procedures—the standard cut, burn and poison. Please consider this "alternative treatment" and remember cancer does not need to be feared...just to be fought and it can be! I did it and so can you."

Irene

Accredited breast thermography is a simple screening procedure to monitor breast health risk. Start implementing this useful tool into your health plan. Ladies, get your daughters and granddaughters imaged; breast health begins after the breasts have fully developed around the age of twenty-five. Early detection is prevention.

## Become Estrogen Free®

Reduce excess estrogen and become hormonally balanced. Excess estrogen increases breast cancer risk, accelerates aging, promotes weight gain, infertility, irritability, fibroids, dense breasts, PMS, and symptoms of menopause Therefore, it's essential to remove all environmental estrogen from diet and lifestyle to reduce risk, be your true weight and "feel" good.

Now it sounds easy, but very few actually do it. It is difficult in the beginning, but you're tough! That's why you bought the book; you're up for a challenge. Besides, once you get your routine down, it will be comfortable.

If you've come this far, it is crystal clear what environmental estrogens are. If you just opened up to this chapter here is a quick recap of what estrogens to avoid.

The Estrogen Free® Lifestyle Shopping List

Avoid Synthetic Estrogens

- Hormone replacement therapy (HRTs)
- Birth Control Pills (BCPs)
- IUD with hormones
- Estrogen injections

- Estrogen patches
- Estrogen vaginal rings
- Estrogen vaginal creams

Avoid these popular estrogenic foods

- Flax – oil, seeds, crackers, chips, cereal and milk (flax is 20 times stronger than soy).
- Soy – tofu, edamame, fermented soy, cereal, milk, cheese and meats
- Eggs labeled Omega 3 (flax) and fed soy
- Garbanzo beans or chick peas
- Hummus
- Sesame - oil, crackers or bread
- Multigrain bread, crackers and cereal
- Doughnuts
- Veggie burgers
- Non-organic meats, cheese and milk

These foods contain smaller amounts of plant estrogens, which are fine a couple times a week just not in large amounts or daily. However, if you have breast cancer these must also be avoided.

- Dried apricots
- Almonds
- Cashews
- Alfalfa sprouts
- Mung bean and sprouts
- Dried dates
- Sunflower seeds
- Chestnuts
- Dried prunes
- Olive oil
- Rye bread
- Walnuts
- Almonds
- Cashews

- Winter squash
- Hazelnuts
- Collard greens
- Peanut butter
- Cabbage
- White beans
- Peaches
- Red wine

Shopping for supplements and herbs:

Avoid these popular women's health supplements and herbs that are estrogenic. Hint: If it's labeled "women's health," or "breast health" drop it and run. It usually contains a form of estrogen.

- Bioidentical estrogen
- Any women's supplement starting with "Est" for estrogen or "Phyto" for plant or "Meno" for menopause.
- Aloe (A. barbadensis Mill)
- Ashwagandha/Indian ginseng (Withania somnifera)
- Asian ginseng (Panax ginseng, Ren Shen)
- Astragalus/Huang qi (Astragalus membranaceus)
- Black Cohosh (Cimicifuga racemosa, Sheng Ma)
- Burdock root (Arctium lappa)
- Chasteberry (Vitex agnuscastus)
- Dong Gui/Dong Quai (Angelica sinensis)
- Fo-Ti/Ye Jiao Teng (Polygonum multiflorum)
- Hops (Humulus lupulus)
- Kudzu root (Pueraria montana)
- Lavender (Lavandula angustifolia, L. officinalis)
- Licorice (Glycyrrhiza glabra, Gan Cao)
- North American ginseng (Panax quinquefolius, Xi Yang Shen)
- Milk thistle (Silybum marianum)
- Mistletoe (Viscum album)
- Red Clover (Trifolium pretense)
- Rhubarb (Rheum rhabarbarum)

- Turmeric (Curcuma longa)
- Xiang Fu (Rhizoma Cyperi Rotundi)

Avoid these estrogenic essential oils:

- Aniseed
- Basil
- Chamomile
- Cinnamon
- Clary sage
- Coriander
- Cypress
- Evening Primrose
- Fennel
- Geranium
- Lavender
- Oregano
- Peppermint
- Rose
- Rosemary
- Sage
- Tea Tree
- Thyme

Shopping for bed, bath and body:

Avoid these little extras no one ever thinks about:

- BPA – is a synthetic pseudo estrogen
- BPA Free – contains more harmful product – BSA
- Hand sanitizers or wipes, including baby wipes, contain Triclosan – is a synthetic pseudo estrogen
- Anything labeled anti-bacterial – the medical establishment has finally recognized the damage of anti-biotic overuse. These products are causing the same harmful effects.
- Canned foods – contains BPA in the lining
- Plastic bottles, cups, plastic wrap, cookware – BPA

- Teflon cookware – is carcinogenic
- Baby formula – contains soy
- Styrofoam
- Microwaves

Also, be on the lookout for these toxic non-organic or "natural" products:

- Skincare
- Cosmetics
- Hair care
- Conventional deodorants
- Bath and body products
- Fabric softener
- Laundry soap
- Perfume
- Air fresheners

Debriefing:

"I cannot say enough great things about Pink Image, especially Wendy Sellens. Almost a year ago, I had pain off and on in my left breast that sometimes would throb so much it would wake me up in the middle of the night. I did research and was intrigued by thermography as a non-invasive way to detect abnormalities. There were many options for thermography, but chose Pink Image because of their advisor and qualified staff. I was unsure what to expect, but Wendy instantly put me at ease walking me through the process the entire way.

"Wendy immediately saw an unusual hypervascular pattern in the area I was experiencing pain (I could see it as well on the screen). I subsequently had an ultrasound in which everything checked out fine, but at Wendy's suggestions, I made some lifestyle changes. Wendy informed me I was estrogen dominant/progesterone deficient and needed to make changes to the products I was using and food I was eating. Things I thought were good for me, such as flax and soy, were actually perpetuating my imbalance.

"Wendy armed me with a lot of data and provided me with links to other sites to do research. I have to admit I was overwhelmed at first, but it was so nice to hear Wendy tell me change did not need to occur overnight. I'm probably 70/30 (70 percent good ... 30 percent not so good!) now in the lifestyle changes we have incorporated based on Wendy's suggestions and I have to say, I feel sooooo much better! I have not had the pain in my left breast since making the changes and I know it is directly correlated to the products and food choices made.

"Thanks Wendy and Pink Image!!"

Erika


You will also need to remove all petrochemical and ecoestrogens products from your house to reduce exposure. It is not necessary to dump everything into the trash. Take your time. When a product is finished, replace it with an estrogen free or petrochemical free product. This may take a few months, so don't be in a rush.

Only use petrochemical free or organic products and avoid "natural" body and household products. To be certified organic, a product has to be 95 percent organic. To be called "natural," a product only has to contain one natural product, which usually isn't organic. If you eat organic, why would you use non-organic products on your skin which are delivered directly into the blood stream? I highly recommend that pregnant women, nursing mothers, and children should only use organic body and household products to reduce exposure to petrochemicals and ecoestrogens.

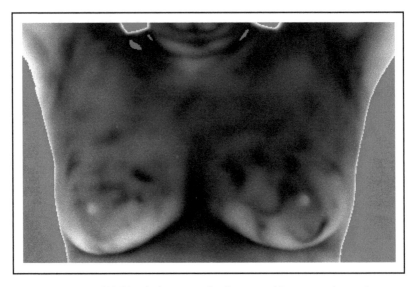

Woman reports use of bioidentical estrogen for five years. Note unusual vascular pattern. Progesterone deficiency imbalance. "At risk" thermogram.

Debriefing:

"Pink Image is the best! I have family history of breast cancer so it has always been a concern of mine. A friend of mine has been in to see Wendy and suggested that I go to find out the health of my breasts and what I can do to prevent the possibility of breast cancer. I made my appointment with Wendy and I can't say enough great things about her and how informative she was. I am amazed at the amount of products that contain estrogen and are very unsafe. Every woman should have breast thermography."

Alicia

#1 Rule at Breast Cancer Boot Camp, *no estrogen therapies or products!* Live estrogen free®!

# Progesterone Therapy

Women should be hormonally balanced, but due to rising environmental estrogens, synthetics such as BCPs and HRTs, phytoestrogens (flax, soy, bioidentical estrogens) and ecoestrogens (commercial estrogens in household products), women have excess estrogen. This increases risk of breast and uterine cancer, and causes symptoms of PMS and menopause. Even though many women experience symptoms of PMS and menopause, they are not normal; they are medical pathology. Progesterone therapy is a simple and effective treatment to balance hormones and treat symptoms of PMS and menopause, while reducing the risk of breast and uterine cancer.

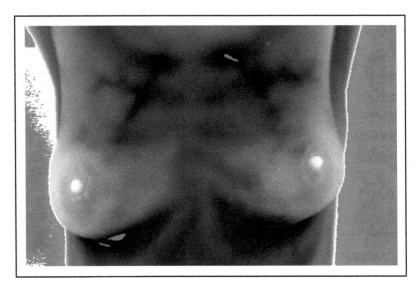

Initial thermogram. Woman reports six years of progesterone use.
Note slight vascular pattern. Normal thermogram.

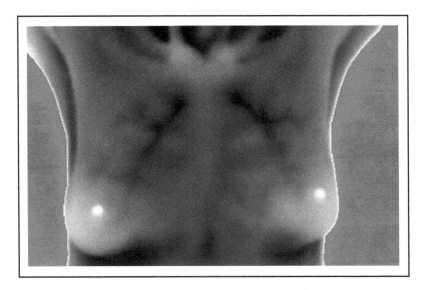

Repeat thermogram. Woman reports continued use of progesterone.

Side effects of PMS and menopause can be successfully treated with progesterone and/or testosterone. Dr. Hobbins was one of the original bioidentical researchers and spent much time in France where bioidentical research was popular in the 70s and 80s. Dr. Hobbins proved the importance of progesterone in reducing vascularity and risk through his years of extensive research monitoring the effects of progesterone with thermograms. This can be seen in his study, "Double Blind Study of Effectiveness Transcutaneous Progesterone in Fibrocystic Breast Conditions Monitored by Thermography." He attempted to combine progesterone with niacin, B3, to increase progesterone circulation. Dr. Hobbins observed that the niacin increased circulation and that progesterone wasn't able to accumulate in the breasts in order to reduce vascularity and create a hormone balance. His study and years of thermographic evidence demonstrate that progesterone cream is the most effective delivery system.

Progesterone receptors are found in the breasts, so apply progesterone cream directly to the breasts to reduce vascularity and create hormone balance. To the breasts, ladies! Do not waste money applying progesterone anywhere else, as application elsewhere results in it dissipating to areas without receptors. Think about it. Why would you apply progesterone cream to your thighs, abdomen or wrists when the receptors are in your breasts? Doesn't make any sense. *Apply it daily*. Many doctors believe that application should take place during the leutal phases, the last fourteen days of the cycle. Due to the high amount of environmental estrogens women are exposed to, this recommendation doesn't suffice; daily application is required. When breasts are normal or nonvascular thermographically, then application can be decreased.

Dr. Hobbins also experimented with other forms of progesterone to observe their effect on vascularity in the breasts. Pills are ineffective as they get destroyed in the gut; sublingual and rectal administration is ineffective as it is not local and dissipates in the circulatory system. A cream is fat soluble—the skin acts as a reservoir and allows the progesterone to build up and fight excess estrogen, creating a balance while decreasing risk and symptoms of PMS or menopause.

Do not use progesterone cream made with any other ingredients! Most likely those ingredients are estrogenic. Time and time again I see women come in with their specially made cocktail cream and their breasts are high risk. Avoid "natural" or wild yam as these are estrogenic. Be careful buying something over the counter or at wellness centers as most contain wild yam, black cohosh, and red clover which are all phytoestrogens. Only use compounded progesterone cream.

The amount of progesterone differs for each woman according to breast size. Work with a physician who understands this concept since pharmacies only have one application amount for *every* woman. Application is twenty swipes across each breast from sternum to lateral side of breast and back to sternum. This equals one swipe. Do *both* breasts daily.

Certified breast thermography clinics will evaluate each woman and grade her progesterone deficiency on a level from one to three. Each woman is given a different percentage, 3 percent, 6 percent, and 10 percent according to progesterone deficiency mild to severe. Progesterone strength and length of usage will be determined by repeat thermograms and patient feedback. Most women will have to be on progesterone for most of their lives due to exposure from environment and diet.

Progesterone deficiency grade 1 (relative)—Mild progesterone deficiency

Progesterone deficiency grade 2 (relative)—Moderate progesterone deficiency

Progesterone deficiency grade 3 (relative)—Severe progesterone deficiency

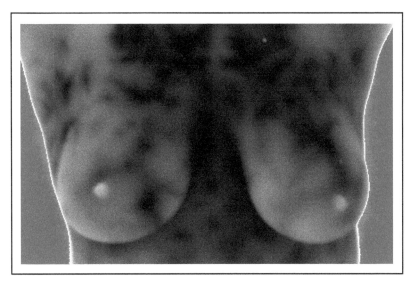

Initial thermogram for woman sharing her experience with progesterone cream below. No hormones. Note unusual vascular pattern. Normal thermogram.

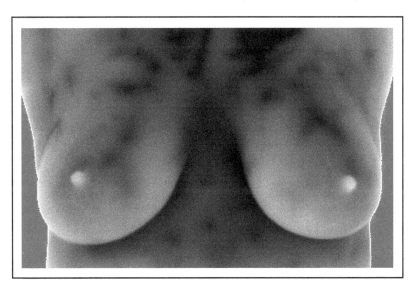

Repeat thermogram one year. Woman reports continued use of progesterone. Thermogram demonstrates decrease in vascularity by removing estrogenic foods and applying progesterone cream (no estrogen) daily to the breasts.

Debriefing:

"I found out about thermograms by accident and was surprised to find Pink Image right here in Solana Beach. Dr. Sellens spent a lot of time educating me over the phone about thermography before I decided to make my appointment. I was frustrated with extreme PMS symptoms, weight gain, fatigue, and having my period every 3 weeks. Not cool! After my first thermogram, Dr. Sellens made some suggestions for how to balance my hormones [including progesterone cream] so that I could return to a regular cycle and to help alleviate my other symptoms as well. After following her advice, I am happy to say that it worked and I now have normal periods and those annoying other issues have improved. My second thermogram showed significant change for the better. I am thankful to Dr. Sellens for all her hard work and dedication in educating women in this field of study. I will definitely continue coming back and learning the truth about breast health."

Janie

Progesterone cream is one of the fundamental treatments in Breast Cancer Boot Camp. Learn it! Use it! Love it! Progesterone will create hormone balance, reduce breast risk, and decrease your symptoms of menopause and PMS. Imagine no more cramps?! Some women even loose weight since estrogen causes the body to hold on to fat around the belly and thighs. Weight loss is a side effect of Breast Cancer Boot Camp. Nice, huh? However, be careful, when you are hormonally balanced you are going to be fertile, so take precautions. Progesterone cream—*Use it, ladies!*

## Testosterone Therapy

Testosterone is antagonistic to estrogen, not progesterone. What this means if you have excess estrogen and their symptoms testosterone treats these symptoms effectively. Dr. Hobbins prescribed testosterone to menopausal women since the 1970's to treat night sweats, hot flashes, and low libido with great success. The number one symptom of low testosterone is low libido. Women *love* their testosterone. It is important to balance the levels of testosterone in the body for optimum breast health as well. Chinese medicine's basic principle is a balance between yin and yang. Testosterone is yang. Yang is active and energetic, and as women, we require the correct amount of testosterone to function correctly.

Dr. Hobbins' years of bioidentical research has found that the most beneficial application of testosterone is by injection (100 mg every couple of months) for post-menopausal women. The female body requires a jolt to the system, while levels slowly decrease, until the next shot. However, since most doctors are not familiar with hormone therapy, they do not prefer to use injections and therefore prescribe a cream. In this case, Dr. Hobbins advises post-menopausal women to get a very high percentage cream in order to jolt their deficient system. Again, many doctors don't understand hormones that well and won't prescribe this. Apply testosterone cream directly to the clitoris. Don't mix testosterone cream with other ingredients; each hormone must be applied separately to the appropriate areas of the body to be effective.

Testosterone is primarily used by post-menopausal women, but women in their forties and above can experiment to see if they like it. You have to experiment with the dose to see what is effective for you; each of us requires a different dose. With most post-menopausal women they can handle daily dosing. With testosterone cream, Dr. Hobbins said it is difficult for post-menopausal women to overdose, so I tried to. I applied large amounts for ninety days to observe any side effects. It altered my period and created some mild flesh colored acne. My nurse practitioner actually prescribed a 5 percent cream for me and the compounding pharmacy *refused* to fill it! When these obstacles occur, find another doctor and pharmacy willing to work with you. Remember, you are in charge of your body. Have an open dialogue with your doctor to find the dose that is right for you. Many doctors and compounding pharmacies don't recognize that everyone is different. They want everyone to fit into a box and follow very strict guidelines. Find a doctor willing to work with you to determine the appropriate amount. Since blood tests can't accurately show true levels, listen to your body to find the dose that works for you.

For those of you who require it—knock yourself out, ladies, enjoy your testosterone.

## Holistic Therapy

Dr. Hobbins recognized the importance of prevention in decreasing illness and disease, and strongly supports proven alternative therapies. In 1978, he was a founding member of the American Holistic Medical Society. In 2000, the American Board of Holistic Medicine held its first certification exam, and Dr. Hobbins became the eighty-fourth certified physician in the United States.

To reduce the risk of breast cancer and other diseases with prevention, go to a holistic doctor. They offer medical prevention and antiaging medicine diagnoses by treating imbalances and illnesses before they become a disease. Westerners have been programmed to believe when you get sick you go to the doctor. In holistic medicine, you go to the doctor to prevent illness, disease, and premature aging. To age correctly and healthfully, individuals must always treat imbalances before they become severe issues.

Holistic doctors treat the entire body at once and don't chase symptoms. They use customized herbal formulations—essentially polypharmacies that treat the "whole" body. All the herbs interact synergistically to maximize the effectiveness of a formulation. Each herb has a particular property. They are warming, cooling, create circulation, reduce pain, dissolve accumulations, phlegm, and dampness while targeting and strengthening organs, muscles, skin, and hair. Holistic medicine is customized for each patient. Two patients may both present with a cough, but receive two different treatments as they present differently due to the underlying condition, so the medicine is tailored for each individual patient. Holistic doctors include Chinese medical physicians, homeopathic and Ayurvedic doctors.

With more than five thousand years of history and use, ten thousand, if including medical Qi Gong, Chinese medicine is the oldest in the world. It has stood the test of time due to hundreds of years of extensive research conducted by Chinese medical schools on the combined effects of herbs. It took Chinese herbalists hundreds of years to document adverse effects of each herb and adverse effects of each herbs reaction to each other. Western supplementation is only just realizing the antagonistic effects that supplements have on each other in the body. On the other hand, this may be the reason studies show that Western herbs and supplements increase some cancers and may be ineffective is due to the lack of similar long-term scientific research. Western supplements have not received the scientific scrutiny required to be properly dispersed as medicine. Supplementation and pharmaceuticals treat one problem while herbal formulas can treat the entire body and are customized for each patient. It is very rare to prescribe one herb, that is not considered medicine. When combined, herbs strengthen the effects of other herbs or decrease toxicity of another herb with the ability to treat several different pathologies at one time.

Chinese herbs are parts of actual plants which are alive and have vitality. A formula is brewed which allows the plants to synergistically work together and is fresh. (Avoid herbs that contain Sulphur, a toxin and we rarely prescribe pills due to possibility of contamination). Supplements are synthetic replications or if they are whole foods, contain toxic preservatives for shelf life. Herbal formulas' degrade.

If a certain doctor is not mentioned in this section it is because they do not treat the body "wholly." They cannot "read" the body; they must rely on lab work, which can be inaccurate. They also have to prescribe a supplement for *each* deficiency the patient has, so they sell several noncustomized, questionable supplements versus one specifically tailored formula of several herbs.

Most health issues can be treated successfully with holistic medicine without the side effects that can come with supplements, vitamins, and pharmaceuticals. The key is to begin treatment early. The longer or more chronic the issue, the longer treatment is required. If you have had a problem for twenty years, don't give holistic medicines two weeks. It might take months to a year to resolve. However, you should be noticing improvements to determine if it is working for you. Children respond the quickest with holistic medicine. I had a friend tell me her five year old was recently diagnosed with asthma. I told her not that it was treatable at the age and refereed her to an herbalist. Willing to try anything she took her daughter and was amazed at the results and how much she learned about her daughter's health that Western doctors were never able to explain.

Since most women are progesterone deficient, we experience many gynecological disorders, long, heavy periods, cramps, headaches, fatigue, bloating, endometriosis, infertility, and amenorrhea (no period). All of these disorders can be treated successfully with holistic medicine. I had been on BCPs since I was fifteen for painful periods. I was experiencing amenorrhea for three years and the gynecologists were constantly telling me this was fine. Not getting your period at the age of thirty is *not* fine! Do not believe doctors that tell you this acceptable. They just don't have the tools to fix these health issues. Their treatment is to throw more estrogen at the problem. I stopped taking my BCPs, started acupuncture three times a week with daily herbs, and in only three months my periods began again *without* the pain I had experienced my entire menstruating years.

Debriefing:

"Wendy at Pink Image Breast Thermography and her Breast Cancer Boot Camp are a wonderful resource for me. I have a strong family history of breast cancer. Doctors have recommended for years for me to remove my healthy breasts. Undergoing surgery, while I am healthy, does not sit right with me and I am focused on prevention. Wendy encourages regular MRIs along with thermography. I feel very supported by having complimentary options. I love thermography because I can actually see what is going on in my breasts. I have been having thermography with Wendy for the past couple of years. I am so grateful for Wendy's recommendations for breast health based on her research. I avoid flax and soy, apply progesterone cream, watch what products I buy, and go to acupuncture regularly. With thermography, Wendy is able to show me the positive changes in my breasts since I have shifted my life style. I am very grateful to have this valuable information and education."

Leanne

In traditional Chinese medicine, a good doctor could aid his patients' recovery, but a great doctor's patients never fell ill. Many aliments that Western medicine can't explain, holistic medicine can treat effectively. I recommend making a holistic doctor your primary care or secondary care physician in addition to your Western medical doctor. Balance is a key and integration of both is ideal.

## Proper Digestion

Might sound funny to talk about this so early in the chapter, but I am amazed at the people who do not have proper digestion. Many people may eat properly, but if their digestion system is not efficient, they may not be obtaining the adequate amount of nutrients from food and are therefore depriving their body of the ability to perform optimally.

Correct digestion must be obtained. This can be achieved with the help of a holistic doctor who can determine if the patient is troubled by dampness, heat, cold, poor circulation, or disharmony. Signs of poor digestion: constipation, diarrhea, loose or soft stool, inconsistency in bowel movements, unusual foul odor of bowel movements, tenesmus ("feeling" of constantly need to pass stool even if bowels are empty), usual belching or flatulence, regurgitation, abdominal distension or bloating, borborygmos (rumbling), and pain.

What the heck is healthy? A "healthy" digestion consists of two to three bowel movements a day, usually after every meal. Classic Chinese medical text states that when the stomach is full, the bowels are empty. Watch a dog—it eats, and then it immediately needs to go outside to "take care of business." If you do not have at least one per day, this is considered constipation. If you are constipated, you reabsorb toxins back into your body due to the delayed transit time and the absorptive properties of the intestines. It is not okay to have only one or two a week; that is very toxic.

If you suffer from constipation, try drinking ice cold beverages. The cold stimulates the digestive tract to warm up the body and increase bowel movements.

Constipation smoothie: Blend very ripe bananas (I mean very ripe, the ones you would use for banana bread mix) with walnuts and strawberries. All of these aid bowel movements. Blend these with ice and a little raw milk. Since the ice is cold, it will shock the gut into working harder to compensate and therefore increase peristalsis. Please take note that the addition of ice is treatment is not suggested as a regular practice.

However, it's the opposite with diarrhea—if you drink too many ice cold beverages, this may cause diarrhea (though it may not be the only cause), so instead try warm-to-hot drinks. This will not stimulate the gut and may decrease diarrhea. If you experience a lot of diarrhea or loose stools, you are not absorbing the proper amount of nutrients. In this case, stop drinking any cold or iced beverages. Only drink hot or room temperature drinks as this more closely matches the temperature of the gut and will not create overstimulation.

To decrease the "leakage," we call upon our ally the banana once again. Only this time, it must be very unripe, with a green peel. Now this is the part that most do not care for, but the entire banana, peel and all, needs to be consumed. It is the astringent properties of the inner pith-like layer of the peel that assists in binding the stool. The best approach is to slice one-fourth to one-half slices so that they resemble silver dollars. The first slice will be difficult due to the saliva being astringed, but the mouth quickly adjusts and difficulty should decrease. This astringing feeling is what is also happening in the digestive tract! It is also beneficial to cook with banana flower.

Ladies, functional digestion is a key component in Breast Cancer Boot Camp and must be addressed. Once your digestion is strengthened, you will absorb nutrients more efficiently, which strengthens your body. If you have any of the abovementioned signs or symptoms and are spending a ton of money on organic food, you are literally flushing your money down the drain, as minimal amounts of nutrients are taken in.

## Nutrition: Eat Your Medicine

"Shouldn't live to eat, you eat to live." William Hobbins M.D.

Nutrition is the key to health! You are what you eat! Many people do not want to subscribe to this simple theory, but many patients fix their aliments simply by adjusting their diet. To prevent disease and be healthy, you have to invest time, energy, and money into your food. If you are unwilling to alter your diet, you will not obtain optimum health. Either do your own research or see a specialist, but whatever you do, eat your medicine, health can't be found in a pill.

At Breast Cancer Boot Camp we have the quarter rule. Be good 75 percent of the time and enjoy or have fun the other quarter. I keep only Breast Cancer Boot Camp foods in my house, so I can't cheat. When I go out to eat is when I get to enjoy comfort foods, cravings, or desserts. Find a technique that works for you. Listen to your body. If you need a day off, take it, don't deprive yourself by sticking to a strict regiment all the time. Rules can be broken sometimes, especially around holidays.

Many doctors are not familiar with true nutrition. During four years of medical school, the average student takes only one course in nutrition. During these limited hours of nutritional education, students are heavily propagandized by agricultural and pharmaceutical interests. In addition, few have interest in continued education with regard to nutrition. Therefore, false and old misinformation becomes the current misinformation.

Enjoy your food! Flavor is an important property of both food and herbs. The Chinese medical tradition involves much emphasis on flavors and how they react with the body and particular organs. Without going into a study of specific flavors, it is important that flavor be recognized and incorporated into one's diet. It is also important that the flavor of foods be present when one eats them. Food should be invoking emotions of pleasure, joy, etc. Enjoying what keeps us alive is important and seeking out those foods, even if not so "healthy" on occasions, which are enjoyed and are fulfilling. Flavor creates joy, so you enjoy your food. If you don't enjoy your food, your body will not respond and will not receive the amount of nutrients versus something you enjoy. That's why it is ok to eat desserts sometimes. Your body is craving chocolate and you enjoy eating it. When you are on a balanced diet of meat, fruit and veggies, your body will not want to consume just junk food, it finds a balance.

It is also important to note that when one's diet is well balanced and full of flavor, there is going to be much less of a craving for those "junk-food" products. Think about it. Most "junk-food" is packed with flavor (typically sweet) and such a craving is telling the body that something is lacking in the regular diet. Make the appropriate adjustments and the cravings decrease or go away entirely. Junk food junkies can break the cravings, it just takes time.

The body does know best...but are we listening to it?

Debriefing:

"Pink Image has changed the way I take care of myself. I went there for a simple thermogram over a year ago, but ended up getting life changing advice that I decided to take to minimize my chances of becoming a breast cancer statistic like my mom and grandmother. Wendy was insistent that my hormonal IUD was contributing to high estrogen levels showing up in my left breast and said the only way I can get that to change is to replace the IUD with the non-hormonal one. I was very resistant, as I sure liked not having any periods on the Mirena. But after my 2nd thermogram in 8 months showing no changes even after I made drastic diet and changes in the body products I was using (switched to non-paraben and more natural), I decided it was time to get the hormones out of my body. I wish I would have done it much sooner as I didn't know I would start dropping that extra weight off without hardly any extra effort! I've dropped 5 pounds very easily in 3 months where it used to be a battle to lose half a pound and then it would come back as soon as

I ate a large dinner. I still have to have to get a follow up thermogram in the next few months, but the pain I used to get in my left breast has almost left me thankfully.

Wendy's simple advice on changing the types of foods I eat and the type of products I put on my body every day has been the first step in being proactive in my continued well being. It doesn't have to be hard. I just have to make the extra effort to research the products I am buying, and making the conscious effort to eat the better foods, including organic. She truly has been wonderful to work with. I highly recommend Pink Image and Wendy Sellens!"

Maria

## The Organic Argument

Food, water, and air—those are the essentials. These three must be addressed to optimize health. Let us look at food as medicine, in the sense that it maintains health.

"Organic" is a great choice. Sadly, I have personally heard physicians say that they "try to eat healthy and organic, but it's so expensive," and in the next breath mention the cost of raising children as an excuse. This is a serious problem—if you are not willing to sacrifice luxury for health, especially for your children, then what business do you have "practicing medicine?" But I digress. Yes, organic is more expensive, but the benefits far outweigh the costs. That's what we face every day: cost-benefit analysis. Is that job worth the pay, is that coffee worth five dollars?

Before I begin, let me stress the difference between the farmers market and organics in the grocery store. To be labeled organic does not mean that the fertilizer and pesticides must be as well. Loophole with the FDA: anything before 1940's can be labeled organic, according an acquaintance that is a chemist at one of the nation's largest pesticide and fertilizer plants. The farmers rotate crops, may or may not use pesticides and many make their own fertilizer. Produce from the farmers market comes from nutrient rich soil, thus producing a higher quality organic versus at the grocery store.

Imagine the typical apple that you purchase at your average grocery store. It is most likely genetically modified, grown on pesticide-rich and nutrient-deficient soil, sprayed with chemicals, picked before ripening, and wax coated with a pretty glue-backed sticker. *Mmmmmmm*, sounds great. On the other hand, "organic" has strict requirements allowing for confidence in the product. In no way do I advocate complete or any trust in government regulation, but the market does have high quality providers of produce that are typically, but not limited to, USDA organic certified. Furthermore, if you are a "farmers' market" shopper, the produce that you find out that day was most likely picked within the last twenty-four hours. This is a huge nutritional benefit, as the produce is ripe and has had less time to denature or oxidize.

That organic apple is most likely going to provide you significantly more nutritional content at the same caloric value. This means that the enzymes, vitamins, and other nutrients in that apple may take perhaps two or three nonorganic apples in order to match it. You would have to consume two to three times the calories just to achieve the same nutritional value, and believe me, Americans are not calorie-deprived.

Imagine your body responding to these two separate diets. If your body obtains what it needs on a daily basis, your hunger or appetite should be quelled. Therefore, an organic diet provides the nutritional needs at a lower caloric intake, while the nonorganic diet provides less nutritional quality and thereby requires more calories to achieve nutritional needs. This leads to overconsumption, usually accomplished through high-carb foods. With organic you get more nutrients per item therefore consume less.

The specific mathematics involved in choosing organic or nonorganic diets are probably quite difficult and extensive. Instead, try this: dedicate one full month of say 90 percent organic (no one's perfect) diets for the entire family and see how everyone feels. I am sure you'll be pleasantly surprised.

# Fruit: Nature's Present

Think of fruit as a present. A tree or bush surrounds its seed (or future progeny) with the best possible gift it can exchange in hopes that that seed finds a viable site to flourish and continue the genetic game of gift-giving. The fruit is therefore going to be most beneficial in its natural form. It will contain an optimal balance of enzymes, vitamins, sugars, and water. However, a problem arises with the juicing fad. There are bad and not so bad ways to juice, but neither should become a habitual substitute for meals.

Some of the worst habits include drinking juice that contains no protein and is separated from the pulp or flesh, and using it to replace a meal. This is basically sugar overload—the juice bypasses the normal breakdown of food during digestion, causing rapid absorption and therefore a huge insulin response. Not good. What does sugar turn into if not used right away? That's right, *fat*. Also, when juices replace meals, there is a false sense that nutritional requirements have been met. In reality, the person has only supplied enough sugar to get the day started and going until they have a "sugar crash" and need another fix.

Many mothers are giving their children juice thinking they are being "healthy, this is the similar to Kool-Aid, but not synthetic. Dilute the juice with three-fourths water.

# Vegetables: Do as Your Mother Says—Eat Them!

Vegetable are basically components of plants, excluding seeds and fruit. This may include roots, stems, leaves, and even flowers. While we want to seek out "organic" products, we should not neglect the vitality a fruit or vegetable presents with. The vegetable should have a vibrant color relative to its tone, as if it's crying out, "Pick me, eat me!" Keep in mind that some vegetables are meant to be eaten raw, others require cooking, and some can be consumed either way. For example, spinach should not be heated, as its nutrients become altered and diminished. Rather than cook the spinach, place the warm food accompanying the dish onto the spinach to slightly wilt it. Lycopene cannot be acquired from a raw tomato, it must be heated. Many people prefer raw vegetables, which is healthy, but too many cold foods can create issues in the body according to Chinese medicine. So try supplementing with ginger or pepper, they have warming properties, to neutralize the temperature.

## Estrogen-Free® Meat: The Foundation

This is a case where "organic" might not be enough. Organic-raised livestock is a healthy option, but there are some issues to be aware of. Let's examine chicken, for example. The best chicken to eat is free-range and organic-fed. Cage-free is meaningless, due to the fact that the cage is only required by regulation to be opened for a certain amount of time, while the chicken may or may not actually leave the cage. The real problem, though, is what the chickens are fed. Producers often promote vegetarian-fed, but this too can be of concern.

Chickens are omnivores and naturally eat the bugs, mice and grass around the farm, as well as leftover veggies. In addition, smart farmers feed their chickens leftover shells, as this increases the calcium in their eggs. Return your egg cartons and shells to the farmer every week, and they might give you a discount. But if a farm relies on vegetarian feed, that may include soy and flax. As we have well established in this book, that is a problem. This is why it is important to research your sources of meat and animal-based products like milk, cheese, eggs, etc. Contact the source of the product and ask what their feed contains. If there is an element in their feed that contains estrogen, such as soy or flax, inform them why you cannot purchase their item. Industries are at the whim of the consumer, and if enough people demand a specific product, the market will eventually provide it.

Cows are grass eaters and should therefore be labeled as organic, grass-fed, free-range, and nonhormone. Avoid grain-fed cows. Presently, organic grass-fed beef is the safest, most easily available meat to purchase. Hopefully, in the near future, this will change. This will only happen by demand, so get loud!

Fish is a tricky one. While it typically has very good nutritional value, the problem with fish stems from its possible toxicity, mercury, micorplastics and even radiation. Many people have tested with unheard of levels of mercury, as was seen in a patient of mine who was a pescatarian and diagnosed with cancer. Her levels of mercury were a hundred times that of normal levels; her doctor stated that he had never seen levels that high. Some scientific sources report that fish is sixteen times more toxic than nonorganic beef—we're better off eating a nonorganic hamburger than fish. Now, micro-fibers and micro-plastics fleece, nylons, spandex, polyester from our clothes, toys and household products are getting washed out to the oceans are also contaminating our seafood. These biologist are reporting that most shellfish contain plastics due to record numbers, 200 – 9,000 particles per cubic meter of sea water, which we are consuming. What is interesting is that plastics act like a magnet to toxins. If you do wish to eat fish, stay with wild and not farm raised fish. Farmed fish tend to have much more elevated toxicity levels, due to the enclosed environment as well as some genetic modifications (creepy, huh?). Try to always eat wild-caught fish. Keep in mind that, as the oceans grow more polluted, this becomes more difficult.

Wild game is the optimum choice of meat, as it has the strongest vitality. For those who live in the rural to wild regions, take advantage of this opportunity—hunt for your own meat or purchase it from local processing plants. I grew up in Alaska, and my father was a hunter, so we ate very well. I attribute my strong constitution to eating fresh wild salmon, moose, and caribou. I currently live in California, where I have access to wild fowl. Quail, pheasant, duck, and dove are wonderful choices as well. For those with an ethical problem with hunting, remember, few animals die of old age in the wild.

## Healthy Age Old Wisdom

Everyone complains about controversy with all this access to information now. Well, let me set you straight. When were we, as a society, the healthiest? "They" claim we are living longer, but research has debunked this myth, as the body can only live a maximum amount of years, around 120. I believe what they mean to say is more people are living longer, but at what cost? Lying in a bed for five years waiting to die is not living. In 1939, Weston A. Price published "Nutrition and

Physical Degeneration," which was a study of primitive diets from population that were isolated from civilization to observer their development and health. Surprisingly, these populations were almost completely free of disease and illness. Another shock was that the diet of these primitive peoples had little in common other than the main staple of their food was animal fat, even with very low fresh produce available disease and illness were virtually non-existent. Interestingly, he never found a healthy population that lived solely on a plant diet.

Our ancestors utilized whole-animal nutrition for strength and the ability to revitalize the body. Our grandparents led a healthy lifestyle in "the modern world" because they ate a balanced diet, like liver on Thursdays, ate from the garden, no supplements, enjoyed the outdoors and had access to medicine, only as needed, by the family doctor. The building blocks of a strong body include bone broth, organ meat and lard.

Bone broth, especially grass fed beef, is an excellent way to strengthen the body and I strongly suggest that all my cancer patients drink it daily to nourish them back to health. For thousands of years' cultures all over the world used natural remedies to cure disorders by using the idea of like for like. If you had bad digestion you would eat menudo, intestines to heal the digestive tract or Pho, which is tendons for weak muscles and tendons. Muscles, skin and organs need blood for its nutrients and hydration. As we age our blood slowly shunts inward to protect our organs. As the blood leaves our appendages we see the damage in wrinkling of the skin, gray hair, brittle nails and stiff muscles. Blood is what hydrates the skin, hair, nails and muscles. Bone broth *is* anti-aging!

Bone broth is promoted as "the cure of a thousand diseases." We are brainwashed to believe there is a magic pill and people are always asking me to name a magic herb or supplement. I always state eating a balanced diet, but if they try to pin me down I'd go with bone broth with eggs being a strong second.

Bone broth contains collagen, which supports hair, keeps skin smooth, reduces wrinkles and nail health. It is an excellent source of several essential amino acids that are often difficult to get from diet alone, proline glycine, arginine, glutamine, which heal wounds, build collagen, and support the kidneys, arteries, heart and digestive tract.

I suggest for cancer patients and women over 35 consume 6-8 ounces of grass fed beef or bison bone broth daily. Try to avoid chicken due to possible plant estrogen feed. For everyone else 6-8 ounces at least 3 times a week. Don't use the powdered form, don't substitute convenience for quality. Consume high quality *real* organic grass fed bone both. Make it yourself or buy it.

Organ meats are nature's multi-vitamin and are richer than muscle meats. Adding a small amount to ground meat recipes will deliver a nutrient dense meal. They contain fatty acids, EPA and DHA, also fat soluble vitamins A, D, E and K, along with minerals like iron, copper, magnesium, iodine, and the B vitamins, B1, B2, B6, B12 and folic acid. Try a little pate with your champagne next time.

Want a healthy liver? Eat it! Did you know liver is richer in vitamin C than carrots or apples? An incredible bio-available form of iron, liver makes us strong. An excellent source of quality protein and is nature's most concentrated source of vitamin A. Also contains all the B vitamins in quite abundance, especially vitamin B12 and one of our best sources of folate. Trace elements such as copper, zinc and chromium; liver is our best source of copper CoQ10, a nutrient that is vital for cardio-vascular function.

Lard is making a comeback as the "new" coconut oil, why? We have recently learned the medical establishment lied to us concerning saturated fats, saying they were unhealthy, in fact, they are quite beneficial to our health. Lard has 40 percent saturated fat, 50 percent monounsaturated fat, and 10 percent polyunsaturated fat. Lard is heat stable, unlike olive oil that becomes rancid, which makes it ideal for cooking and baking. Healthy cholesterol, which is the precursor and needed to produce our hormones. Lard is one of the highest foods for vitamin D, second to cod liver oil, which is especially important after learning about the contamination of our seafood from micro-plastics.

## Milk and Cheese: If You are in the Moood

Much of the negative publicity against milk is based off hormone laden and over cooked milk products. Dairy is a wonderful source of fat and protein. Many people and physicians believe dairy creates phlegm in the body. This can be true for some people who are lactose intolerant, but grains may also be the issue. Try removing all grains (grains also cause phlegm), and then slowly add dairy back into your diet. If you are still having problems, then find a holistic doctor to address the issue.

Not all people wish to consume milk, or dairy for that matter, but for those who do, there is an important issue to address: homogenized and pasteurized milk are toxic to the body as both are processed with heat. Allows us to clear up some arguments. This heat reduces the size of the healthy milk molecules to a tenth of a micron, which is small enough to escape through the intestines before full digestive processes can occur. These acidic molecules travel freely into our bloodstream, reaching our organs and causing unforeseen health issues, including the hardening of the arteries or atherosclerosis. It is advised to consume only raw organic milk and cheese.

Another argument is the protein molecule is too big. I always wonder if this was true then how the heck have people survived for thousands of years consuming dairy, but for the researchers here you go. A study by Salentinig et al. (2013), looked at the process of milk fat digestion and the results are surprising. Digestion of milk fat requires the molecule to be broken down with a digestive enzyme called lipase. Here is the problem lipase are water soluble, meaning they can only work on the surface of the molecule and in the digestive tract which is aqueous. The answer to this problem is bile. Through emulsification bile breaks down these large molecules making it easier for lipase to digest them. Yes, the smaller the better. This is where the study got interesting. "Instead of grouping together to form larger fat masses, milk fat self-assembled into even smaller emulsion droplets. These nanometer-sized structures (or nanostructures) have a high internal surface area, facilitating the action of lipase. The key phrase…"self-assembled." Although smaller fat molecules are usually formed by the action of bile, Salentinig et al.

observed the formation of these nanostructures even in simulations of milk fat digestion that lacked the addition of bile acids."

No bile? No problem for milk fats! "Salentinig et al. propose an adaptive explanation. Newborns and infants have reduced bile production, but are also dependent upon milk fats for brain growth and development, immunity and even skeletal growth. The self-assembly of nanometer-sized milk fats may have evolved as a compensatory mechanism to ensure the delivery of fatty acids, fat-soluble vitamins and other bioactive components from milk to the developing infant's circulatory system. This is an exciting evolutionary hypothesis, suggesting that milk fat digestion may be adapted to the digestive chemistry of the infant gut." Milk can provide essential fat and fat-soluble vitamins to people with low bile production infants, elderly, and people with gallbladder or liver disease.

If you're in the *mooood* raw milk does the body good. Raw milk is high in vitamins including B12, all 22 essential amino acids, natural enzymes, including lactase, natural probiotics and good fatty acids. Due to this nutrient rich milk it creates a stronger immune system, reduces allergies, increases bone density, builds lean muscle, plus healthy skin and nails and aids with weight loss.

## Estrogen-Free® Eggs: The Perfect Food

It is now possible to buy soy-free eggs, which is a giant step. However, many consumers buy eggs that are high in omegas. Unfortunately, most of these chickens are fed flax. Between flax and soy, it is nearly impossible to have estrogen-free eggs. In fact, it is no different than eating normal eggs from hormonally supplemented, estrogenic, old school chickens, except for the price. Yes, that is right, people buy organic eggs supplanted with soy or flax for triple the price when they can buy traditional eggs with synthetic estrogen that have the same hormonal effect on the body. Try to buy eggs at a farmers market. They usually feed their chickens leftovers from the market and let them roam free.

Seriously, eat the whole egg! The white is just the pretty wrapping for all the good stuff. The majority of the nutrition is found in the yolk, such as the good cholesterol, healthy fat, vitamin A, B1, B2, B5, B9, calcium, some of the protein, plus lots more. Let's compare the yolk versus the egg white. The yolk contains Vitamin A 245 IU, vitamin D 18.3 IU, vitamin E .684 mcg, vitamin K .119 IU, omega 94 IU, protein 2.7 g, folate 24.8 mcg versus the egg white which has no vitamin A, D, E, K, omegas, protein is 3.6 g and folate is 1.3 mcg. The nutrients are in the yolk!

Dr. Hobbins believes the most perfect food is an egg. Being "healthy" is eating the entire egg; eating just egg whites is not. Give it a try—eat two to four eggs a day. Dr. Hobbins even had a woman cure her breast cancer by eating a dozen eggs a day.

# Fat Doesn't Make You Fat!

## The Skinny on Being Skinny

In 2003, the Cochrane Collaboration reviewed low-fat diets with low-calorie diets and found that "fat-restricted diets are not better than calorie-restricted diets in achieving long-term weight loss." In the *American Journal of Medicine*, Walt Willet of the Harvard School of Public Health wrote: "Diets high in fat do not appear to be the primary cause of the high prevalence of excess body fat in our society, and reduction in fat will not be the solution."

This may seem contradictory, but a diet high in fat actually promotes fat loss, or rather, fat stabilization. Not everyone requires fat loss to create a healthier body; some actually need more fat. But how does eating fat not make you fat? It curbs your appetite by releasing cholecystokinin, a hormone that causes a feeling of fullness. When the digestive system has proteins and fat accompanying the sugars (carbohydrates), the insulin response in the bloodstream slows. This decreases the amount of sugar stored in the body as fat, while reducing the inflammatory response due to high levels of insulin in the bloodstream. A helpful hint: if you overeat at meals, try including a nice amount of fatty food—your appetite will be satiated before you overconsume.

The big thing to differentiate here is fat and sugar. Fat is stored energy for the body, ready to burn. Think of fat as charcoal; it must be burned and used by the body. It cannot be stored in this form, as fat or lard cannot hold structure. On the other hand, sugar can form hard crystals that get stored and produce fat in our body.

Sugar is meant to be stored as fat for future use if it's not burned at that very moment. If you run around all day long like a five-year-old, you will not have trouble burning the sugar that you eat. But any sugar not used, and especially at rest, will be stored as fat. High school football players often "carb-load" the night before a game with huge pasta meals. Why? Because it's stored as fat that can be used as energy during the game the next day, when they lack the luxury of taking a meal-break during such high-level activity.

Let's step back and look at the human body as an organism meant to survive the conditions of its environment. Imagine that you are an early human engaged in an everyday struggle to find food. Remember, there wasn't always a fast food restaurant on every corner. If you struggle to achieve a proper caloric intake, anytime that your body gets more than it can use, it will be stored as fat, because you have been telling the body that it's been hard to get enough lately. On the other hand, if you and the tribe score some huge kills and foraging pays off, both with animal products and seeds that are high in fat content, the body is told, "Hey, we're doing pretty good right now. Why don't you burn up this fat so I can hunt more and look good?" Humans are meant to be active, and if you drop below a certain level, we start to store fat. But if we give our bodies the right signals while maintaining proper eating habits, we can reduce the excess storage.

Basically, it comes down to this: fat is used, sugar is stored. Fat has to be broken down and then used, just like sugars have to be broken down and stored, if not used immediately.

## Micronutrients: Units of Rank and File

## The Cholesterol Myth

Biosynthesis is a term used to describe how our body and its cells produce complex molecules. Hormone production is very detailed, with lots of difficult names to pronounce and remember; so since I want you to continue reading, I made it very simple. Estrogen and progesterone are produced from pregalone, which is derived from cholesterol. That's pretty simple, right? This pathway actually creates twenty-six different estrogens that are classified as one hormone out of convenience. All steroid hormones are made from cholesterol, which is why it is crucial that we eat foods rich in healthy fat and cholesterol. Therefore, eliminating cholesterol from the diet, coupled with eating "nonfat" or even "low-fat" diets can create hormone imbalances and weight gain.

Not only is cholesterol important for hormone synthesis, it is also essential for serotonin receptors to function and for synaptic transportation in the nerves. Many mental disorders are caused by deficiencies in serotonin, known as the "happy neurotransmitter," hence SSRI medications. (Might be a good idea to make sure that the cholesterol levels are good as well, huh?). Cholesterol is also a precursor for vitamin D; foods high in vitamin D are also typically high in cholesterol. The majority of these foods come from animals. To sum up a possible scenario, ladies that eliminate cholesterol from their diet and thus diminish their ability to produce vitamin D may therefore create a hormone imbalance that contributes to depression and increased cancer risk.

Without doubt, the largest myth in regards to cholesterol is that it causes arteriosclerosis, which leads to heart attacks/disease, usually due to red meat consumption. This is completely false; there is no evidence or clinical studies to draw this conclusion from. Once again, modern science has incorrectly jumped to conclusions in the fashion of "correlation is causation." Cholesterol is constantly in the bloodstream, as it is vital to nearly every cell in the body. Arteriosclerosis, and diabetes for that matter, is largely attributed to grains.

Here's how this works: the liver makes cholesterol, so the more cholesterol that is consumed throughout the day, the less the liver produces. HDL is so famous because it transports the excess cholesterol in the body back to the liver, where it is either excreted or reutilized. The reason HDL is seen as the "good" lipoprotein is that if arteriosclerosis occurs as a result of cholesterol, the HDL collects it and returns it to the liver. In the expected dichotomy of the body (and universe), the LDL transports cholesterol from the liver to the tissues of the body. This is why it has a bad reputation, despite the fact that it performs an equally important function. It is the equivalent of praising the local waste management company while vilifying your family for creating trash. Once again, it is balance that matters.

Triglycerides (fat transporters) circulate fat in the body; this number should be kept low. Fats that are high in triglycerides and low HDL usually yield from a high-carb diet. This is combination should be avoided, as it leads to diabetes and inflammation.

When there is inflammation in the body, it is the job of cholesterol and LDL to lay down a salve, like a scab. However, this becomes a problem when the body has chronic inflammation, which results from the constant insulin response caused by high-carb diets. And where do the majority of our high-carb foods come from? Grains! As a result of this chronic inflammation, cholesterol and LDL are always present, hard at work to cover up the mistakes of a poor diet. Unfortunately, when cholesterol and LDL constantly work in a site of chronic inflammation, oxidation occurs and causes plaque buildup (oxidation is caused by free radicals that are usually carried by trans fats). If one wants to reduce inflammation and cholesterol buildup, all they really need to do is stop eating trans fats and grains, which contain large amounts of carbohydrates. Inflammation causes LDL to rise, not saturated fat. Every time inflammation occurs, LDL strives to treat it; people assume it is the cause when it is actually the treatment.

My father suffered a heart attack in the past, yet he has great numbers now. I had him reduce his carbohydrate intake and switch from margarine to butter. The result: six years later, his numbers are great and his weight has normalized.

So many people get caught up with blood tests and numbers. Please allow me to help you understand your blood tests. It is common to believe that any number over 200 is a bad cholesterol level, but this is not necessarily true. Just as with hormone testing, the numbers must be analyzed in ratio to each other.

Let's look at my numbers as an example. My cholesterol is 233; 200 is considered normal. But my HDL is 74, with 40 being normal. The reason my cholesterol seems high is because there is a lot of healthy cholesterol in my diet. Here's what we do: take the cholesterol level and divide it by the HDL levels, and anything under five is excellent. So 233 divided by 74 is 3, making me excellent, just in case you didn't know already! Next, we compare HDL to LDL. My LDL is 122, with 130 being normal. Compared with my HDL, which is double, my LDLs are good. But don't be concerned with LDL, it is more important to compare HDL with triglycerides, as it is their level that needs to be low. (Normal is 150 and I am sixty-two.)

I consume a lot of butter for protection of the myelin sheath (nerve insulators which assist in proper nerve conduction) to prevent neurological disorders, such as Alzheimer's and dementia, and to keep my skin supple and healthy. After all, cholesterol is a lipid.

Foods containing healthy cholesterol are eggs, butter, and red meat.

An interesting note: the foods highest in Vitamin D, cholesterol and omega-3 are fish. There is a correlation between low cholesterol and omegas levels among dementia and Alzheimer's victims, with low levels in all three correlating to depression.

## Butter Baby

Ayruvedic physicians use ghee or butter in treatment of patients. Patients have reported that they are prescribed to drink up to two cups of butter a day. I thought about the benefits of this from a Western biomedical perspective and for the last few years and suggested Breast Cancer Boot Camp drink to my patients—two tablespoons of butter, milk, and cinnamon.

Butter contains healthy cholesterol. Cholesterol is needed to repair the myelin sheath around our nerves for synaptic transportation or message sending. This reduces risk of dementia and Alzheimer's. I also believe many women cannot lose the weight because they do not consume enough fat every day. If for years you do not eat fat, your body believes you are in a famine and will hold on to your fat. To reduce fat, eat more fat. Fat is the fuel of your body; it will not be stored. Most importantly, as mentioned, cholesterol is the precursor for all your sexual hormones. You have to consume cholesterol to be hormonally balance. Cholesterol is vital for hormone synthesis, it is also essential for serotonin receptors to function. Many mental disorders are caused by deficiencies in serotonin, known as the "happy neurotransmitter" or SSRI. To be healthy, you have to consume fat and cholesterol. Recently a new diet has become popular, *The Bullet Proof Diet*, which understands the same principles, but uses coffee over milk. I do not approve of juice or protein powder starvation diets. However, since the Bullet Proof Diet is providing the body its fuel, drinking up to a stick of butter during the day, many people have lost a lot of weight without malnutrition. I suggest drinking the coffee butter drink with an egg or a few nuts, which allows for full or proper digestion.

## The Omega 3 Woman

Omega-3s are essential fatty acids—DHA, EPA—that are not produced in the body and therefore need to be acquired through diet. Omegas reduce inflammation, a component in heart disease and asthma, lower triglycerides, and are vital to pregnant women for fetal development. Pretty good stuff, huh?

What about flax? Flax, is unfortunately in the form of ALA, alpha-linolenic acid, not the active form of EPA, eicosapentaenoic acid, and DHA, docosahexaenoic acid. ALA is the shortest of the omega 3s. First, it must be elongated, which is called "elongation," and this requires an enzyme – but it doesn't end there. The second requirement is called "increased desaturation." The omega-3 fat gets altered chemically, which provides more reactivity to the fat. All of these processes require the following nutrients: vitamin B3, vitamin B6, vitamin C, zinc, and magnesium, in order, to successfully convert ALA. If someone is deficient in any of these nutrients, then the conversion is unable to be completed. It is strongly recommended to use the active forms of omega 3 EPA and DHA to get the vital nutrient.

The recommended daily supply of omega-3s is 250 mg. Try these dietary alternatives:

- 2 oz of walnuts
- 3 ½ oz of wild caught salmon, herring or sardines

# Why Pay for Vitamin D When the Sun Is Free?

We have already discussed that cholesterol is needed to produce hormones like progesterone and estrogen, but this amazing molecular element is also a precursor to vitamin D. In order to produce vitamin D within the body, cholesterol must be present and therefore consumed. Sunlight is required to transform cholesterol into vitamin D.

Our bodies have a very difficult time absorbing vitamin D supplements correctly because it is insoluble, the result is often the creation of toxicity in our body. Therefore, it is not advisable to take vitamin D supplements. The only proper way to obtain vitamin D is to make it, and that means getting sun and eating right. Some of you are going to argue this point because your vitamin D levels are too low. If this is the case, use a supplement briefly to get your numbers up, while fixing your diet by increasing cholesterol intake and bathing in the sun when you can. For those of you in rainy, cold regions, it is much harder. Only use supplements in the winter months and get outside in the summer.

If you truly want to stimulate vitamin D production, sit in the sun for fifteen-twenty minutes a day, exposing most of your body. Do not wear sunscreen; your body will slowly adjust with short increments of exposure, it is called a tan. Technically, a good diet that is high in antioxidants should be able to protect the skin from the sun for short periods, though extreme climates and very fair skin may be an exception. If you do this, your vitamin D levels should increase. Some of my healthiest patients are the ones that garden. However, if you are going to be in the sun all day, you may want to wear a petrochemical free sunscreen.

Limit the use of sunglasses. Believe it or not, our eyes are meant to be naked to the various rays of the sun. Our eyes need light. Some of the most important rays, or rather spectrums of rays, occur at sunrise. It is at this time when the sun rays arc, or bend, through the Earth's atmosphere, creating a very specific spectrum of light unlike any other time of the day. All the rays, wavelengths, or frequencies that our body needs are in the morning sunrise. We are much sicker globally because we don't wake at sunrise anymore. We are creatures of light, and it is therefore very beneficial for us to bathe in this particular spectrum. If one feels sick or fatigued, they should attempt to watch the sun rise every morning and evaluate how they feel. It may not cure the ailment, but it should help to strengthen. This is why farmers and primitive cultures were so healthy – daily dose of sunlight *only* found in the sunrise.

There is a reason light therapy is starting to gain momentum, it is because sunglasses have blocked out therapeutic wavelengths or spectrums the body requires. We are just like plants, we need sunlight to grow! Imagine putting on sunglasses, it's the same as putting your plants in the cellar.

This man is the expert, Andreas Moritz and in his book *"Heal Yourself with Sunlight"* he goes into more depth, but sunglasses fool your pineal and pituitary gland into thinking it is night or that you are in the dark. When you are outside and wear sunglasses, you don't produce that protective hormone – melanin, which protects your skin. Another interesting topic he also discusses is the importance of sunlight for the myelin sheath and correlates the increase of MS in northern countries versus southern countries. According to research sunglasses make us appear more attractive, but they're making us sick! Ditch the glasses!

A good example of the effect of light on humans occurred in China, where women working in a factory were suffering horrible menstrual periods. The number of complaints was so large that the issue could not be overlooked. The factory finally realized the installed lighting was causing the health issue, and upon changing the bulbs, the health issue lessened.

Seasonal defective disorder is real. I should know; I'm from Alaska. Per capita, we have some the highest crime rates and suicides in the winter months. We see animals respond to the variations of light with seasonal mating and hibernation. There is a change in the amount of light the sun places upon a region of the earth and the animals respond with instinctive actions. Some animals grow or shed their coats while others migrate. All of this is in some part due to sunlight. As we have already stated, vitamin D is made by our bodies due to sun exposure and it's *free*! Stop wasting money on pills and bathe in the light of health, or in this case, the health of light.

To increase vitamin D in the body get daily sun and it is vital to consume foods high in cholesterol and vitamin D. Foods high in vitamin D are the following:

- Fish-salmon, oysters, sardines, shrimp, 3 ½ ounces
- Caviar/roe, 1 ounce
- Lard, 1 tablespoon
- Bacon or Ham, 3 ounces
- Egg yolk, 1 egg is 10 percent daily recommended amount
- Some mushrooms, 1 cup

## Amino Acids: Protein Power

Amino acids are building blocks of proteins, twenty of which are considered essential to the human body. Nonessential amino acids can be produced in the body while essential amino acids must be attained through dietary intake. Unfortunately, plant proteins are usually missing one or two of these much needed amino acids.

Excellent sources of the nine complete amino acids and are highly suggested for daily consumption.

- Eggs
- Red meat
- Chicken,
- Raw dairy
- Wild caught fish

## Iodine: It's Awesome

Iodine is utilized by the thyroid to produce TH3 and TH4, hormones that influence metabolic rate, heart rate, weight, and blood pressure. Those afflicted with hypothyroidism, or an underactive thyroid, often present with weight gain. This is because these hormones help the body maintain its energy level by burning calories efficiently and minimizing fat storage/accumulation. In addition, iodine helps with the body's growth and development, including the reproduction system, health of hair, nails, and teeth, and elimination of toxins. Interestingly, iodine assists in apoptosis (or programmed cell death), which ensures for new cells, and is essential for organs and the removal of diseased or cancerous cells. It may be used as an anticancer agent, as it is capable of shrinking some cancers.

The most readily available source for iodine is regular table salt. Notice the rise in thyroid issues after salt was demonized? Use iodized salt daily to increase the function of your thyroid. Dr. Hobbins emphasizes there is no correlation with high blood pressure.

Once again, do not rely upon toxic supplements. Eat your iodine!

- Iodized table salt
- Seaweed or kelp
- Fish
- Lima beans
- Garlic
- Spinach

## Antioxidants: Ammunition

Vegetables and fruits are high in antioxidants, some more than others, which fight harmful free radicals in the body. Free radicals have the propensity to rob electrons from certain molecules and therefore create an oxidation effect. This oxidation process may cause cancer, so foods with high levels of antioxidants, primarily certain fruits and vegetables, help combat this process.

## Withdrawals: What to Avoid

Limit sugar and grains, legumes (beans) and carbohydrates. When not utilized by the body, they cause inflammation in the digestive tract. Inflammation creates insulin resistance (diabetes), heart disease (nope, it's not from cholesterol) and cancer.

They can also block absorption of nutrients. Think about what carbohydrates or grains such as pasta, oatmeal, bread, and rice look like when cooked—soggy. That is what they do in your gut—create a swamp that stops the absorption of vitamins and minerals.

Eat clean whole foods that move effortlessly through the intestines. Grains, even organic, are carbohydrates that turn into sugar, and remember, cancer feeds off sugar.

What you really need to remember ladies, carbs make you fat! They are sugar. Want to maintain true weight—wake up and realize comfort food is making you fat. We all need to spoil ourselves sometimes, save the bread for those occasions. Put that delicious bread down, step back, and enjoy it as a treat.

A quick lesson on Lectins. Legumes (beans) are naturally toxic, and this is due to lectins, which are a specific protein that bind to carbohydrates and exist in plants as a protective mechanism. When animals who are not adapted to consuming specific types of lectins eat them, they will experience pain or even death. Lectins can harm the lining of the intestines, especially the microvilli, because they bind to the protein receptors. When the intestines are damaged, lectins, and the foods that they bind to, can pass through the intestinal wall and into the blood stream where they can bind to any carbohydrate containing protein cells. It is speculated that lectins may cause insulin and leptin resistance, two major factors in obesity and diabetes. This is the reason that grains, beans, and other lectin containing foods cannot be eaten raw.

Grains are hard on the intestines. The lectins, as discussed are inflammatory, resistant to digestive enzymes, and they have the ability to sneak out of the intestines and have actually been found in the organs. Phytates, also called anti-nutrients, found in grains can block or slow the absorption of minerals, including iron and calcium. Don't worry! All the same nutrients in grains are found in meat, veggies, fruits, and nuts and are more bioavailable than those found in grain. They keep people sick, fat, and at risk for many diseases.

Ladies, I know you're tired, and it's easy to come home after working all day…you're cranky and too tired to think about what to cook. It's easy to dump pasta in a pot and pour sauce over it, throw it on the table and call the kids. Stop! It's making you and your family sick and fat. Being healthy requires planning. Take the time. The results will be your reward.

Limit your consumption of grains, carbohydrates and beans (legumes). Now you know why. Don't make it your family's daily staple.

Avoid these legumes, peanuts and soy, which are considered the most toxic of the legumes. Many people have an allergy to peanuts and soy and this may be a contributing factor. Avoid soy, garbanzo or chickpea and mung bean, which are phytoestrogens.

Avoid nonorganic coffee. Coffee is one of the most highly sprayed crops. It is the pesticides that are harmful. Dr. Hobbins and I have not found organic coffee to increase vascularity or risk in the breasts, so enjoy. Want a sweeter cup? Add *real* organic sugar and raw milk.

Avoid polyunsaturated oils including sunflower, safflower, sesame, cottonseed, peanut and canola oil. These oils have low temperature stability and therefore easily become rancid and toxic to the body by introducing free radicals. Avoid sesame as it is a phytoestrogen.

Only use centrifuge organic coconut oil, all other coconut oil is processed. Do not cook with coconut oil as it may turn rancid. How did Americans thrive for hundreds of years without coconut oil? Butter, it's better for the body.

Avoid cooking with olive oil. Heating olive oil makes it rancid. Only consume olive oil if it is "first cold press." Right now, you're asking, "What can I cook with?" Use butter; it is very healthy for you and can handle high heat along with flavorful organic bacon grease. One question worth asking is, "Why did heart disease go up in the last couple of decades, after the trend to not cook with butter took over?" Grandma was right; it tastes better with more butter!

Avoid soy milk. Its nature is toxic, legume, and contains phytoestrogens.

Avoid almond milk. The processing, heat, yields a rancid product that can increase free radicals and therefore increase the risk of cancer. Most almond milks contain large amounts of sugar for flavoring and other additives.

Avoid rice milk. It is high in sugar or carbohydrates.

Avoid juices. They are high in carbohydrates or sugar.

"What can I drink?" The best answer, and unfortunately the boring one, is water. We will discuss water below as we have already covered, drinking raw milk, "It does the body good!" Organic tea and coffee are also acceptable. Don't drink your calories with sugar drinks.

Avoid smoked nuts due to rancidity from heat.

Avoid dried fruits. They are concentrated sugars.

Avoid all non-fat or low fat products. These can be highly processed. Fat is the body's fuel. If fat isn't consumed, the body will "hold" onto it in order to fuel the body. Lose weight by eating fat.

Avoid protein powders and shakes. Processed products are usually in a toxic lined can, including BPA. Recent studies are finding large amounts of metals, arsenic, mercury and lead in organic plant-based protein powders.

Avoid beer. Hop are phytoestrogens. Grains make you fat and formaldehyde is used in the bottling process. If you are craving a beer go organic.

Finally, let's discuss wine! Love it! Only drink organic. Grapes are sprayed with pesticides. Wine is made by reducing large amounts of grapes to achieve a single glass of wine. That means the pesticides are concentrated into high levels. Go with white wine. Resveratrol is a bioflavonoid that occurs naturally in grapes and red wine, but is a phytoestrogen.

War Story:

I had a patient who went through gastric bypass surgery. For three months, all she could consume was six protein shakes per day, each containing sixty grams of protein. As a result, she lost her hair, and her skin became permanently scaly. It is not possible to substitute healthy protein and nutrients from whole foods with supplements and shakes.

Avoid synthetic sugar products. There is more and more evidence indicating that these substances are highly carcinogenic, meaning they cause cancer and many more issues, including weight gain! If you have to use sugar, use organic raw sugar or honey—something real.

Healthy women should avoid or limit vitamins and supplements. When you are in the elderly stage of your life or during an illness, it is appropriate to use vitamins or supplements. Get your vitamins and minerals from eating whole organic foods. When you meet your body's nutritional needs for the day, you might eat less because you are fulfilling all your daily requirements with wholesome foods which will decrease cravings for comfort foods which are high in calories. One supplement we do suggest is fish oil daily as many women do not consume enough wild fish daily.

Debriefing:

"Pink Image has changed the way I take care of myself. I went there for a simple thermogram over a year ago, but ended up getting life changing advice that I decided to take to minimize my chances of becoming a breast cancer statistic like my mom and grandmother. Wendy was insistent that my hormonal IUD was contributing to high estrogen levels showing up in my left breast and said the only way I can get that to change is to replace the IUD with the non hormonal one. I was very resistant as I sure liked not having any periods on the Mirena. But after my 2nd thermogram in 8 months showing no changes even after I made drastic diet and changes in the body products I was using (switched to non paraben and more natural), I decided it was time to get the hormones out of my body. I wish I would have done it much sooner as I didn't know I would start dropping that extra weight off without hardly any extra effort! I've dropped 5 pounds very easily in 3 months where it used to be a battle to lose half a pound and then it would come back as soon as I ate a large dinner. I still have to have to get a follow up thermogram in the next few months, but the pain I used to get in my left breast has almost left me, thankfully.

"Wendy's simple advice on changing the types of foods I eat and the type of products I put on my body every day has been the first step in being proactive in my continued well being. It doesn't have to be hard. I just have to make the extra effort to research the products I am buying, and making the conscious effort to eat the better foods, including organic. She truly has been wonderful to work with. I highly recommend Pink Image and Wendy Sellens!"

Maria

Eat your medicine! True health can be found in our daily meals. Nutrition is the foundation of Breast Cancer Boot Camp.

## The Animal Diet

Dr. Hobbins created "Eat Like the Animals." This is taken from his *Christian Medical Center Newsletter*, September 2002.

*Eat like the animals*

1. All of God's animals except for the last that He made eat all of God's food exactly as he designed it for them, gave them a taste for it with no processing, no cooking, and no confusion on the animals' part. These animals, as you will observe in nature, are never overweight, rarely have serious diseases secondary to nutrition, and live their full life expectancy without the benefit of any help except the Lord's.
2. All food is perfect. It takes a large human ego to believe that we can make a better fat (margarine) than butter or animal fat, and that we can make any carbohydrates better in the sense of the way they are distributed to the body and rate at which they are converted into a sugar. The excess sugar that is taken in is utilized by insulin, driven into the cell and stored as fat (this is simplified). We are the only one of God's creatures who processes food by grinding, mashing, juicing, or cooking. All of the other animals have to use the oral instruments available to them such as teeth, molars, or muscles to prepare their food.
3. Cooking does not improve food value! When food is cooked, several things are likely to happen. The most important is that the substances the Lord wanted to nourish us with are converted from the complex to the simple in all things. Even during the making of table sugar or baking a potato, it is turned from a complex

starch, which if eaten raw, will not raise blood sugar, whereas if it is baked and made into a baked potato, it has mostly turned the starch into a simpler sugar and you get an elevated blood sugar. This raises the glycemic index (absorption rate) and starts Syndrome X—insulin and hormone burning.

4. Recent evidence initially presented by the Swedes is that any heating of carbohydrates above 140 degrees makes a very strong cancer-producing substance. At 140 degrees steaming, there is a 1 mg per 100 mg of carbohydrate, whereas at boiling, there is a 2 mg per 100 mg. With baking at 350 degrees, there is 1,000 mg; with deep frying or microwaving at 600 degrees, there is a 2,000. This means that, as the temperature increases, the damage and the cancer substance increase exponentially (this substance is an acrylamide).

The processing of all carbohydrates is the biggest problem for humans as far as nutrition and subsequent health problems—obesity, diabetes, hardening of the arteries, and probably some of the dementias. No other animals have fire, grill, frying pans, boiling pots, baking ovens, microwaves, or deep frying pans. Likewise, juicing frees up the sugar from its pulp or sap that is contained within, thus causing more rapid absorption and a higher blood sugar level. This increases your diabetic episode each time you do it.

5. Supplements (raw foods) are needed because of cooking and processing causing maximal loss of enzyme and catalyst in a natural food. There is no such thing as a "complex" carbohydrate after cooking. Only raw foods have all of the supplements that God desired for us to have.

6. Some supplements (pills, powders, etc.) are acid and some are alkali; some are oil-based and some are aqueous (water soluble). This means that they do not mix well when they are purified and then added back together.

7. Multiple vitamins inactivate each other, making salts of each other and blocking absorption. Thus, vitamin supplementation comes from raw food as God's design; however, the individual vitamins should be taken separately and is of no greater cost other than the

inconvenience. An example of what happens in the processing of vitamins is niacin, vitamin B3 = nicotinic acid (side effect of flushing). This is an active supplement. Niacin nonflushing is less than 10 percent effective because this is being given as inactive salt, nicotamide. This form does no particular good!

8. Digestion is a chemical process that should be undertaken under the best of conditions. There are five major stages in this process; each must be protected in this process and timing.
   a. Mastication and saliva (simple sugar).
   b. Gastric mixing and acid preparation, especially of proteins.
   c. Biliary (gallbladder and liver quarts of bile). Emulsification of oils and fats in preparation for digestion.
   d. Pancreatic protein and fat enzymes to prepare the proteins and fats for absorption and our internal use.
   e. Small bowel. The upper three feet is alkaline for special processing of carbohydrates. The lower intestine is for the selective absorption of the processed food.

*Do not take free minerals with meals* (such as calcium, because it makes salt out of the acids and inactivates them).

In summary, God wants us to eat like the rest of his creatures. He wants us to eat the food as he hung it on the tree, grew it in the ground, flew it in the sky, and swam it in the ocean. The least amount of processing will be best assimilated and utilized for our best health.

## Estrogen-Free® Water

Water is vital for life. As many already know, one will die from dehydration before dying of starvation. It is imperative to drink clean water. Below I will go into great detail about the factors needed for perfect drinking water, and I will show you, ladies, how toxic your water sources may be. It will probably scare you, as it did me.

It took me two years to find a good, clean source of water. I am by no means an expert on water, but due to the path in health research I have taken, it was inevitable for me to thoroughly examine such an important element of life. I think many will be surprised at the toxicity of our drinking water, including filtered and bottled, and how it could affect all of us and cause many health concerns. This book was not written to sell water, so for those interested, watch my videos or visit my websites for contact information on the water purification company we use and promote.

Avoid estrogenic water. Nearly all tap water, which includes reverse osmosis, filtrated, and bottled water, contains medical waste. If the water source is not from the ground, which most are not, it is actually filtered water. Every pill that each American consumes has tiny molecules that cannot be absorbed into the body, and as a result, are urinated out. Unfortunately, our sewage treatment plants are not equipped to remove these microscopic particles, and because of this, they are recycled back into the drinking water. What this comes down to is that nearly every American is microdosing the same drugs that the rest of the population consumes. Not only do we consume nanograms of sleeping pills and cholesterol meds, but also birth control pills and hormone replacement therapies. Therefore, without proper filters, the typical individual consumes small doses of estrogen several times a day.

Did you know that fluorine (fluoride) and chlorine are neurotoxins? A neurotoxin is a poison that acts on the nervous system, resulting in interference with neuron communication. Neurotoxin exposure can cause mental retardation, memory impairment, epilepsy, dementia, and Alzheimer's. Fluoride is a toxic waste byproduct of the aluminum production process. It is commercial-grade hydrofluoric acid that *everyone* is ingesting; it is *not* a pharmaceutical-grade fluoride that you can purchase at a pharmacy.

The American Dental Association has announced that it is not appropriate to use fluoride on children under the age of five. Read the warning label on toothpaste containers and you will see that it cautions ingestion by infants.

> WARNING: Keep out of reach of children under 6 years of age. If you accidentally swallow more than used for brushing, seek professional assistance or contact a Poison Control Center immediately.

In fact, New Hampshire mandated a water bill warning of the toxic side effects of fluoride on infants. If this does not disturb you, consider the fact that the average adult is about 60 percent water (as a weight ratio) and an infant can be up to 79 percent.

In order for the thyroid to function, it needs to utilize iodine. Iodine and fluorine are in the same column in the periodic table, meaning they have similar bonding capabilities or affinities. In the event that fluoride is present and iodine is lacking, the thyroid will uptake fluoride at a higher rate than iodine. This is due to the excessive amounts of fluoride and minimal amounts of iodine in our diet. The eventual result is possible thyroid diseases. Yet when people stop ingesting fluoride, symptoms of thyroid disease, allergies, and migraines may disappear. Fluoride is in virtually all water and it takes a special filter to eliminate it. Bottled, reverse-osmosis, filtered, and tap water all have it, meaning it is present in all soups, teas, coffees, and baked goods that use water.

Fluoride also kills good bacteria in the intestines, which causes many digestive issues. Where do you get your water? Better look! Again, a special filter is needed to remove fluoride from your water system. Be warned, some filters claim to remove fluoride and do not, so do your research.

Cancer thrives in an acidic environment, yet struggles in an alkaline environment. All tap, filtered, reverse osmosis, and many bottled waters are acidic. There are many alkaline water systems out there, but unfortunately, most of them use an additive. You know the rules by now, stay away from anything processed. Water that is actually found in a river mixes with rocks or minerals, and it is this interaction that makes the water alkaline. The water system that I personally use does not have an additive, but rather, infuses minerals into the water. Not only does this make the water alkaline, it also allows for these minerals to be incorporated into your diet. One more reason we don't need pills. This water system infuses calcium, magnesium, sodium, and potassium into the water and what your body does not use is excreted. It's similar to drinking water from a river, as it mixes with the rocks and soil.

Alkalinity is mainly achieved by our breath – full deep breaths. Shallow or rapid breathing causes acidity. Your hypothalamus with assistance from your lungs keeps your blood's PH at 7.4 or alkaline. This is why deep breathing, taking three long breaths or mediation with deep breathing is considered effective, it's calming and creating an alkaline environment. Just keep breathing!

When discussing alkalinity, we must dispel this myth - eating acid or alkaline food does not make your body alkaline or acidic! If you are eating a lot of acidic foods your body will have to neutralize it and then discard. That is why your urine tests high for acidity, it was discarded! Certain food products will produce more alkalinity or acidity, as required by the nature of the food, during digestion. When all food comes in contact with the stomach, the gastric acid makes all food acidic, in order to break it down for absorption. The jejunum, pancreatic juices and bile have different PH or alkaline and acidic properties that will neutralize this acidity. To keep it basic the digestive process is one long continuous tube and all the food gets mixed together and is dispelled as feces. Feces should be neutral. All your food becomes neutral or is buffered to protect the body and is controlled by the digestive juices that control the PH which should have an end product that is neutral or buffered. You can't control your digestion by just eating alkaline foods, the body will naturally find a balance and make it neutral. However, if years of poor food choices wears down your body so it is incapable or unable to digests properly, then yes, there will be health issues, but this explanation is for normal healthy people. If want to control or assist your digestion, then eat a balanced diet or eat equal parts acidic and alkaline.

Due to the digestive process in order to receive the benefits of alkaline water, it must be drunk on an empty stomach, or as described above will be mixed with the food and neutralized by the digestive juices.

Drink water all day and still feel unhydrated? That is because tap water, reverse osmosis, filtered, and bottled water is "dead." What does it mean for water to be "dead"? From a biological standpoint, water is not alive, but it is vital to life and should be obtainable. If not completely obtainable, I refer to the water as "dead." Take a look at a strong flowing stream or a running river, and then compare that water to a pond or stagnant pool of water. Which would be the preferred drinking source? Minerals and movement give water vitality, but for a water molecule to enter into a cell, it has to be its natural size. Most natural water is in the form of six molecule clusters. On the other hand, "dead" water is typically found in clusters of twelve to thirteen water molecules. These larger molecule clusters are mostly found in tap, reverse osmosis, filtered, and most bottled waters. These water sources have lost their original cluster size through processing. Exposure to electricity (most alkaline water systems are electrical) and boiling causes the water molecules to break their bonds and increase in size. The twelve to thirteen water molecule clusters cannot fit into our cells, and as a result, we remain unhydrated. *Do not* buy a water filtration system that is "plugged in," the electricity destroys the water and makes it dead or nonhydrating.

Want to be beautiful? Hydrate with real estrogen free water!

## Sweet sweat

It is not healthy to sweat excessively. Hot yoga has become very popular, and though this may be beneficial for the average person once a week, it is not a recommended daily practice. Some people may be able to handle it for a moderate period, but in the long run the body will have difficulty keeping up with the constant need to replenish. Why is this? Because sweat is *not* replenished by just drinking water. Have you tasted sweat? It is salty. With regard to Chinese medicine, it is a precious fluid. It contains not only water, but electrolytes; our bodily processes make this fluid. Keeping our system cool is one of the body's most important duties because if our body temperature exceeds a certain level, proteins (primarily in the brain) begin to denature and destroy cells and tissue. Do not waste such bodily fluids without understanding the expense your body pays. You may end up weaker and less healthy.

As a side note, if you happen to sweat profusely, try not to use the marketed electrolyte drinks, as they most likely contain high amounts of fructose corn syrup. I advise my patients to eat a dill pickle or have a shot or two of dill pickle brine (juice), as there are rich in electrolytes yet contain few processed sugars.

If you are sweating too much, outside of working out, go to a holistic doctor they can fix this issue.

Ladies, save your sweat, it's a precious fluid. Limit your hot yoga and sauna.

# Functional Adrenals

Due to false propaganda, salt consumption has decreased. So why has adrenal exhaustion increased, as seen in the mass influx of coffee shops and energy drinks?

By the time a person is medically diagnosed with adrenal deficiency, 90 percent of adrenal function is gone! No need to worry, as Chinese medicine can observe a deficiency years before a Western diagnosis, and in doing so, can attempt to improve adrenal function. People who use coffee or energy drinks to wake up and make it through the day most likely have adrenal deficiency or exhaustion. Unfortunately, this is the majority, and that is bad news.

The adrenals are little bean-shaped organs that sit on top of the kidneys. They are a part of the endocrine system and release hormones in conjunction with stress. In Chinese medicine, the kidneys (which include the adrenals) are our reserves, and once they run out, we are getting pretty close to "closing the account," if you catch my drift. Essentially, when we overtax ourselves with stress, work, excess exercise, too many drugs, or not enough sleep, we literally take years off our life.

If the adrenals are taxed, one will *not* lose weight. The adrenals will detect that the body is overworked and holds onto fat, or stored energy, no matter how hard a person diets or exercises! If a person does not get what they need from their daily diet and suffers from improper digestion, the body draws from its reserves. The digestive system follows a theory: if the pot is empty, draw from the well, the kidneys. Everything stems from the kidneys; they are the blueprint of your whole system. If you take from the kidneys, you age yourself! The first sign of this appears in our skin, in the form of wrinkles and age spots. The kidneys are the foundation of the body's "essence," and once that is depleted, soon, nothing will remain.

First, let me be clear, salt is NaCl, not sodium, Na. The harmful effects of sodium have caused a lot of confusion and misinformation with the beneficial nutrient, salt. Salt is the raw material needed for the adrenals. Many Chinese physicians will laugh at this because each organ has a flavor, and the kidneys' are salt. The Chinese have known this for over five thousand years—that's why they are smiling. You crave what you are deficient in. Look at the low salt trend of the past couple of decades and the same era's overconsumption of coffee and energy drinks. I am not certain if the correlations actually have a direct link to one another, but nonetheless, I find it very interesting. The point that I really wish to make is that salt intake has *nothing* to do with your blood pressure, despite what modern medicine leads you to believe. In fact, it is an outright lie that salt increases your blood pressure. Let this myth go!

Dr. Hobbins is retired now, but when he was performing surgery, he had a favorite nurse who worked twelve-hour days with him, assisting five to seven complicated surgeries per day. She called in one day because she was literally paralyzed; she couldn't move. At the hospital, she was immediately hooked up to a saline solution. Dr. Hobbins observed her as she slowly moved her fingers, then her hands, and in an hour she was up—he said it was like a miracle. Lack of salt makes you *weak*!

Just recently, one of Dr. Hobbins' former patients called him for advice with regard to her fatigue. She traveled all over the world and saw many specialists, and even went to the Mayo Clinic, but no one could diagnose her problem. Her condition was a complete mystery. Dr. Hobbins asked about her sodium intake, to which she replied "very low," as she had high blood pressure. He told her, "Salt *everything*!" Two weeks later, he received a beautiful card expressing her gratitude for so simply solving the problem that several specialists could not. Dr. Hobbins cannot help but chuckle when he tells that story.

Don't worry about getting any special nine-dollar-a-bottle salt; simply get regular iodized salt. Unfortunately, due to the pollution of our oceans microplastics are now in showing up in our sea salt and it is advised to avoid this once nutritious source.

The information above can be easily tested if you are a skeptic. Measure your blood pressure at least three times per day, as this will give you a more accurate reading. After a few days of establishing your approximate blood pressure, slowly add salt to your diet while continuing to regularly monitor your blood pressure. Please consult your physician if you are on any medications before trying this dietary change.

It is also important to keep in mind that, as you get older, your blood pressure naturally increases. This occurs because your blood vessels harden and lose elasticity as you age. Not only do very few doctors share this with their patients, but they continue to prescribe elderly patients blood pressure medications for having levels above what, say, a thirty-year-old should have. This inevitably results in a systemic pressure increase due to the decreased ability of the arteries and veins to "give" in response to the heart's powerful force. If your BP is 130–150 at 50–70, this is normal for aging.

Functioning adrenals are mandatory for health. Don't exhaust yours, ladies. It will prematurely age you.

## It's Called Beauty Sleep for a Reason

Another secret to a healthy life is sleep. Sounds easy, but I am surprised by the amount of sleep-deprived people there are. Most people need seven to ten hours—if you are not getting enough you need to fix this problem. The only excuse to this Breast Cancer Boot Camp protocol is women with small children, for obvious reasons. Sleep is the time when the body rests and rejuvenates itself from all the taxing activities of the day. It is called beauty sleep for a reason, and if you are not sleeping soundly throughout the night and waking up without an alarm, you are aging yourself.

If you have sleeping problems, are unable to fall asleep, are waking during the night or waking early, go to a holistic doctor, either Chinese, Ayurvedic, or homeopathic. They can treat your sleeping disorder.

If possible, take naps. When your kids take a nap, I know you want to get chores done, but if you are sleep deprived you should also take a nap with them. This will make you stronger mentally and physically. For people who work hard go home and take a nap after work, I do. If you are not a nap person then you need to go to bed early.

Ladies, sleep is another vital protocol to Breast Cancer Boot Camp. If you make this change, you will be surprised how much stronger you will feel. When you awake rested, you can tackle the day with a smile.

# Moderate Exercise: These Boots are Made for Walking

Excessive exercise, including cardio for more than twenty minutes straight, may be too taxing for the adrenals. To maintain proper weight, one should only work out for about twenty to thirty minutes a day. This is obviously different for everybody and these twenty minutes of working out, heavy lifting, whether through weights, resistance training, or body weight exercises.

It is also important to run and walk to maintain an active lifestyle. If a person exercises every day, but then sits in front of a computer for the rest of it that is not considered active. Notice that I said "run" and "walk," not "jog." It surprises me that every "jogger" refers to themselves as a "runner." This will step on many people's toes, but running and jogging are as different as running and walking. Furthermore, most of the joggers that I come across have horrible stride and form, and cannot actually run at all.

Jogging is very hard on the joints, as it creates a hard collision contact with the ground without much forward momentum. When I say run, I actually mean sprint. Sprint till you can't run anymore. Your body easily finds a correct functional stride, versus jogging which I consider just falling forward. If you start sprinting you will feel the difference in your legs. You are engaging your muscles in a full stride, lifting high, and pushing off. This engages your tendons and ligaments in your knees and ankles which minimizes injury versus jogging. Sprinting is hard, jogging is easy. Sprinting creates strength. Jogging drains energy. Sprint just a couple blocks, start with one, maybe two, and build up. Just run for a few minutes. I do a fifteen-minute walk sprint. Some days, I sprint more, some days I walk more, listen to your body and what it is capable of daily. I think you will be surprised at how strong you feel switching to correct cardio.

If a person exercises beyond their ability, they are most likely taxing their adrenals. The adrenals are primitive; they register that the body is overworking, and in response, they initiate fat retention and storage to preserve energy. You may know, or be, a person who works out like crazy, thirty or more minutes of cardio, but to no effect. This is the reason why—over taxation. Take it easy, move often, and when working out, make the time count with intense but short exercise.

Why do we seem to gain weight in our late thirties? Because we don't go out dancing like we did when we were younger. Ahhh…remember those nights, well, some of them anyways? Ladies, drop book club and form dance club! Get the girls together and dance, it is fun exercise. You don't have to always go out. Play DJ and stay in.

## Become a Wild Child

Become a wild child again. Play outside, breathe, soak in the sun and laugh, especially around trees and the water. Studies have found trees emit oils, called phytoncides, that assist our immune system. Love the water? There is a new term – "blue mind." The Journal of Environmental Psychology says within 3 hours of being by a body of water people report feeling refreshed and revitalized.

Time outdoors has also been proven to lower stress, which will strengthen your immunity, naturally. Besides, who doesn't love a little time with Mother Nature. Soak up that sun and is the perfect way to get a daily dose of vitamin D. While you're at it get in a little exercise, walk, sprint, or stretch and just breathe in the fresh air. For the busy ladies, kill two birds with one stone – exercise outside.

The sun nourishes and strengthens us. At the Karolinska Institute in Sweden they conducted a study with 30, 000 women for over twenty years, which found that "women who avoided lying out in the sun were twice as likely to die compared to those who make sunbathing a daily ritual."

More research is proving the sun doesn't cause cancer, but the chemicals in sunscreen are carcinogenic. Elizabeth Plourde, Ph.D., "has shown that malignant melanoma and all other skin cancers increased significantly with ubiquitous sunscreen use over a 30-year period." When we are outside the wavelengths from the light is absorbed into the eyes and sends signals to the pituitary gland which triggers hormones to be released for skin protection. This is another reason why it is imperative to not wear sunglasses.

As we discussed in the vitamin D section wearing sunglasses is unhealthy. It is because sunglasses have blocked out therapeutic wavelengths or spectrums the body requires. We are just like plants, we need sunlight to grow! Well, shoes do the same thing, they insulate us from the earth or ground. We live and grow from the earth and sun, just like plants, shoes and sunglass keep us from growing and being healthy because they shield us from the electrical impulses, frequencies and wavelengths.

Clint Ober, grounding pioneer, discovered in the 1960's the importance of grounding electrical cable wires into the ground, which is simply called grounding. If lightening would strike the cable wires in the neighborhood grounding them to the earth would prevent electrical appliances in the houses from being destroyed. He thought if wires need grounding what about humans?

The human body has electrical impulses that uses frequencies for communication and health benefits. The earth is also electrical, and when we have contact with it through our bare feet or skin we absorb the healing electrons supplied by the earth to support specific functions of the organs and systems of the body. This is called "Grounding" or "Earthing." Research has shown grounding reduces inflammation, increases better sleep and benefits the heart. Walk, sit, stand on sand, grass, dirt, or concrete, and if possible, wet surfaces which are better at conduction. Wood, asphalt, and vinyl are not conductive.

Get outside every day to stay healthy. Kick off your shoes and ditch the sunglasses and sunscreen. Holistic breast health provided by Mother Nature.

## Bra Basics

Do bras increase risk of breast cancer? Dr. Ray Lawson, Dr. Hobbins' teacher, attempted to study the thermographic effects of bras on the native population in Canada in the 60s. His hypothesis for the study was that bras increased risk for cancer and wanted to monitor changes with thermography. He distributed bras to the women of one village and had a control group with another village where no bras were distributed. He didn't realize the culture of trading and when he returned the bras had been traded to the control group, so the study was tainted.

Dr. Hobbins and I believe bras cause stagnation and don't allow for proper circulation in the upper body, especially to the lymph located under the arm. From a Chinese medical standpoint, there are meridians that run alone the breasts, bras may cause an obstruction.

In the US, it is socially proper to wear a bra, if you do not have a problem with social norms then be free. For those of us who aren't that brave, remove your bra as soon as you return home from work or outside activities. Do not wear a bra to bed! This includes sports bras. Try not to use an underwire if possible.

Get fitted when buying bras. The cup should enclose all of the breast tissue and not cut off the sides of the breast. Use the straps to adjust the top of the cup. It should not be too tight that the breast bulge over or too loose and cause a gap. The band should be on the loosest hook and should not be too tight that it pinches. A perfect fit should be comfortable. I suggest having an everyday comfortable bra for long work hours and then have a "party" bra or push-up or sexy bra for special occasions. Heck, every girl needs one to feel special or sexy.

## Massage: Hand to Hand Combat

Massage cannot reduce vascular stimulation in the breasts! We have not been able to prove that massage can reduce vascularity with thermography. Massage is extremely beneficial to the breasts, but cannot reverse the underlying condition. Breast massage can aid lymph drainage, reduce cysts and promote circulation. I suggest a quick self-breast massage everyday when applying progesterone cream. This is also a good time to familiarize yourself with your breasts, so any changes are noticed early.

Many women have told me that they don't like to massage their breasts. I have a couple of alternatives. First, have your partner massage your breasts; just like when you need a back rub, request a breast massage. Grab some coconut oil and have them rub small circles with their fingertips or softly knead the breasts for just a couple minutes once or twice a week. Gentle shaking or vibration is also beneficial. Warning: This could be fun and sometimes leads to lovemaking, which also strengthens passion or libido and more importantly, your relationship.

Gua Sha is an incredible form of alternative massage that can benefit the breasts. This is holistic breast health from Chinese medicine. Gua Sha is scraping of the skin, translated to combing the sand, with a smooth tool to bring blood flow or circulation to areas in need. It is *not* bruising, that is the Sha, which looks like sand. If you don't need it, then it won't turn red; that is how you know what areas need increased circulation and healing. This is an alternative to increase blood flow, circulation and possibly decrease fibroids or stagnation. Yes, I do it and love it. Watch videos on my You Tube channel on how to do it, what you need, and what to avoid.

For women who want to decrease cysts, fibroids, and masses in the breasts, I suggest castor oil massaged into the breasts then apply a heating pad to increase circulation. This can be done daily if desired for 15-20 minutes. Castor oil has properties that breakdown accumulations in the breasts.

If imaging before and after a massage to "see" changes in breasts, images *have* to be in reverse gray, since color does not display the blood vessels. Color will detect differences created by creams and oils which are reflective to the infrared camera so don't trust color images. Another issue with color is, massage will create increased circulation which will increase heat in the breasts. To get a correct image, the breasts have to be exposed to the cold stress challenge, which will cool the breasts. So if imaging before and after massage without use of oils, the breasts are required to be properly cooled for thermography with the cold stress challenge.

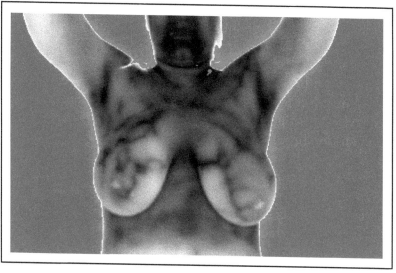

This thermogram is from a physician who teaches a specialized "weekly self breast massage" protocol to her patients and other physicians. Note unusual vascular pattern.

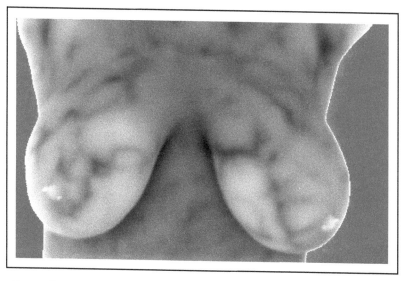

Repeat thermogram two years later. Note persistent unusual vascular pattern after two years of weekly self massage.

# Self-Exam: Self Reliance

Self-exam in the is still the best way to personally monitor your breast health, feeling for anything that is new or unusual. So, let's make it simple and easy!

Self-exam should be done once a month after the corpus leuteum phase, or right after your period when estrogen is decreasing also reducing stimulation to the breasts. For post-menopausal women they should have no estrogen stimulation, since the body stopped creating estrogen, and anytime of the month is fine.

Frist, and this is key, look for any changes in the skin, dimpling, thickening or nipple inversion. These are what are called yellow flags and you need to see your gynecologist for their assistance.

The best time in is the shower where you can make a slick barrier for your fingers to slide across with soap. For the breast you are going to check put your arm above your head or rest on shower wall, this will lift and stretch the tissue, optimizing the exam. Start at the fringe or edge of your breasts using the tips of your second, third and fourth fingers and gently apply pressure or press down, since you are soaped up move slowly in a spiraling circle starting at the edge of your breasts moving inwards, still spiraling in a circle till you reach your nipple and areola, which you will also want to press gently down on this area too.

Many women have found their breast cancers with self-exam when mammograms missed them. It is considered preventive care.

# Honorable Discharge

Though simple and easy, once incorporated into your life, *Breast Cancer Boot Camp* is effective and life-saving. I hope that this book helps to change your life just as Dr. Hobbins changed mine. My goal is to reach as many women as possible, young and old, so that they can be given a fighting chance against this horrible disease. Take up arms of knowledge, recruit your fellow woman, and start a revolution for life. Restore the confidence of a healthy life, enjoy yourself along the journey, and remember that there is no reason for any of us to lay down our weapons, retreat, or become another fallen soldier...after all, our breasts are meant to nourish life, not be the end of it!

# Appendix A: Collateral Damage

L ist of side effects taken from pharmaceutical companies. Names of drugs are not revealed just the side effects, so may differ with each name brand.

## 1. Progestin: synthetic form of progesterone

*Contraindications*

Thrombophlebitis, thromboembolic disorders, cerebral apoplexy; liver dysfunction or disease; known or suspected malignancy of breast or genital organs; undiagnosed vaginal bleeding; missed abortion; known or suspected pregnancy.

*Precautions*

Because progestin may cause some degree of fluid retention, conditions which might be influenced by this factor, such as epilepsy, migraine, asthma, cardiac or renal dysfunction, require careful observation.

May cause breakthrough bleeding or menstrual irregularities.

May cause or contribute to depression.

The effect of prolonged use of this drug on pituitary, ovarian, adrenal, hepatic, or uterine function is unknown.

May decrease glucose tolerance; diabetic patients must be carefully monitored.

May increase the thrombotic disorders associated with estrogens.

*Adverse Reactions*

Breast tenderness and galactorrhea
Sensitivity reaction such as urticaria, pruritus, edema, or rash
Acne, alopecia, and hirsutism (excess hair growth)
Edema, weight changes

Cervical erosions and changes in cervical secretions
Cholestatic jaundice
Mental depression, pyrexia, nausea, insomnia, or somnolence
Anaphylactoid reaction and anaphylaxis
Thrombophlebitis and pulmonary embolism
Break through bleeding, spotting, amenorrhea, or changes in menses
Fatigue, backache, itching, dizziness, nervousness, loss of scalp hair

*When taken with Estrogens, the Following Have Been Observed*

- Rise in blood pressure, headache, dizziness, nervousness, and fatigue
- Change in sex drive, hirsutism and loss of scalp hair, decrease in T3 uptake values
- PMS like syndrome, change in appetite
- UTIs
- Erythema multiforme, erythema nodosum, hemorrhagic eruption, and itching

*Side Effects Taken from the Mayo Clinic*

Along with their needed effects, progestins used in high doses sometimes cause some unwanted effects such as blood clots, heart attacks and strokes, or problems of the liver and eyes. Although these effects are rare, some of them can be very serious and cause death. It is not clear if these problems are due to the progestin. They may be caused by the disease or condition for which progestins are being used.

The following side effects may be caused by blood clots. Although not all of these side effects may occur, if they do occur they need immediate medical attention.

Get emergency help immediately if any of the following side effects occur:

*Rare*

Symptoms of blood clotting problems, usually severe or sudden, such as:

- Headache or migraine
- Loss of or change in speech, coordination, or vision
- Numbness of or pain in chest, arm, or leg
- Unexplained shortness of breath

Check with your doctor as soon as possible if any of the following side effects occur:

*More Common*

- Changes in vaginal bleeding (increased amounts of menstrual bleeding occurring at regular monthly periods, lighter vaginal bleeding between menstrual periods, heavier vaginal bleeding between regular monthly periods, or stopping of menstrual periods)
- Symptoms of blood sugar problems (dry mouth, frequent urination, loss of appetite, or unusual thirst)

*Less Common*

- Mental depression
- Skin rash
- Unexpected or increased flow of breast milk

*Rare For Megestrol—During Chronic Treatment*

- Backache
- Dizziness
- Filling or rounding out of the face
- Irritability
- Mental depression
- Nausea or vomiting
- Unusual decrease in sexual desire or ability in men
- Unusual tiredness or weakness

Some side effects may occur that usually do not need medical attention. These side effects may go away during treatment as your body adjusts to the medicine. Also, your health care professional may be able to tell you about ways to prevent or reduce some of these side effects. Check with your health care professional if any of the following side effects continue or are bothersome or if you have any questions about them:

*More Common*

- Abdominal pain or cramping
- Bloating or swelling of ankles or feet
- Blood pressure increase (mild)
- Dizziness
- Drowsiness (progesterone only)
- Headache (mild)
- Mood changes
- Nervousness
- Pain or irritation at place of injection site
- Swelling of face, ankles, or feet
- Unusual or rapid weight gain

*Less Common*

- Acne
- Breast pain or tenderness
- Brown spots on exposed skin, possibly long-lasting
- Hot flashes
- Loss or gain of body, facial, or scalp hair
- Loss of sexual desire
- Trouble in sleeping

Not all of the side effects listed above have been reported for each of these medicines, but they have been reported for at least one of them. All of the progestins are similar, so any of the above side effects may occur with any of these medicines.

After you stop using this medicine, your body may need time to adjust. The length of time this takes depends on the amount of medicine you were using and how long you used it. During this period of time check with your doctor if you notice the following side effects:

- Delayed return to fertility
- Stopping of menstrual periods
- Unusual menstrual bleeding (continuing)

*For Megestrol*

- Dizziness
- Nausea or vomiting
- Unusual tiredness or weakness

Other side effects not listed may also occur in some patients. If you notice any other effects, check with your healthcare professional.

Call your doctor for medical advice about side effects.

## 2. Estrogen Patch Side Effects Provided by Manufacturer

Estrogens have been reported to increase the chance of womb (endometrial) cancer.

Estrogen containing products should not be used to prevent heart disease or dementia.

Estrogen given alone or in combination with another hormone (progestin) for replacement therapy may increase your risk of:

- Heart disease (e.g., heart attacks)
- Stroke
- Serious blood clots in the legs (deep vein thrombosis) or lungs (pulmonary embolism)
- Dementia
- Breast cancer

These risks appear to depend on the length of time patch is used and the amount of estrogen per dose. Therefore patch should be used for the shortest possible length of time at the lowest effective dose, so that you obtain the benefits and minimize the chance of serious side effects from long term treatment. Consult your doctor or pharmacist for details.

Do not use patch if:

- You are allergic to any ingredient in the patch
- You have known or suspected breast cancer or other cancer that is estrogen dependent
- You have blood clots, circulation disorders, liver problems, or the blood disease porphyria
- You have had a recent heart attack or stroke
- You are pregnant, or suspect you may be pregnant, have recently given birth or are breast feeding, have vaginal bleeding of abnormal or unknown cause or have cancer of the uterus

## 3. IUD with Hormones Side Effects for the Consumer Provided by Manufacturer

Acne, back pain, breast pain, or tenderness, changes in menstrual bleeding (e.g., spotting), changes in sex drive, dizziness, lightheadedness, bleeding or cramping during placement, headache, nausea, vomiting, weight gain.

Seek medical attention right away if any of these *severe* side effects occur when using IUD with hormones:

- Severe allergic reactions (rash, hives, itching, difficulty breathing, tightness of the chest, swelling of the mouth face, lips, or tongue)
- Breast lumps
- Changes in vision
- Chills and fever
- Genital sores
- Mental or mood changes (e.g., depression)
- Missed menstrual period
- Numbness of an arm or leg
- Painful sexual intercourse
- Prolonged heavy menstrual bleeding,
- Severe pain or tenderness in the abdomen or pelvis
- Sharp or crushing chest pain
- Sudden leg pain

- Sudden severe headache
- Vomiting
- Dizziness or fainting
- Sudden shortness of breath
- Unusual or odorous vaginal discharge
- Unusual vaginal swelling or bleeding
- Yellowing of the skin or eyes.
- This is not a complete list of all side effects that may occur.

## IUD with Hormones Side Effects for the Professional Provided by Manufacturer

The following most serious adverse reactions associated with the use of the IUD with hormones are discussed in greater detail in the warnings and precautions sections:

- Ectopic pregnancy
- Intrauterine pregnancy
- Group A streptococcal sepsis
- Pelvic Inflammatory Disease
- Embedment
- Perforation
- Breast cancer
- The most common adverse reactions (>5 percent users)
- Uterine/vaginal bleeding alterations (51.9 percent)
- Amenorrhea (23.9 percent)
- Intermenstrual bleeding and spotting (23.4 percent)
- Abdominal/pelvic pain (12.8 percent)
- Ovarian cysts (12 percent)
- Headache/migraine (7.7)
- Acne (7.2 percent)
- Depressed/altered mood (6.4 percent)
- Menorrhagia (6.3 percent)
- Breast tenderness/pain (4.9 percent)
- Vaginal discharge (4.9 percent)
- IUD expulsion (4 percent)

# 4. Estrogen Shot/Injectable Suspension Manufacture Is Currently Involved in a
## Class Action Suit. Information Below
## Taken From Law Firm:

The most serious problems are long term adverse side effects of osteoporosis, hip joint fracture, loss of bone density, or loss of height or shrinking. Less serious side effects are:

- Menstrual irregularities, including bleeding and spotting
- Amenorrhea or not having any periods
- Spotty darkening of the skin, usually around or on the face
- Weight gain due to increased appetite from shot
- Pregnancy-like symptoms which include sore breasts, nausea, fatigue, abdominal discomfort, that may occur after first 4 injections, but usually go away
- After a year of the injections, 57 percent of women are not menstruating
- After 2 years of the injections, 68 percent of women are not menstruating
- After stopping injections, period may return within 3-10 months, some may never get period again
- After the last injection, a significant side effect is that it takes an average of 9-12 months to become pregnant

Researchers in England found that women using long term injections for birth control are more likely to have low bone mass density that women who opt for other birth control methods.

Another study conducted in Italy found that more than 40 percent of women who had injections for 12 months or more had the side effect of a lower that average bone density. The expected rate of low bone mass density in women of a young age is only 18 percent.

Both studies conclude that young women taking birth control injections show a decrease in bone mass density at an age when it should be increasing. Low bone density is associated with osteoporosis, a disease that causes the bones to become so thin that they can break with just a minor bump or fall.

## Estrogen Shot/Injectable Suspension Side Effects for the Consumer Provided by Manufacturer

Acne, dizziness, drowsiness, fever, headache, hot flashes, nausea, pain, redness and swelling at injection site, sleeplessness, and weakness.

Seek medical attention right away if any of these *severe* side effects occur when using estrogen shot/injectable suspension:

- Severe allergic reactions (rash, hives, itching, difficulty breathing, tightness in the chest, swelling of the mouth, face, lips or tongue)
- Blood clots
- Changes in menstrual flow including breakthrough bleeding, spotting, or missed periods
- Chest pain
- Mental or mood changes
- Partial or complete loss of vision or change in vision
- Severe dizziness or fainting
- Severe stomach pain
- Shortness of breath
- Slurred speech
- Sudden loss of coordination
- Sudden or severe headache or vomiting
- Swelling of fingers or ankles
- Unusual weight gain or loss
- Weakness, numbness, or pain in the arms or legs
- Yellowing of the skin or eyes
  This is not a complete list of all side effects that may occur

## Estrogen Shot/Injectable Suspension Side Effects for the Professional Provided by Manufacturer

The following important adverse reactions observed with the use of estrogen shot are discussed in greater detail in the warning and precautions section:

- Loss of bone mineral density
- Thromboembolic disease (blood clots)
- Breast cancer
- Anaphylaxis and anaphylactiod reactions
- Bleeding irregularities
- Weight gain

## 5. Estrogen Vaginal Ring Was FDA Approved as Safe. Now, More Than 100 Lawsuits Have Been Filed Alleging the Ring Side Effects Caused Serious Health Problems

## Estrogen Vaginal Ring Side Effects for the Professional Provided by Manufacturer

- Blood clots
- Strokes and heart attacks
- High blood pressure and heart disease

*Breast Cancer and Reproductive Organs*
Breast cancer has been diagnosed with slightly more often in women who use the pill than in women of the same age who do not use the pill. This small increase in the number of breast cancer diagnoses gradually disappears during the 10 years after stopping use of the pill. It is not known whether the difference is caused by the pill. It may be that women taking the pill are examined more often, so that breast cancer is more likely to be detected.

Women who have currently have or have had breast cancer should not use hormonal contraceptives, including the ring, because breast cancer is usually a hormone sensitive tumor.

Some studies have found an increase in the incidence of cancer of the cervix in women who use oral contraceptives. However, this finding may be related to factors other than the use of oral contraceptives.

- Gallbladder disease
- Liver tumors/cancer
- Lipid metabolism and inflammation of the pancreas

The common side effects reported by the ring users are as reported by the manufacturer:

- Vaginal infections and irritation
- Vaginal secretion
- Headache
- Weight gain
- Nausea
- Vomiting
- Change in appetite
- Abdominal cramps
- Breast tenderness or enlargement
- Irregular vaginal bleeding or spotting
- Changes in menstrual cycle
- Temporary infertility after treatment
- Fluid retention
- Spotty darkening of the skin, particularly on the face
- Rash
- Weight changes
- Depression
- Intolerance to contact lenses
- Nervousness
- Dizziness
- Loss of scalp hair

Call your doctor right away if you get any of the symptoms listed below. They may be signs of a serious problem.

- Sharp chest pain, coughing blood, or sudden shortness of breath (possible clot in lung)
- Pain in the calf (possible clot in the leg)
- Crushing chest pain or heaviness in the chest (possible heart attack)
- Sudden severe headache or vomiting, dizziness or fainting, problems with vision or speech, weakness, or numbness in an arm or leg (possible stroke)
- Sudden partial or complete loss of vision (possible clot of the eye)
- Yellowing of the skin or whites of the eyes (jaundice), especially with fever, tiredness, loss of appetite, dark colored urine, or light-colored bowel movements (possible liver problems)
- Severe pain, swelling, or tenderness in the abdomen (gallbladder or liver problems)
- Sudden fever (usually 102 degrees F or more), vomiting, diarrhea, dizziness, fainting, or a sunburn-like rash on the face or body (very rarely toxic shock syndrome)
- Breast lumps (possible breast cancer or benign breast disease)
- Irregular vaginal bleeding or spotting that happens in more than 1 menstrual cycle or lasts for more than few days
- Urgent, frequent, burning and/or painful urination, and cannot locate the ring in the vagina (rarely accidental placement of ring in the urinary bladder)
- Swelling of your fingers and ankles
- Difficulty sleeping, weakness, lack of energy, fatigue, or a change in mood (possible severe depression)

# 6. Vaginal Cream Side Effects Provided by Manufacturer

Important safety information:

Using estrogen-alone may increase your chance of getting cancer of the uterus. Report any unusual vaginal bleeding right away while you are using vaginal cream. Vaginal bleeding after menopause may be a warning sign of cancer of the uterus. Your healthcare provider should check any unusual vaginal bleeding to find the cause. Do not use estrogen alone or estrogens with progestin to prevent heart disease, heart attacks strokes or dementia. Using estrogen-alone may increase your chances of getting strokes or blood clots.

Possible side effects of vaginal cream

- Breast cancer
- Cancer of the uterus
- Stroke
- Heart attack
- Blood clots
- Dementia
- Gallbladder disease
- Ovarian cancer
- High blood pressure
- Liver problems
- High blood sugar
- Enlargement of benign tumors

Some of the warning signs of these serious side effects include:

- Breast lumps
- Unusual vaginal bleeding
- Dizziness and faintness
- Changes in speech
- Severe headaches
- Chest pain
- Shortness of breath

- Pains in your legs
- Changes in vision
- Vomiting
- Yellowing of the skin, eyes, or nail beds

Call your health care provider right away if you get any of these warning signs, or any other unusual symptoms that concern you. Less serious, but common side effects include:

- Headache
- Breast pain
- Irregular vaginal bleeding or spotting
- Stomach/abdominal cramps, bloating
- Nausea and vomiting
- Hair loss
- Fluid retention yeast infection
- Reactions from inserting Vaginal Cream, such as vaginal burning, irritation and itching.

# Appendix B

Estrogens and Breast Cancer: A Chronology by Carol Ann Rinzler

1929:   The first estrogen (estrone) is isolated and identified

1931:   First American woman given first injection of estrogen

1932:   Estrogen injections produce malignant breast tumors in male laboratory mice

1934:   First use of estrogens to treat symptoms of menopause

1937:   Natural female hormones used to suppress ovulation in laboratory rabbits at Penn State University

*The incidence of breast cancer in the United States is 67 cases per 100,000 (white) women*

1938:   Chemists at Schering Company produce estrogen pills

1940:   The first oral estrogens for ERT go on sale

Scientists at the National Cancer Institute find synthetic estrogen diethylstilbestrol (DES) produces breast tumors in male and female laboratory mice

The leading causes of cancer deaths among American women are cancer of the uterus and cancer of the stomach

*The incidence of breast cancer in the United States is 59 cases for every 100,000 women*

*An American woman's lifetime risk of breast cancer in 1-in-20*

1941: More than a dozen brands of estrogen are available for treatment of menopausal and menstrual disorders

1944: Syntex, a pharmaceutical company, created to manufacture and sell synthetic progesterone

1945: Cancer researcher discovered that a chemical's ability to stimulate unregulated cell growth is one measure of its potential carcinogenicity

1950: *The incidence of breast cancer in the United States is 65 cases for every 100,000 women*

*An American woman's lifetime risk of breast cancer in 1-in-15*

1951: Birth control pioneer Margaret Sanger makes first donation to support Gregory Goodman Pincus' research on chemical contraceptives

Syntex steroid chemist Carl Djerassi patents nonethindrone, the first effective oral progestin

1955: More than thirty brands of estrogen products on the market: injectable solutions, pills, ointments, suppositories, and nasal sprays

1956: G.D. Searle and Planned Parenthood begin trials of the estrogen/progestin birth control pill in Puerto Rico

1957: FDA approves use of estrogen/progestin combination for medical conditions such as menstrual disorders

1960: FDA grants permission for Searle to market an estrogen/progestin product, Enovid-10 as an oral contraceptive

*The Merck Index* publishes its first warning of a link between estrogen and cancer of the breast and reproductive organs

*The incidence of breast cancer in the United States is 72 cases for every 100,000 women*

*An American woman's lifetime risk of breast cancer is now 1-in-15*

1961:   800,000 American women fill their first prescription for an oral contraceptive

1962:   FDA approves a second oral contraceptive, Ortho Pharmaceuticals' Ortho-Novum

1963:   1.2 million American women are using the Pill

Robert Wilson meets "Mrs. P.G.," the woman whose use of Enovid-10 keeps her "young" at age fifty

1965:   1-in-4 married American women have used or is using birth control pills

1966:   Robert Wilson publishes *Feminine Forever*; estimates that in 1967 the number of "sexually restored, post-menopausal women" will pass 14,000

1969:   British Committee on Safety of drugs recommends banning oral contraceptives containing more that 50 mcg estrogen

The First National Conference on Breast Cancer, sponsored by the American Cancer Society (ACS) and the U.S Public Health Service, convenes in Washington D.C.

*The ACS predicts 29,000 female breast cancer deaths*

*The incidence of breast cancer in the United States is 72.5 cases for every 100,000 white; 60.1 cases for every 100,000 black women*

1970:   First warning (blood clots) included in package insert for oral contraceptives

8.5 million American women are using birth control pills; 65 percent of them are "high dose" products with more that 50 mcg of estrogen

The American Medical Association's Council on Drugs says that estrogen may stimulate existing breast tumors to malignant activity

*The incidence of breast cancer in the United States is 74 cases for every 100,000 women*

*An American woman's lifetime risk of breast cancer is now 1-in-13*

1971:   Synthetic estrogen (DES) reported to cause vaginal cancers in daughter of women who took the drug while pregnant

Second National Conference on Breast Cancer convenes in Los Angeles

1972:   *Breast cancer is now the leading cause of cancer deaths among American women*

1973:   10 million American women, including 36 percent of all married women, are using birth control pills

1974:   70 percent of all married American women have a "favorable view" of the Pill

5 million American women are using estrogen to relieve menopausal symptoms

*The ACS predicts 90,000 new cases of female breast cancer and 33,000 female breast cancer deaths*

1975:   An NCI study shows a six- to elevenfold increase in incidence of breast cancer among women with prior history of benign breast disease who had used the Pill for more than six years

Four separate studies show an increase as high as 50 percent in the incidence of endometrial cancer among women using estrogen products

1976:   22.3 percent of all fertile American women are using oral contraceptives

Approximately 6 million women are using ERT

Study of one doctor's practice in Kentucky show an overall 30 percent increased risk of breast cancer among women using ERT

1977:   *The incidence of breast cancer in the United States is 81 cases for every 100,000 women*

1980:   19 percent of American women of childbearing age use the Pill

17 percent of all birth control pills sold in the United States still contain more than 50 mcg estrogen

A study in two Los Angeles retirement communities shows an 80 percent higher risk of breast cancer among women who take a cumulative lifetime dose of 1,500 mcg estrogen

*The incidence of breast cancer in the United States is 90 cases for every 100,000 women*

*An American woman's lifetime risk of breast cancer is now 1-in-11*

1981:   Research at the University of Southern California finds a significant increase in the incidence of breast cancer among women who use oral contraceptives before a first full-term pregnancy

Researchers from the National Institute of Health publish study of 1,600 women in twenty-nine cancer centers across the country showing that use of ERT may raise a woman's risk of breast cancer to nearly seven times higher than normal

1982:   Following publicity about acute effects of oral contraceptives (blood clots, migraine, heart attacks, stroke), the percentage of American married women using the Pill falls to 19.8

1983:   17 million prescriptions are written for estrogen

Second California study shows that women who use the Pill for more than four years before their first full-term pregnancy or before age twenty-five are four times more likely to develop breast cancer before age forty-five

1984:   *New England Journal of Medicine* reports a 47 percent higher incidence of breast cancer among 4 million women who used DES while pregnant

*The ACS predicts 115,000 new cases of female breast cancer*

1985:   11.8 million American women age eighteen to forty-four are using the Pill, the leading reversible method of birth control in the United States; 25 percent of them are using it longer that five years

1986:   Nearly 12.5 million American women age fifteen to forty-four are using the Pill

FDA approves Estraderm, CIBA Pharmaceutical's new patch that delivers continue allow doses of estrogen through the skin for post-menopausal ERT

*The ACS predicts 123,000 new cases of female breast cancer and 39,900 deaths*

1987: CASH study shows a more-than-200 percent increase in risk of breast cancer among fifty- to fifty-four-year-old women whose ovaries have been removed or who have a family history of breast cancer and who use ERT

*An American woman's lifetime risk of breast cancer is now 1-in-10*

1988:   Approximately 14 million American women age fifteen to forty-four are using the Pill

Nineteen years after the British have acted, the FDA recommends removing from the market all oral contraceptives containing more than 50 mcg estrogen

*The ACS predicts 135,000 new cases of female breast cancer and 42,300 deaths*

1989: Nurses Health Study (121,000 married female nurses) show that women currently using oral contraceptives are 60 percent more likely than nonusers to develop breast cancer

3.5 million American women are using ERT

*The incidence of breast cancer in the America is 105 cases per 100,000 women*

1990: 26 percent of American women of childbearing age are using the Pill

Nurses Health Study shows that women who use ERT are 30 to 40 percent more likely than nonusers to develop breast cancer

Incidence of ER+ tumors among American women is increasing five times faster than incidence of ER-negative tumors

*The ACS predicts 150,000 new cases of female breast cancer and 44,300 deaths*

1991: 16 million American women ager fifteen to forty-four are using The Pill; 37 percent of them for five years or longer

15 percent of all post-menopausal American women are using ERT

A meta-analysis from the U.S. Centers of Disease Control attributes 4, 708 new cases of breast cancer and 1.468 deaths a year to use of ERT

*An American woman's lifetime risk of breast cancer is now 1-in-9*

*The ACS predicts 175,000 new cases of female breast cancer and 44,500 deaths*

1992:   *The National Cancer Institute predicts 180,000 new cases of female breast cancer and 46,000 deaths*

*An American woman's lifetime risk of breast cancer is now 1-in-8*

## Chronology continued by Wendy Sellens, DAOM

2000:   *The AAFP predicts 182,800 new female cases of breast cancer and 48,800 deaths*

2005:   *The ACS predicts 211,240 new cases of female invasive breast cancer and 58, 490 of in situ breast cancer and 40,410 deaths*

*The ACS predicts 1,690 cases of breast cancer in men and 460 deaths*

2011:   *The ACS predicts 230,480 new cases of female invasive breast cancer and 57,650 of in situ breast cancer and 39,520 deaths.*

*The ACS predicts 2,140 cases of breast cancer in men and about 1 percent of breast cancers and 450 deaths]*

2017:   *The ACS predicts an estimated 252,710 new cases of female invasive breast cancer with approximately 40,610 deaths.*

*The ACS predicts 2,470 cases of bresat cancer in MEN and 460 men are expected to die from breast cancer in 2017.*

# Appendix C

Phytoestrogen Content of Fruits & Vegetables by Gunter G.C. Kuhnle, et.al. Comprised by Paleo for Women.

| Food (taxonomic name) | Preparation | Variety | Family | Phytoestrogens | Isoflavones | Lignans |
|---|---|---|---|---|---|---|
| Apple (*Malus domestica*) | Cored | Cox | Rosaceae | 4 | 2 | 2 |
| Apple (*Malus domestica*) | Cored | Golden Delicious | Rosaceae | 5 | 2 | 3 |
| Apple (*Malus domestica*) | Cored | Granny Smith | Rosaceae | 4 | 2 | 2 |
| Apple (*Malus domestica*) | Cored | Red dessert | Rosaceae | 3 | 1 | 2 |
| Apple (*Malus domestica*) | Peeled, cored & cooked | Cooking apple | Rosaceae | 9 | 7 | 2 |
| Apple (*Malus domestica*) | Peeled & cored | Cooking apple | Rosaceae | 5 | 3 | 2 |
| Apple (*Malus domestica*) | Peeled & cored | Cox | Rosaceae | 5 | 2 | 2 |
| Apple (*Malus domestica*) | Peeled & cored | Golden Delicious | Rosaceae | 5 | 3 | 2 |
| Apple (*Malus domestica*) | Peeled & cored | Granny Smith | Rosaceae | 4 | 2 | 2 |
| Apple (*Malus domestica*) | Peeled & cored | Red dessert | Rosaceae | 2 | <1 | <1 |
| Apricot (*Prunus armeniaca*) | Stoned | | Rosaceae | 53 | 1 | 52 |
| Apricot (*Prunus armeniaca*) | Dried | | Rosaceae | 443 | 12 | 431 |
| Apricot (*Prunus armeniaca*) | Tinned in syrup, drained | | Rosaceae | 24 | 2 | 22 |
| Asparagus (*Asparagus officinalis*) | Cooked | | Asparagaceae | 154 | 2 | 152 |
| Aubergine (*Solanum melongena*) | Raw | | Solanaceae | 9 | <1 | 8 |
| Aubergine (*Solanum melongena*) | Cooked | | Solanaceae | 8 | <1 | 8 |

_Wendy Sellens, DACM, LAc_

| | | | | | | |
|---|---|---|---|---|---|---|
| Avocado (*Persea americana*) | Peeled & stoned | | Lauraceae | 43 | 9 | 34 |
| Banana (*Musa* sp.) | Peeled | | Musaceae | 3 | 2 | 1 |
| Beans, baked (*Phaseolus vulgaris*) | Cold | | Fabaceae | 28 | 5 | 22 |
| Beans, baked (*Phaseolus vulgaris*) | Heated | | Fabaceae | 25 | 6 | 19 |
| Beans, Broad beans (*Vicia faba*) | Fresh, podded | | Fabaceae | 21 | <1 | 21 |
| Beans, Broad beans (*Vicia faba*) | Cooked | | Fabaceae | 22 | <1 | 21 |
| Beans, Butter beans (*Phaseolus limensis*) | Dried | | Fabaceae | 196 | 51 | 143 |
| Beans, Butter beans (*Phaseolus limensis*) | Cooked from dried | | Fabaceae | 36 | 13 | 22 |
| Beans, French beans (*Phaseolus vulgaris*) | | | Fabaceae | 147 | 50 | 94 |
| Beans, French beans (*Phaseolus vulgaris*) | Cooked | | Fabaceae | 159 | 48 | 109 |
| Beans, Haricot beans (*Phaseolus vulgaris*) | Dried | | Fabaceae | 132 | 21 | 106 |
| Beans, Haricot beans (*Phaseolus vulgaris*) | Cooked from dried | | Fabaceae | 29 | 6 | 22 |
| Beans, Kidney beans (*Phaseolus vulgaris*) | Dried | | Fabaceae | 172 | 73 | 89 |
| Beans, Kidney beans (*Phaseolus vulgaris*) | Cooked from dried | | Fabaceae | 41 | 14 | 26 |
| Beans, Runner beans (*Phaseolus coccineus*) | Trimmed & strung | | Fabaceae | 201 | 164 | 26 |
| Beans, Runner beans (*Phaseolus coccineus*) | Trimmed, strung & cooked | | Fabaceae | 156 | 132 | 18 |
| Beansprouts (*Vigna radiata*) | Pre-washed | | Fabaceae | 798 | 351 | 86 |
| Beetroot (*Beta vulgaris*) | Raw, peeled | | Chenopodiaceae | 8 | 1 | 7 |
| Beetroot (*Beta vulgaris*) | Cooked | | Chenopodiaceae | 10 | <1 | 10 |
| Beetroot (*Beta vulgaris*) | Pickled | | Chenopodiaceae | 5 | 1 | 4 |
| Beetroot (*Beta vulgaris*) | Precooked | | Chenopodiaceae | 8 | 1 | 7 |
| Blackberries (*Rubus* sp.) | Fresh | | Rosaceae | 57 | <1 | 56 |
| Blackberries (*Rubus* sp.) | Stewed from fresh | | Rosaceae | 221 | <1 | 220 |

| | | | | | | |
|---|---|---|---|---|---|---|
| **Blackcurrant** (*Ribes nigrum*) | Fresh | | Grossulariaceae | 109 | 2 | 107 |
| **Blackcurrant** (*Ribes nigrum*) | Tinned in juice and syrup, drained | | Grossulariaceae | 69 | <1 | 69 |
| **Broccoli** (*Brassica oleracea*) | Fresh, thick stalks removed | | Brassicaceae | 71 | <1 | 71 |
| **Broccoli** (*Brassica oleracea*) | Cooked, thick stalks removed | | Brassicaceae | 96 | 3 | 90 |
| **Broccoli, sprouting** (*Brassica oleracea*) | Tough stalks removed | | Brassicaceae | 68 | 1 | 66 |
| **Broccoli, sprouting** (*Brassica oleracea*) | Cooked from fresh | | Brassicaceae | 41 | 3 | 38 |
| **Brussel sprouts** (*Brassica oleracea*) | | | Brassicaceae | 75 | <1 | 74 |
| **Brussel sprouts** (*Brassica oleracea*) | Cooked | | Brassicaceae | 59 | <1 | 58 |
| **Cabbage, green** (*Brassica oleracea*) | | | Brassicaceae | 11 | <1 | 10 |
| **Cabbage, green** (*Brassica oleracea*) | Cooked | | Brassicaceae | 8 | <1 | 7 |
| **Cabbage, January King** (*Brassica oleracea*) | | | Brassicaceae | 14 | 4 | 10 |
| **Cabbage, January King** (*Brassica oleracea*) | Cooked | | Brassicaceae | 6 | 1 | 5 |
| **Cabbage, red** (*Brassica oleracea*) | | | Brassicaceae | 7 | <1 | 6 |
| **Cabbage, red** (*Brassica oleracea*) | Cooked | | Brassicaceae | 4 | <1 | 4 |
| **Cabbage, Savoy** (*Brassica oleracea*) | | | Brassicaceae | 30 | 4 | 26 |
| **Cabbage, Savoy** (*Brassica oleracea*) | Cooked | | Brassicaceae | 15 | 3 | 12 |
| **Cabbage, white** (*Brassica oleracea*) | | | Brassicaceae | 12 | <1 | 11 |
| **Cabbage, white** (*Brassica oleracea*) | Cooked | | Brassicaceae | 8 | <1 | 8 |
| **Carrots** (*Daucus carota*) | | | Apiaceae | 125 | 4 | 121 |
| **Carrots** (*Daucus carota*) | Cooked | | Apiaceae | 114 | 3 | 111 |
| **Carrots** (*Daucus carota*) | Tinned | | Apiaceae | 49 | <1 | 48 |
| **Cauliflower** (*Brassica oleracea*) | | | Brassicaceae | 15 | <1 | 14 |
| **Cauliflower** (*Brassica oleracea*) | Cooked | | Brassicaceae | 12 | <1 | 11 |

| | | | | | | |
|---|---|---|---|---|---|---|
| Celeriac (*Apium graveolens*) | Peeled | | Apiaceae | 14 | 2 | 13 |
| Celeriac (*Apium graveolens*) | Peeled, cooked | | Apiaceae | 36 | <1 | 35 |
| Celery (*Apium graveolens*) | | | Apiaceae | 7 | <1 | 7 |
| Celery (*Apium graveolens*) | Cooked | | Apiaceae | 8 | <1 | 8 |
| Cherries (*Prunus* sp.) | Stoned | | Rosaceae | 27 | 20 | 6 |
| Cherries (*Prunus* sp.) | Glace | | Rosaceae | 7 | 4 | 3 |
| Chestnuts (*Castanea sativa*) | | | Fagaceae | 217 | 2 | 214 |
| Chestnuts (*Castanea sativa*) | Cooked | | Fagaceae | 283 | 2 | 280 |
| Chick peas (*Cicer arietinum*) | Dried | | Fabaceae | 609 | 607 | 2 |
| Chick peas (*Cicer arietinum*) | Cooked from dried | | Fabaceae | 420 | 416 | 4 |
| Chick peas, as Houmous | | | | 169 | 135 | 34 |
| Chicory (*Cichorium intybus*) | | | Asteraceae | 19 | <1 | 19 |
| Chinese leaves (*Brassica rapa*) | | | Brassicaceae | 12 | 1 | 11 |
| Clementine (*Citrus reticulata*) | Pith and skin removed | | Rutaceae | 6 | <1 | 5 |
| Coconut (*Cocos nucifera*) | Fresh | | Arecaceae | 42 | 10 | 32 |
| Coconut (*Cocos nucifera*) | Desiccated | | Arecaceae | 26 | 3 | 23 |
| Courgette (*Cucurbita pepo*) | | | Cucurbitaceae | 35 | <1 | 35 |
| Courgette (*Cucurbita pepo*) | Cooked | | Cucurbitaceae | 46 | 3 | 43 |
| Cranberries (*Vaccinium* sp.) | | | Ericaceae | 93 | 3 | 88 |
| Cucumber (*Cucumis sativus*) | | | Cucurbitaceae | 12 | <1 | 12 |
| Cucumber (*Cucumis sativus*) | w/o Skin | | Cucurbitaceae | 13 | <1 | 13 |
| Curly kale (*Brassica oleracea*) | Cooked | | Brassicaceae | 8 | 2 | 6 |
| Dates (*Phoenix dactylifera*) | Boxed, stones removed | | Arecaceae | 168 | 4 | 163 |
| Dates (*Phoenix dactylifera*) | Dried | | Arecaceae | 599 | 14 | 584 |

| Dates, medjool (*Phoenix dactylifera*) | Stones removed | | Arecaceae | 192 | 35 | 157 |
|---|---|---|---|---|---|---|
| Fennel (*Foeniculum vulgare*) | | | Apiaceae | 72 | <1 | 72 |
| Fennel (*Foeniculum vulgare*) | Cooked | | Apiaceae | 85 | <1 | 85 |
| Figs (*Ficus* sp.) | | | Moraceae | 389 | 12 | 376 |
| Figs (*Ficus* sp.) | Dried | | Moraceae | 129 | 14 | 114 |
| Garlic (*Allium sativum*) | Peeled | | Alliaceae | 99 | 2 | 97 |
| Gooseberries (*Ribes uva- crispa*) | | | Grossulariaceae | 72 | <1 | 71 |
| Gooseberries (*Ribes uva- crispa*) | Stewed with sugar | | Grossulariaceae | 121 | <1 | 121 |
| Grapefruit (*Citrus x paradisi*) | Peel, pith and pips removed | | Rutaceae | 39 | 17 | 21 |
| Grapefruit (*Citrus x paradisi*) | Tinned in juice | | Rutaceae | 21 | 13 | 4 |
| Grapes, black (*Vitis* sp.) | Seeds removed | | Vitaceae | 19 | 5 | 14 |
| Grapes, dried as Currants (*Vitis* sp.) | Dried | | Vitaceae | 87 | 17 | 70 |
| Grapes, dried as Raisins (*Vitis* sp.) | Dried | | Vitaceae | 88 | 7 | 81 |
| Grapes, red, seedless (*Vitis* sp.) | | | Vitaceae | 21 | 6 | 15 |
| Grapes, white, seedless (*Vitis* sp.) | | | Vitaceae | 18 | <1 | 17 |
| Green beans (*Phaseolus vulgaris*) | Frozen, sliced | | Fabaceae | 58 | 19 | 38 |
| Green beans (*Phaseolus vulgaris*) | Frozen, sliced, cooked | | Fabaceae | 46 | 16 | 30 |
| Greengage (*Prunus* sp.) | Stoned | | Rosaceae | 105 | 2 | 103 |
| Kiwi (*Actinidia delicosa*) | Skin removed | | Actinidiaceae | 111 | <1 | 111 |
| Leek (*Allium ampeloprasum*) | | | Alliaceae | 66 | 1 | 65 |
| Leek (*Allium ampeloprasum*) | Cooked | | Alliaceae | 61 | 9 | 52 |
| Lemon (*Citrus x limon*) | Freshly juiced | | Rutaceae | 4 | 1 | 2 |
| Lemon (*Citrus x limon*) | Peeled | | Rutaceae | 29 | 4 | 25 |
| Lentils, red (*Lens culinaris*) | Dried | | Fabaceae | 54 | 51 | 3 |

483

| Lentils, red (Lens culinaris) | Cooked | | Fabaceae | 14 | 13 | <1 |
|---|---|---|---|---|---|---|
| Lettuce, cos (*Lactuca sativa*) | | | Asteraceae | 5 | <1 | 4 |
| Lettuce, iceberg (*Lactuca sativa*) | | | Asteraceae | 7 | <1 | 7 |
| Lettuce, little gem (*Lactuca sativa*) | | | Asteraceae | 7 | 1 | 6 |
| Lettuce, round (*Lactuca sativa*) | | | Asteraceae | 8 | <1 | 8 |
| Lychees (*Litchi chinensis*) | Tinned in syrup | | Sapindaceae | 4 | 3 | <1 |
| Mandarin (*Citrus reticulata*) | Tinned | | Rutaceae | 5 | 2 | 2 |
| Mangetout (*Pisum sativum*) | Cooked | | Fabaceae | 47 | 38 | 9 |
| Mango (*Magnifera* sp.) | Skinned & stoned | | Anacardiaceae | 20 | 1 | 19 |
| Mango (*Magnifera* sp.) | Tinned in syrup | | Anacardiaceae | 4 | 3 | <1 |
| Marrow (*Cucurbita* sp.) | | | Cucurbitaceae | 9 | <1 | 9 |
| Marrow (*Cucurbita* sp.) | Cooked | | Cucurbitaceae | 8 | <1 | 8 |
| Melon, cantaloupe (*Cucumis melo* ssp.) | Skin & seeds removed | | Cucurbitaceae | 16 | <1 | 16 |
| Melon, galia (*Cucumis melo* ssp.) | Skin & seeds removed | | Cucurbitaceae | 11 | <1 | 11 |
| Melon, honeydew (*Cucumis melo* ssp.) | Skin & seeds removed | | Cucurbitaceae | 25 | 3 | 22 |
| Melon, water (*Citrullus lanatus*) | Skin & seeds removed | | Cucurbitaceae | 35 | <1 | 34 |
| Mung beans (*Vigna radiata*) | Dried | | Fabaceae | 323 | 32 | 289 |
| Mung beans (*Vigna radiata*) | Cooked from dried | | Fabaceae | 50 | 8 | 42 |
| Mushrooms (*Agaricus bisporus*) | Wiped & trimmed | | Agariaceae | n/a | n/a | <1 |
| Mushrooms (*Agaricus bisporus*) | Cooked | | Agariaceae | 2 | 2 | <1 |
| Mushrooms (*Agaricus bisporus*) | Microwaved | | Agariaceae | <1 | <1 | <1 |
| Nectarine (*Prunus persica*) | Stones removed | | Rosaceae | 25 | 1 | 24 |
| Okra (*Abelmoschus esculentus*) | Topped & tailed | | Malvaceae | 86 | 2 | 84 |

484

| | | | | | | |
|---|---|---|---|---|---|---|
| **Olives, black, pitted** (*Olea europaea*) | Tinned in brine, drained in jar of brine, | | Oleaceae | 16 | 2 | 14 |
| **Olives, green** (*Olea europaea*) | stoned, drained | | Oleaceae | 33 | 1 | 32 |
| **Onion rings** (*Allium cepa*) | Breaded/battere d | | Alliaceae | 55 | 44 | 11 |
| **Onions** (*Allium cepa*) | | | Alliaceae | 31 | <1 | 31 |
| **Onions** (*Allium cepa*) | Cooked | | Alliaceae | 21 | <1 | 20 |
| **Orange** (*Citrus sinensis*) | peel & pith removed | | Rutaceae | 36 | 12 | 21 |
| **Orange** (*Citrus sinensis*) | Longlife juice | | Rutaceae | 9 | <1 | 4 |
| **Papaya** (*Carica papaya*) | Peel & seeds removed | | Caricaceae | 4 | 2 | 2 |
| **Parsley** (*Petroselium crispum*) | Leaves | | Apiaceae | 197 | 59 | 137 |
| **Parsnip** (*Pastinaca sativa*) | | | Apiaceae | 65 | 5 | 60 |
| **Parsnip** (*Pastinaca sativa*) | Cooked | | Apiaceae | 66 | <1 | 65 |
| **Passion Fruit** (*Passiflora edulis*) | Juice & seeds | | Passifloraceae | 71 | 43 | 26 |
| **Peach** (*Prunus perica*) | Stoned | | Rosaceae | 43 | <1 | 42 |
| **Peach** (*Prunus perica*) | Tinned in syrup, drained | | Rosaceae | 2 | 2 | <1 |
| **Pear** (*Pyrus communis*) | w/o Skin | Comice | Rosaceae | 19 | 2 | 17 |
| **Pear** (*Pyrus communis*) | w/o Skin | Conference | Rosaceae | 6 | <1 | 5 |
| **Pear** (*Pyrus communis*) | w/o Skin | Williams | Rosaceae | 6 | 6 | <1 |
| **Pear** (*Pyrus communis*) | Tinned, drained | | Rosaceae | 1 | <1 | <1 |
| **Pear** (*Pyrus communis*) | w/o skin | Comice | Rosaceae | 8 | <1 | 7 |
| **Pear** (*Pyrus communis*) | w/o Skin | Conference | Rosaceae | 3 | <1 | 3 |
| **Pear** (*Pyrus communis*) | w/o Skin | Williams | Rosaceae | 3 | 3 | <1 |
| **Peas** (*Pisum sativum*) | Tinned, processed, drained | | Fabaceae | 2 | 2 | <1 |
| **Peas, fresh** (*Pisum sativum*) | | | Fabaceae | 3 | 2 | 1 |

| | | | | | | |
|---|---|---|---|---|---|---|
| Peas, fresh (*Pisum sativum*) | Cooked | | Fabaceae | 1 | 1 | <1 |
| Peas, frozen (*Pisum sativum*) | | | Fabaceae | 3 | 1 | 2 |
| Peas, frozen (*Pisum sativum*) | Cooked | | Fabaceae | 2 | 1 | 1 |
| Peas, garden (*Pisum sativum*) | Tinned, drained | | Fabaceae | 2 | 1 | 1 |
| Peas, marrowfat (*Pisum sativum*) | Tinned, drained | | Fabaceae | 51 | 50 | <1 |
| Peas, mushy (*Pisum sativum*) | Tinned/frozen | | Fabaceae | 15 | 14 | 1 |
| Peas, petit pois (*Pisum sativum*) | Frozen | | Fabaceae | 8 | 6 | 2 |
| Peas, split, dried (*Pisum sativum*) | | | Fabaceae | 15 | 11 | 4 |
| Peas, split, dried (*Pisum sativum*) | Cooked | | Fabaceae | 13 | 12 | <1 |
| Peas, sugar snap (Pisum sativum) | Cooked | | Fabaceae | 44 | 31 | 13 |
| Peas, whole, dried (*Pisum sativum*) | | | Fabaceae | 29 | 28 | <1 |
| Peas, whole, dried (*Pisum sativum*) | Cooked | | Fabaceae | 10 | 9 | <1 |
| Pepper, green (*Capsicum annuum*) | | | Solanaceae | 11 | <1 | 11 |
| Pepper, red (*Capsicum annuum*) | | | Solanaceae | 16 | 5 | 11 |
| Pepper, yellow (*Capsicum annuum*) | | | Solanaceae | 11 | 6 | 5 |
| Pineapple (*Ananas comosus*) | | | Bromelidaceae | 38 | 21 | 17 |
| Pineapple (*Ananas comosus*) | Tinned in juice, drained | | Bromelidaceae | 14 | 2 | 12 |
| Plum, red (*Prunus domestica*) | | | Rosaceae | 8 | 2 | 6 |
| Plum, Victoria (*Prunus domestica*) | | | Rosaceae | 26 | 2 | 24 |
| Plum, yellow (*Prunus domestica*) | | | Rosaceae | 72 | 2 | 69 |
| Plum, yellow *Prunus domestica*) | Cooked | | Rosaceae | 152 | 2 | 150 |
| Pomegranate (*Punica granatum*) | Flesh & seeds | | Lythraceae | 304 | <1 | 304 |
| Potato, chips (*Solanum tuberosum*) | From chip–shop | | Solanaceae | 11 | 7 | 3 |

| Potato, chips (*Solanum tuberosum*) | Oven chips | | Solanaceae | 15 | 11 | 4 |
|---|---|---|---|---|---|---|
| Potato, crisps (*Solanum tuberosum*) | | | Solanaceae | 22 | 5 | 17 |
| Potato, for baking (*Solanum tuberosum*) | Boiled | | Solanaceae | 3 | 2 | 1 |
| Potato, for baking (*Solanum tuberosum*) | w/o Skin, boiled | | Solanaceae | 2 | 1 | <1 |
| Potato, mashed, instant (*Solanum tuberosum*) | | | Solanaceae | 4 | 2 | 1 |
| Potato, new (*Solanum tuberosum*) | | | Solanaceae | 18 | 16 | 2 |
| Potato, new (*Solanum tuberosum*) | Boiled | | Solanaceae | 5 | 2 | 3 |
| Potato, new (*Solanum tuberosum*) | w/o Skin | | Solanaceae | 4 | 2 | 2 |
| Potato, new (*Solanum tuberosum*) | w/o Skin, boiled | | Solanaceae | 3 | 3 | <1 |
| Potato, old (*Solanum tuberosum*) | | | Solanaceae | 10 | 8 | 2 |
| Potato, old (Solanum tuberosum) | Baked | | Solanaceae | 3 | 2 | 1 |
| Potato, old (*Solanum tuberosum*) | Boiled | | Solanaceae | 1 | <1 | <1 |
| Potato, old (*Solanum tuberosum*) | w/o Skin, baked | | Solanaceae | 3 | 1 | 2 |
| Potato, red (*Solanum tuberosum*) | w/o Skin | | Solanaceae | 10 | 1 | 8 |
| Potato, red (*Solanum tuberosum*) | w/o Skin, boiled | | Solanaceae | 20 | 5 | 15 |
| Potato, waffle (*Solanum tuberosum*) | Cooked | | Solanaceae | 9 | 5 | 4 |
| Prune (*Prunus domestica*) | Dried | | Rosaceae | 363 | 6 | 357 |
| Prune (*Prunus domestica*) | Cooked from dried | | Rosaceae | 108 | 2 | 106 |
| Prune (*Prunus domestica*) | Semi–dried, ready to eat | | Rosaceae | 284 | 3 | 281 |
| Prune (*Prunus domestica*) | Tinned in syrup & juice, not drained | | Rosaceae | 75 | 3 | 72 |
| Pumpkin (*Cucurbita* sp.) | | | Cucurbitaceae | 154 | <1 | 154 |
| Quince (*Cydonia oblonga*) | Stewed | | Rosaceae | 9 | 2 | 7 |
| Radish (*Raphanus sativus*) | | | Brassicacea e | 3 | <1 | 3 |

| | | | | | | |
|---|---|---|---|---|---|---|
| Raspberries (*Rubus idaeus*) | | | Rosaceae | 26 | 2 | 24 |
| Raspberries (*Rubus idaeus*) | Tinned in syrup, drained | | Rosaceae | 21 | 5 | 15 |
| Redcurrants (*Ribes rubrum*) | | | Grossulariaceae | 47 | <1 | 46 |
| Rhubarb (*Rheum* sp.) | | | Polygonaceae | 1 | 1 | <1 |
| Rhubarb (*Rheum* sp.) | Cooked | | Polygonaceae | 3 | 2 | <1 |
| Salad cress (*Lepidium sativum*) | | | Brassicacea e | 18 | 3 | 15 |
| Satsuma (*Citrus unshiu*) | | | Rutaceae | 24 | 2 | 12 |
| Sharon fruit (*Diospyros* sp.) | | | Ebenaceae | 11 | 6 | 5 |
| Soya bean (Glycine max) | Cooked | | Fabaceae | 17556 | 17544 | 11 |
| Soya bean (*Glycine max*) | Frozen, cooked | | Fabaceae | 10687 | 10621 | 64 |
| Soya bean, Tofu (*Glycine max*) | Microwaved | | Fabaceae | 10619 | 10609 | 10 |
| Soya flour (*Glycine max*) | | | Fabaceae | 124727 | 124381 | 345 |
| Soya mince granules (*Glycine max*) | Cooked | | Fabaceae | 20850 | 20745 | 101 |
| Spinach (*Spinacia olearcea*) | | | Amaranthaceae | 7 | 2 | 5 |
| Spinach (*Spinacia olearcea*) | Cooked | | Amaranthaceae | 4 | <1 | 3 |
| Spring green (*Brassica oleracea*) | | | Brassicaceae | 56 | 11 | 45 |
| Spring green (*Brassica oleracea*) | Cooked | | Brassicaceae | 43 | 13 | 30 |
| Spring onion (*Allium* sp.) | | | Alliaceae | 62 | 9 | 53 |
| Strawberries (Fragaria × ananassa) | | | Rosaceae | 8 | <1 | 7 |
| Strawberries (Fragaria × ananassa) | Tinned in syrup, drained | | Rosaceae | 40 | 2 | 38 |
| Sultanas (*Vitis* sp.) | | | Vitaceae | 54 | 11 | 44 |
| Swede (*Brassica napobrassica*) | | | Brassicaceae | 6 | 1 | 5 |
| Swede (*Brassica napobrassica*) | Cooked | | Brassicaceae | 2 | <1 | 2 |

| | | | | | | |
|---|---|---|---|---|---|---|
| **Sweet potato** (*Ipomoea batatas*) | | | Convolvulaceae | 259 | 1 | 258 |
| **Sweet potato** (*Ipomoea batatas*) | Cooked | | Convolvulaceae | 251 | 1 | 249 |
| **Sweetcorn** (**Zea mays**) | Boiled on the cob | | Poaceae | 9 | 2 | 7 |
| **Sweetcorn** (**Zea mays**) | Frozen, tinned, drained | | Poaceae | <1 | <1 | <1 |
| **Sweetcorn** (**Zea mays**) | Frozen, tinned, drained, heated | | Poaceae | 3 | <1 | 2 |
| **Sweetcorn** (**Zea mays**) | Kernels from the cob | | Poaceae | 2 | <1 | 1 |
| **Sweetcorn, baby** (**Zea mays**) | | | Poaceae | 6 | <1 | 5 |
| **Tomato** (*Solanum lycopersicum*) | | | Solanaceae | 6 | 1 | 4 |
| **Tomato** (*Solanum lycopersicum*) | Grilled | | Solanaceae | 7 | <1 | 6 |
| **Tomato** (*Solanum lycopersicum*) | Pureed | | Solanaceae | 9 | 5 | 5 |
| **Tomato** (*Solanum lycopersicum*) | Tinned | | Solanaceae | 3 | 1 | 2 |
| **Tomato ketchup** | | | | 14 | 7 | 8 |
| **Turnip** (*Brassica rapa*) | | | Brassicaceae | 12 | <1 | 12 |
| **Turnip** (*Brassica rapa*) | Cooked | | Brassicaceae | 8 | <1 | 8 |
| **Watercress** (*Nasturtium* sp.) | | | Brassicaceae | 45 | <1 | 45 |
| **Vegetable grills** | Cooked | | | 43 | 16 | 27 |
| **Brown sauce** | | | | 214 | 46 | 168 |
| **Fruit cocktail** | Tinned in syrup, drained | | | 3 | <1 | 3 |
| **Mixed peel** | | | | 38 | 32 | 6 |
| Pate vegetarian assorted | | | | 581 | 488 | 92 |
| Pate vegetarian chick pea based (*Cicer arietinum*) | | | Fabaceae | 1494 | 1444 | 49 |
| Pate, mushroom (*Agaricus bisporus*) | | | Agariaceae | 17 | 8 | 8 |

# Glossary

Antagonistic: 1: opposition in physiological action; especially: interaction of two or more substances such that the action of any one of them on living cells or tissues is lessened 2: opposition of a conflicting force, tendency, or principle

Benign: 1: of a mild type or character that does not threaten health or life 2: having a good prognosis: responding favorably to treatment

Bilateral: a: of, relating to, or affecting the right and left sides of the body or the right and left members of paired organs b: having bilateral symmetry

Bioavailability: the degree and rate at which a substance (as a drug) is absorbed into a living system or is made available at the site of physiological activity

Bioidentical: having the same molecular or chemical structure as a substance produced in the body, but not an exact copy

Biosynthesis: 1: a process during which an enzyme converts a product into a complex product 2: production of a chemical compound by a living organism

Carcinogen: a substance or agent causing cancer

Delta T: temperature difference; regarding breast thermography, temperature difference between the breasts

Ecoestrogen: John Mclachland has coined this term, "estrogens found in the environment," that are bioidentical to the body's estrogen; in this book it refers to chemical estrogens found in daily household, commercial and body products

Endogenous: caused by factors inside the organism or system

Environmental estrogen: estrogens originating outside of the body; which include synthetic estrogens, ecoestrogens, and phytoestrogens, which mimic the body's estrogen

Exogenous: 1: caused by factors (as food or a traumatic factor) or an agent (as a disease-producing organism) from outside the organism or system 2: introduced from or produced outside the organism or system; specifically: not synthesized within the organism or system

Feminization: 1: to give a feminine quality to 2: to cause (a male or castrate) to take on feminine characters (as by implantation of ovaries or administration of estrogens

Free Radicals: an unchanged molecule, typically highly reactive and short lived, having an unpaired valence electron; the body can handle free radicals, but if antioxidants are unavailable, or if the free-radical production becomes excessive, damage can occur; free radical damage accumulates with age

Follicles: are structures that develop to enclose and protect a single egg each, they mature along with the egg until ovulation happens, which is when the follicle ruptures and the egg is released

Follicular Phase: is the first phase of the menstrual cycle during which follicles in the ovary mature, it ends with ovulation

Genetically modified organisms (GMOs): refer to crop plants created for human or animal consumption using the latest molecular biology techniques, these plants have been modified in the laboratory by genetic engineering to enhance desired traits such as increased resistance to herbicides or improved nutritional content; adverse reactions and side effects have been associated with GMOs and some countries have banned them

In situ: 1: in the natural or original position or place, concerning breast cancer in its original place or ducts

In vitro: outside the living body and in an artificial environment

In vivo: in the living body of a plant or animal

Leutal Phase: the second half or last fourteen days of the menstrual cycle after ovulation; the corpus luteum secretes progesterone which prepares the endometrium for the implantation of an embryo; if fertilization does not occur then menstrual flow begins

Malignant 1: tending to produce death or deterioration: tending to infiltrate, metastasize, and terminate fatally 2: of unfavorable prognosis: not responding favorably to treatment

Metastasis: 1: a. change of position, state, or form b: the spread of a disease-producing agency (as cancer cells) from the initial or primary site of disease to another part of the body; also: the process by which such spreading occurs 2: a secondary malignant tumor resulting from metastasis

Metastasized: to spread or grow

Neoangiogenesis: new blood vessels or new blood growth

Parity: 1: the state or fact of having borne offspring 2: the number of times a female has given birth counting multiple births as one and usually including stillbirths 3: age at time of first child

Pescatarian: one whose diet includes fish but no other meat

Phytoestrogen: a chemical compound that occurs naturally in plants and has estrogenic properties, that mimic the body's estrogen

Premenstrual Syndrome (PMS): which is not "normal" but a pathology or disorder that symptoms may include migraines, headaches, abdominal, back and leg cramps, bloating, diarrhea, irritability, mood swings, fatigue, breast tenderness, breast or abdomen distention and weight gain

Progestin: a synthetic form of progesterone, not originating form the body which has serious adverse side effects.

Rancid.: having a rank smell or taste usually from chemical change or decomposition; with regards to oils, when an oil is heated, it undergoes a partial or complete chemical breakdown, which leads to it becoming somewhat rancid, this heat-induced process transforms formerly healthy oils into dangerous oils, which are most often carcinogens; this happens regardless of their original nutrient content

Synthetic estrogen: estrogens produced in a lab that mimic the body's estrogen, but have been altered chemically in order to be patented and sold; which include ERTs, HRTs, BCPs, IUDs, estrogen patches, rings and injections

Thermal radiation: is electromagnetic radiation generated by the thermal motion of charged particles in matter, all matter with a temperature greater than absolute zero emits thermal radiation

Thermogram: a record made by a thermograph.

Thermography: the use of thermograms to study heat distribution in structures or regions.

Vascularity: stimulation of the existing blood vessels

Vasoconstriction: narrowing of the lumen of blood vessels

# References

## 2. Intel

"About Breast Cancer." *Susan G. Komen for the Cure Puget Sound*. Puget Sound Affiliate of Susan G. Komen for the Cure, n.d. Web. <http://www.komenpugetsound.org/understanding-breast-cancer/about-breast-cancer/>.

Boschert, Sherry. "Teenage Menstruation: What's Normal and What's Not?." *Internal Medicine News*. 01 Feb 2009: n. page. Web.

"Breast cancer: Prevention and control." *World Health Organization*. World Health Organization. Web. <http://www.who.int/cancer/detection/breastcancer/en/index5.html>.

"Breast Cancer Statistics." *Susan G. Komen for the Cure*. Susan G. Komen for the Cure, n.d. Web. <http://ww5.komen.org/breast-cancer/statistics.html>.

DeSantis, Carol. *Breast Cancer Facts & Figures 2007-2008*. 1st Ed. Atlanta, Ga.: American Cancer Society, 2007. Print.

DeSantis, Carol. *Breast Cancer Facts & Figures 2009-2010*. 1st Ed. Atlanta, Ga.: American Cancer Society, 2009. Print.

DeSantis, Carol. *Breast Cancer Facts & Figures 2009-2010*. 1st Ed. Atlanta, Ga.: American Cancer Society, 2009. Print.

DeSantis, Carol. *Breast Cancer Facts & Figures 2009-2010*. 1st Ed. Atlanta, Ga.: American Cancer Society, 2009. Print.

DeSantis, Carol. *Breast Cancer Facts & Figures 2011-2012*. 1st Ed. Atlanta, Ga.: American Cancer Society, 2011. Print.

"Estimated Breast-Cancer Mortalities, Incidence, and I/M Ratios, U.S.A *." *CA - A Cancer Journal for Clinicians* n.pag. *American Cancer Society*. Database.

"Fast Stats." *Surveillance Epidemiology and End Results*. National Cancer Institute, n.d. Web. <http://seer.cancer.gov/faststats>.

Forouzanfar, Mohammad. "Breast and cervical cancer in 187 countries between 1980 and 2010: a systematic analysis." *Lancet*. 378.9801 (2011): 1461-84. Print.

"Menstrual Cycle." *Natural Family Planning Teachers Association of Ireland*. Natural Family Planning Teachers Association of Ireland, n.d. Web.

"Menstruation in Girls and Adolescents: Using the Menstrual Cycle as a Vital Sign." *Journal of the American Academy of Pediatrics*. 118.5 (2006): 2245-2250. Web. <http://pediatrics.aappublications.org/content/118/5/2245.abstract?sid=72292d5a-a247-4ef9-8ba1-87c4035d586f>.

Nakamoto, Jon. "Menarche: Myths and variations in normal pubertal development." *Western Journal of Medicine*. 172.3 (2000): 182-185. Web. <http://www.ncbi.nlm.nih.gov/pmc/articles/PMC1070801/>.

Powell, Alvin. "Breast cancer danger rising in developing countries." *Harvard Gazette* [Cambridge, Mass.] 16 April 2009, n. pag. Web. <http://news.harvard.edu/gazette/story/2009/04/breast-cancer-danger-rising-in-developing-world/>.

Scowcroft, Henry. "Why are breast cancer rates increasing?." *Cancer Research UK*. Cancer Research UK, 04 Feb 2011. Web. <http://scienceblog.cancerresearchuk.org/2011/02/04/why-are-breast-cancer-rates-increasing/>.

Smigal, Carol. *Breast Cancer Facts & Figures 2005-2006.* 1st Ed. Atlanta, Ga.: American Cancer Society, 2005. Print.

Stewart, Sherri, Jessica King, et al. United States. Department of Health and Human Services. *Cancer Mortality Surveillance - United States - 1990-2000.* Washington, DC: U.S. Government Printing Office, 2004. Print.

Warren, Barbour, and Carol Devine. "Breast Cancer in Men." *Program on Breast Cancer and Environmental Factors* (2010): n.pag. Web. Cornell University, College of Veterinary Medicine. <http://ecommons.library.cornell.edu/handle/1813/14300>.

"What are the key statistics about breast cancer?" *Surveillance Epidemiology and End Results.* National Cancer Institute, n.d. Web. <http://seer.cancer.gov >.

"What Is Hormonal Therapy?." *Breastcancer.org.* N.p., 17 Sep 2012. Web. <http://www.breastcancer.org/treatment/hormonal/what_is>.

# 3. Artillery

Netter, Frank. *Ciba Collection of Medical Illustrations - Reproductive.* Washington, DC: Library of Congress, 1975. Print.

# 4. Chemical Warfare

Anderson, G.L., M. Limacher, A.R. Assaf, et al. "Effects of Conjugated Equine Estrogen in Postmenopausal Women With Hysterectomy." *Journal of the American Medical Association.* 291.14 (2004): 1701-1712. Web. <http://jama.jamanetwork.com/article.aspx?a rticleid=198540>.

Chilvers, CED, and JM Deacon. "Oral contraceptives and breast cancer." *British Journal of Cancer*. 61. (1990): 1-4. Print.

Chilvers, CED, and SJ Smith. "The effect of patterns of oral contraceptive use on breast cancer risk in young women." *British Journal of Cancer*. 69.5 (1994): 922-923. Web. <http://www. ncbi.nlm.nih.gov/pmc/articles/PMC1968892/>.

Chlebowski, Rowan, Garnet Anderson, Margery Gass, et al. "Estrogen Plus Progestin and Breast Cancer Incidence and Mortality in Postmenopausal Women." *Journal of the American Medical Association*. 304.15 (2010): 1684-1692. Web. <http:// jama.jamanetwork.com/article.aspx?a rticleid=186747>.

Collins, John, Jennifer Blake, et al. "Breast cancer risk with postmenopausal hormonal treatment." *Human Reproduction Update*. 11.6 (2005): 545-560. Web. <http://humupd.oxford-journals.org/gca?g ca=humupd;11/6/545&submit=Go&allch= &action=Get All Checked Abstracts>.

Elstein, M., and K. Ferrer. "The Effect Of A Copper-Releasing Intrauterine Device On Sperm Penetration In Human Cervical Mucus In Vitro." *Reproduction*32, no. 1 (1973): 109-11. doi:10.1530/jrf.0.0320109.

Heiss, Gerardo, Robert Wallace, Garnet Anderson, et al. "Health Risks and Benefits 3 Years After Stopping Randomized Treatment With Estrogen and Progestin." *Journal of the American Medical Association*. 299.9 (2008): 1036-1045. Web. 14 Mar. 2013. <http://jama.jamanetwork.com/article.aspx?a rticleid=1108397>.

Hulley, S, D Grady, et al. "Randomized trial of estrogen plus progestin for secondary prevention of coronary heart disease in postmenopausal women." *Journal of American Medical Association*. 280.7 (1998): 605-613; 671-672. Print.

"IUDs Block Fertilization." United Nations. Published Winter 1996. http://www.un.org/popin/popis/journals/network/network162/blck162.html.

Lacey, James, Pamela Mink, Jay Lubin, et al. "Menopausal Hormone Replacement Therapy and Risk of Ovarian Cancer." *Journal of the American Medical Association*. 288.20 (2002): 2544. Web. <http://jama.jamanetwork.com/article.aspx?a rticleid=195119>.

Lee, John. *What your doctor may not tell you about menopause*. New York, NY: Grand Central Publishing, 1996. Print.

"Oral Contraceptives and Cancer Risk." *National Cancer Institute*. National Institutes of Health, 21 Mar 2012. Web. <http://www. cancer.gov/cancertopics/factsheet/Risk/oral-contraceptives>.

"Overview: Breast Cancer and the Pill." *The Polycarp Research Institute*. The Polycarp Research Institute. Web. <http://www. polycarp.org/overviewbreastcanceroralcontraceptives.htm>.

Pike, MC, BE Henderson, JT Casagrande, et al. "Oral Contraceptive Use and Early Abortion as Risk Factors for Breast Cancer in Young Women." *British Journal of Cancer*. 43.72 (1981): n. page. Print.

Rossouw, JE, GL Anderson, et al. "Risks and benefits of estrogen plus progestin in healthy postmenopausal women: principal results." *Journal of American Medical Association*. 288.3 (2002): 321-333. Print.

"The Estrogen-Plus-Progestin Study." *Women's Health Initiative*. National Institutes of Health. Web. <http://www.nhlbi.nih.gov/ whi/estro_pro.htm>.

What are the risk factors for breast cancer?. (2013, February 26). Retrieved from http://www.cancer.org/cancer/breastcancer/ detailedguide/breast-cancer-risk-factors

# 5. Biological Warfare

Almada, Anthony. "SDG precision standardized Flaxseed Extract Scientific Research Monograph." *Brevail*. 2003: n. page. Print.

Bergman Jungeström, Malin, Lilian Thompson, and Charlotta Dabrosin. "Flaxseed and Its Lignans Inhibit Estradiol-Induced Growth, Angiogenesis, and Secretion of Vascular Endothelial Growth Factor in Human Breast Cancer Xenografts In vivo." *Clinical Cancer Research*. 13.3 (2007): 1061-1067. Web. <http://clincancerres.aacrjournals.org/content/13/3/1061.long>.

Daniel, Kaayla. *The Whole Soy Story - the dark side of America's favorite health food*. Washington, DC: New Trends Publishing, 2005. Print.

Duffy, Christine, Kimberly Perez, and Ann Partridge. "Implications of Phytoestrogen Intake for Breast Cancer." *Clinical Cancer Research*. 57. (2007): 260-277. Print.

Fallon, Sally, and Mary Enig. "Cinderella's Dark Side."*Nexus*. Apr 2000: n. page. Web. <http://www.mercola.com/article/soy/avoid_soy3.htm>.

Iguchi, Taisen, and Tomomi Sato. "Endocrine Disruption and Developmental Abnormalities of Female Reproduction." *American Zoologist*. 40.3 (2000): 402-411. Print.

Kuhnle, Gunter G. C., Caterina Dell'Aquila, Sue M. Aspinall, Shirley A. Runswick, Angela A. Mulligan, and Sheila A. Bingham. "Phytoestrogen Content of Foods of Animal Origin: Dairy Products, Eggs, Meat, Fish, and Seafood." *Journal of Agricultural and Food Chemistry*56, no. 21 (2008): 10099-0104. doi:10.1021/jf801344x.

Lee, John, Zava, David, and Virginia Hopkins. *What your doctor may not tell you about breast cancer*. New York: Warner Books, Inc., 2005. Print.

Lee, John, and Virginia Hopkins. *What your doctor may not tell you about menopause*. New York: Warner Books, Inc., 1996. Print.

Saika, Kumiko, and Tomotaka Sobue. "Epidemiology of Breast Cancer in Japan and the US." *Japan Medical Association Journal*. 52.1 (2009): 39-44. Print.

Selchell, KDR. *Discovery and Importance of Lignans*. 92-93. Print. [Unable to further source this reference.]

Thompson, Lilian U., Beatrice A. Boucher, Zhen Liu, Michelle Cotterchio, and Nancy Kreiger. "Phytoestrogen Content of Foods Consumed in Canada, Including Isoflavones, Lignans, and Coumestan." *Nutrition and Cancer* 54, no. 2 (2006): 184-201. doi:10.1207/s15327914nc5402_5.

Valentzis, LS, MM Cantwell, C Cardwell, et al. "Lignans and breast cancer risk in pre- and post-menopausal women: meta-analyses of observational studies." *British Journal of Cancer*. 100.9 (2009): 1492-1498. Print.

Zava, David T., Charles M. Dollbaum, and Marilyn Blen. "Estrogen and Progestin Bioactivity of Foods, Herbs, and Spices." Hypertension (High Blood Pressure). Accessed September 03, 2018. http://www.cancersupportivecare.com/estrogenherb.html.

# 6. Ecoterrorism

Arnold, SF, Peter Vonier, et al. "In vitro synergistic interaction of alligator and human estrogen receptors with combinations of environmental chemicals." *Environmental Health Perspectives*. 105. (1997): 615-618. Print.

Colborn, Theo. "TEDX The Endocrine Disruption Exchange." Overdose: How Drugs and Chemicals in Water and the Environment are Harming Fish and Wildlife. Committee on Natural Resources. 1324 Longworth House Office Building, Washington, DC. 9 Jun 2009. Address.

"Effects of Pollutants on the Reproductive health of Male Vertebrae Wildlife- Males Under Threat." *Chemtrust*. 2007-2009: n. page. Web. <http://www.chemtrust.org.uk/documents/ Male Wildlife Under Threat 2008 full report.pdf>.

"Endocrine Disruptor Screening Program."*Environmental Protection Agency*. Environmental Protection Agency, 11 August 2011. Web. <http://www.epa.gov/endo/pubs/edspover-view/primer.htm>.

Golden, R, J Gandy, and G Vollmer. "A review of the endocrine activity of parabens and implications for potential risks to human health." *Critical reviews in toxicology*. 35.5 (2005): 435-458. Web. <http://www.ncbi.nlm.nih.gov/ pubmed/16097138>.

Long, M, A Stronati, et al. "Relation between serum xenobiotic-induced receptor activities and sperm DNA damage and sperm apoptotic markers in European and Inuit populations." *Reproduction*. 133.2 (2007): 517-530. Print.

McLachlan, John, and Steven Arnold. "Environmental Estrogens." *American Scientist*. 84. (1996): 452-461. Print.

Newbold, RR, RB Hanson, et al. "Proliferative lesions and reproductive tract tumors in male descendants of mice exposed developmentally to diethylstilbestrol." *Carcinogenesis*. 19.9 (1998): 1655-1663. Web. <http://carcin.oxfordjournals.org/con-tent/19/9/1655.short>.

"PANNA: New Evidence That Endocrine Disruptors Block Sperm Function." *Pesticide Action Network Updates Service.* (2002): n. page. Web. <http://www.panna.org/legacy/panups/panup_20020802.dv.html>.

Steinmetz, Rosemary, Natasha Mitchner, et al. "The Xenoestrogen Bisphenol A Induces Growth, Differentiation, and c-fos Gene Expression in the Female Reproductive Tract." *Endocrinology.* 139.6 (1998): 2741-2747. Web. <http://endo.endojournals.org/content/139/6/2741.full.pdf>.

## 7. Breast Canswers to Estrogen Lies

Ahmed, SA, BD Hissong, et al. "Gender and Risk of Autoimmune Diseases: Possible Role of Estrogenic Compounds." *Environmental Health Perspectives.* 107.5 (1999): 681-686. Print.

Daniel, Kaayla. *The Whole Soy Story - the dark side of America's favorite health food.* Washington, DC: New Trends Publishing, 2005. Print.

Duffy, Christine, Kimberly Perez, and Ann Partridge. "Implications of Phytoestrogen Intake for Breast Cancer." *Clinical Cancer Research.* 57. (2007): 260-277. Print.

Fallon, Sally, and Mary Enig. "Cinderella's Dark Side."*Nexus.* Apr 2000: n. page. Web. <http://www.mercola.com/article/soy/avoid_soy3.htm>.

Gerson, Joel. *Milad'ys Standard Textbook for Professional Estheticians.* 8. Albany, NY: Delmar, 1998. 77. Print.

Graham, J Dinny, and Christine Clarke. "Physiological Action of Progesterone in Target Tissues."*Endocrine Reviews.* 18.4 (1997): 502. Web. 25 Mar. 2013. <http://edrv.endojournals.org/content/18/4/502.abstract>.

Haapasaari, KM, T Raudaskoski, et al. "Systemic therapy with estrogen or estrogen with progestin has no effect on skin collagen in postmenopausal women."*Maturitas*. 27.2 (1997): 153-162. Print.

Harvey, et al. "Cholesterol and health Uncovering the truth about America's demonized nutrient."*Biochemistry*. (2005): 235-238. Print.

Heiss, Gerardo, Wallace, Robert, et al. "Health Risks and Benefits 3 Years After Stopping Randomized Treatment With Estrogen and Progestin." *Journal of the American Medical Association*. 2008; 299(9): 1036-1045

Hulley, Stephen, Deborah Grady, et al. "Randomized Trial of Estrogen Plus Progestin for Secondary Prevention of Coronary Heart Disease in Postmenopausal Women." *Journal of the American Medical Association*. 280.7 (1998): 605-. Web. <http://jama.jamanetwork.com/article.aspx?articleid=187879>.

Iguchi, Taisen, and Tomomi Sato. "Endocrine Disruption and Developmental Abnormalities of Female Reproduction." *American Zoologist*. 40.3 (2000): 402-411. Print.

Jick, H, B Dinan, and KJ Rothman. "Oral contraceptives and non-fatal myocardial infarction." *Journal of the American Medical Association*. 239.14 (1978): 1403-1406. Print.

Lee, John, and Virginia Hopkins. *What your doctor may not tell you about menopause*. New York: Warner Books, Inc., 1996. Print.

Lee, John, and David Zava. *What your doctor may not tell you about breast cancer*. New York: Warner Books, Inc., 2002. Print.

Maheux, R, F Naud, M Rioux, et al. "A randomized, double-blind, placebo-controlled study on the effect of conjugated estrogens on skin thickness."*American Journal of Obstetrics and Gynecology*. 170.2 (1994): 642-649. Print.

Netter, Frank. *Ciba Collection of Medical Illustrations - Reproductive*. Washington, DC: Library of Congress, 1975. Print.

Nicodemus, Kristin, Aaron Folsom, and Kristin Anderson. "Menstrual History and Risk of Hip Fractures in Postmenopausal Women The Iowa Women's Health Study." *Amrican Journal of Epidemiology*. 153.3 (2001): 251-255. Print.

Patriarca, MT, KZ Goldman, JM Dos Santos, et al. "Effects of topical estradiol on the facial skin collagen of postmenopausal women under oral hormone therapy: a pilot study." *Eur J Obstet Gynecol Reprod Biol*. 130.2 (2006): 202-205. Print.

Piérard-Franchimont, C, C Letawe, et al. "Skin water-holding capacity and transdermal estrogen therapy for menopause: a pilot study." *Maturitas*. 22.2 (1995): 151-154. Web. <http://www.maturitas.org/article/0378-5122(95)00924-A/abstract>.

Prior, JC. "Progesterone as a bone-trophic hormone."*Endocrine Reviews*. 11.2 (1990): 386-398. Print.

Rickard, David, Urszula Iwaniec, Glenda Evans, et al. "Bone Growth and Turnover in Progesterone Receptor Knockout Mice." *Endocrinology*. 149.5 (2008): 2383–2390. Print.

Rinzler, Carol Ann. *Estrogen and Breast Cancer: A Warning to Women*. New York: Macmillan Publishing Company.1993. Print

Rossouw, JE, GL Anderson, et al. "Risks and benefits of estrogen plus progestin in healthy postmenopausal women: principal results From the Women's Health Initiative randomized controlled trial.." *Journal of the American Medical Association.* 288.3 (2002): 321-333. Web. <http://jama.jamanetwork.com/article.aspx?a rticleid=195120>.

Saika, Kumiko, and Tomotaka Sobue. "Epidemiology of Breast Cancer in Japan and the US." *Japan Medical Association Journal.* 52.1 (2009): 39-44. Print.

Schmidt, JB, M Binder, et al. "Treatment of skin aging with topical estrogens." *International Journal of Dermatology.* 35.9 (1996): 669-674. Print.

Selchell, KDR. *Discovery and Importance of Lignans.* 92-93. Print. [Unable to further source this reference.]

Son, ED, and JY Lee. "Topical application of 17beta-estradiol increases extracellular matrix protein synthesis by stimulating tgf-Beta signaling in aged human skin in vivo." *Journal of Investigative Dermatology.* 124.6 (2005): 1149-1161. Web. <http://www.nature.com/jid/journal/v124/n6/full/5602843a.html>.

"Uterus." *The Free Dictionary.* Dorland's Medical Dictionary for Health Consumers. Web. <http://medical-dictionary.thefreedictionary.com/uterus>.

"Vagina." *The Free Dictionary.* Dorland's Medical Dictionary for Health Consumers. Web. <http://medical-dictionary.thefreedictionary.com/vagina>.

Varila, E, I Rantala, et al. "The effect of topical oestradiol on skin collagen of postmenopausal women." *British Journal of Obstetrical Gynaecology.* 102.12 (1995): 985-989. Print.

Valentzis, LS, MM Cantwell, C Cardwell, et al. "Lignans and breast cancer risk in pre- and post-menopausal women: meta-analyses of observational studies." *British Journal of Cancer*. 100.9 (2009): 1492-1498. Print.

# 8. Supplements

Baggott, JE, RA Oster, and T Tamura. "Meta-analysis of cancer risk in folic acid supplementation trials." *Cancer Epidemiology*. 36.1 (2012): 78-81. Print.

Brody, Jane. "Puzzle in a Bottle – A special report; In Vitamin Mania, Millions Take a Gamble on Health."*New York Times* [New York] 26 October 1997, Health. Print.

Carmel, Ralph. "Is testing for clinical cobalamin deficiency truly unreliable?." *Journal of the American Society of Hematology*. 106.3 (2005): 1136-1138. Web. 25 Mar. 2013. <http://blood-journal.hematologylibrary.org/content/106/3/1136.2.full>.

Klein, Eric, Ian Thompson, et al. "Vitamin E and the Risk of Prostate Cancer The Selenium and Vitamin E Cancer Prevention Trial." *Journal of the American Medical Association*. 306.14 (2011): 1549-1556. Web. <http://jama.jamanetwork.com/article.aspx?a rticleid=1104493>.

Larsson, SC, A Akesson, L Bergkvist, and A Wolk. "1.Multivitamin Use and Breast Cancer Incidence in a Prospective Cohort of Swedish Women."*American Journal of Clinical Nutrition*. 91.5 (2010): 1268-1272. Print.

Lawson, KA, ME Wright, et al. "Multivitamin Use and Risk of Prostate Cancer in the National Institutes of Health–AARP Diet and Health Study." *Journal of the National Cancer Institute*. 99.10 (2007): 754-764. Print.

Omenn, Gilbert, Gary Goodman, et al. "Full Effects of a combination of beta carotene and vitamin A on lung cancer and cardiovascular disease." *New England Journal of Medicine*. 334. (1996): 1150-1155. Web. 25 Mar. 2013. <http://www.nejm.org/doi/full/10.1056/NEJM199605023341802>.

Patterson, Ruth. *Functional Foods and Nutraceuticals*. June 2003: n. page. Print. [Further source information is not available.]

"The Effect of Vitamin E and Beta Carotene on the Incidence of Lung Cancer and Other Cancers in Male Smokers." *New England Journal of Medicine*. 330.15 (1994): 1029-1035. Web. <http://atbcstudy.cancer.gov/pdfs/atbc33010291994.pdf>.

"What are the risk factors for breast cancer?." *American Cancer Society*. American Cancer Society, 26 Feb 2013. Web. <http://www.cancer.org/cancer/breastcancer/detailedguide/breast-cancer-risk-factors>.

# 9. Progesterone

Hobbins, William, and Joseph Riina. "Double-Blind Study of Effectiveness Transcutaneous Progesterone in Fibrocystic Breast Conditions Monitored by Thermography." *[Unk]*. (1986): n. page. Print.

Lee, John, and Virginia Hopkins. *What your doctor may not tell you about menopause*. New York: Warner Books, Inc., 1996. Print.

Lee, John, and David Zava. *What your doctor may not tell you about breast cancer*. New York: Warner Books, Inc., 2002. Print.

Netter, Frank. *Ciba Collection of Medical Illustrations - Reproductive*. Washington, DC: Library of Congress, 1975. Print.

# 10. Breast Cancer

"Breast Cancer Types." *National Breast Cancer Foundation, Inc.*. National Breast Cancer Foundation, Inc.. Web. <http://www. nationalbreastcancer.org/types-of-breast-cancer>.

"Breast Cancer Types: What Your Type Means." *Mayo Clinic*. Mayo Clinic, 02 Oct 2012. Web. <http://www.mayoclinic.com/ health/breast-cancer/HQ00348>.

Cooke, Robert. *Dr. Folkman's War: Angiogenesis and the struggle to defeat cancer*. 1st Ed. New York: Random House, 2001. Print.

Gonzalez, Nicholas, and Linda Isaacs. *The Trophoblast and the Origins of Cancer: One solution to the medical enigma of our time*. 1st Ed. New York: New Spring Press, 2009. Print.

"What are the risk factors for breast cancer?." *American Cancer Society*. American Cancer Society, 26 Feb 2013. Web. <http://www.cancer.org/cancer/breastcancer/detailedguide/ breast-cancer-risk-factors>.

# 11. Certified Breast Thermography Survival Guide

For more breast thermography studies, around 1,100, please visit the *research* page of our website: womensacademyofbreast-thermography.com

Gros, C, Gauthrie, M. "Breast Thermography and Cancer Risk Prediction". Cancer 45:51-56 1980.

Haberman J, Goin J, Love T, Ohnsorg F, Aggarwal R. Breast cancer detection by absolute temperature thermography and computer techniques. In: Ring EFJ Phillips B eds. Recent Advances in Medical Thermology. Plenum Press, New York. 1984; pp. 557-569. [#877]

Hobbins, W.B. To Mammogram or Not - 5 years Practical Experience"

Presented: Wisconsin Surgical Society Milwaukee, WI, 1969

Hobbins, W.B. Seven Year Mammography Survey in Private Practice.

Presented: Wisconsin Surgical Society Door County, WI, 1971
11th Annual Early Breast Cancer Detection San Diego, CA, 1971

Non-Mutilating Treastment for Bresat Cancer Strasbourg, France, 1972

Hobbins, W.B. Thermography in General Surgery Practice, Proceedings, American Thermographic Society, AGA, 1973

Hobbins. W. B. Mass Breast Cancer Screening by Thermography (1,100 women in 53 hours).

Presented: First European Thermographic Society Meeting Amsterdam, Netherlands, 1974

American Thermographic Society Chicago, IL 1974

Hobbins, W.B. What Is a Day of Life Worth, RN Magazine, April, 1975

Hobbins. W.B. Mass Breast Cancer Screening with Thermography 25,000 cases.

Presented: American Thermographic Society Atalnta, GA 1975

Wisconsin Surgical Society Telemark WI 1975

Hobbins, W.B. Mass Breast Cancer Screening with Thermography, Applied Radiology, November-December 1976 5:57-62

Hobbins, W.B. Experiences with Thermographic Breast Cancer Screening in the State of Wisconsin, Proceedings, Breast Disease in Gynecological and Medical Primary Care Practice, pp. 267-281, April, 1977

Hobbins, W.B. Thermography, Highest Risk Marker in Breast Cancer, Proceedings, Gynecological Society for the Study of Breast Disease, pp. 267-282;59, 1977.

Presented: 3rd International Symposium on Detection and Prevention of Cancer New York, NY, 1976.

American Thermographic Society Washington, D.C., 1976

The Canadian Thermographic Society Annual Meeting Montreal, Quebec, Canada, 1976.

The Second Annual Mid-American Breast Cancer Symposium Madison, WI, 1976

Gynecological Society for Study of Breast Diseases Washington, D.C., 1977

American Thermographic Society Boston, MA, 1978

French Thermographic Society Lyon, France, 1980

Hobbins, W.B. Who Has Breast Cancer? Lets Find Out, Clinical Medical, December 1977

Hobbins, W.B. Thermography – The Decision Maker

Presented: The American Gynecological Society for the Study of Breast Disease – Washington, D.C. April 1977

Hobbins, W.B. A Community Screening for Breast Cacner with Physical Exam and Thermography. Proceedings-Breast Disease in Gynecological and Medial Preamry Care Practice, April, 1977

Presented: American Thermographic Society Boston, MA, 1988

Hobbins, W.B. Thermal Signal in Breast Disease Sympathetic Nervous Infulence.

Presented: American Thermographic Society Boston, MA, 1977

Hobbins, W.B. Thermography, Highest Risk Marker (Mobile Mass Breast Cancer Screening). Medical Thermology, 1978

Hobbins, W.B. Mobile Mass Breast Cancer Screening; Thermography; Highest Risk Marker, Medical Thermography, European Press, Ghent, Belgium, pp. 61-67, 1978

Hobbins, W.B. Thermography and Pain, Medical Thermography, European Press, Ghent, Belgium, pp. 273-274, 1978

Hobbins, W.B. Thermography and Assessment of Breast Cancer (letter), JAMA 242:2761, 1979

Hobbins, W.B. B.J. King, Report of Thermographic Breast Biopsy Correlation ACTA Thermographica, Vol. 5, No. 1, pp.43-45, 1980

Hobbins, W.B. Comparison of Telethermography and Contact Thermography in Breast Thermal Examinations, ACTA Thermographica, Vol. 5, No. 1, pp. 51-53, 1980

Presented: European Thermographic Society Barcelona, Spain, 1978

Society for Study of Breast Disease Boston, MA 1979.

Hobbins, W.B. Thermography: highest risk marker. Presented, 8th Seminaire de Telethermographie, Lyon, June 26-28 (abstract). Acta Thermographica 1980; 5(3) 153.

Hobbins, W.B. Report of Thermographic Breast Biopsy Correlation. ACTA Thermographica, 1980

Hobbins, W.B. Significance of an Isolated Abnormal Colorgram, La Nouvelle Presse Medicale, Vol. 10, No. 38, pp. 3153-3155, 1981

Presented: Hungarian Medical Society Sarasota, FL, October 1981

American Thermographic Society Washington, D.C. May 1982

Fourth Symposium on Thermogrammatry Budapest, Hungary, March, 1983

Hobbins, W.B. The Physiology of the Breast by Cholesteric Plate Analysis, in Gordon F. Schwartz and Douglas Marchant (eds), Breast Disease Diagnosis and Treatment, Elsevier/North-Holland, New York, pp. 87-98, 1981

Presented: Society for Study of Breast Disease Philadelphia, PA, 1980

Association for the Advancement of Medical Instrumentation San Francisco, CA, 1980

4th International Symposium in Detection and Prevention of Cacner London, England 1980.

Hobbins, W.B. A New Beginning for Thermography, RNM Images, pp. 43-45, October 1982

Hobbins, W.B. Thermography and Pain, in Michel Gautherie and Ernest Albert (eds), Biomedical Thermology, Alan R. Liss, Inc. New York, pp. 361-375, 1982

Hobbins, W.B. New Horizons in Thermography, Far East Health, January 1983

Hobbins, W.B. Thermography of the Breast Revisited 1982, Modern Medicine of Canada, March, 1983

Hobbins, W.B. Thermography (letter), CA, 372-376;33, 1983

Hobbins, W.B. The Combined Use of Thermography & Ultrasonography, in Jack Jellins and Toshiji Kobayashi (eds), Ultrasonic Examinations of the Breast, pp. 335-339, June, 1983

Hobbins, W.B. Thermography of the Breast A Skin Organ in Harry Rein (ed), The Primer on Thermography, pp 37, July, 1983

Hobbins, W.B. Thermography of the Breast A Skin Organ, in Gautherie M, Albert E, Keith L et al., Thermal Assessment of Breast Health. Chapter 5. MTP Press, Ltd. Lancaster, England, pp 37-48, July 1984

Presented: Argentinean Society of Mastology Buenos Aires, Argentina, April 1984.

Chilean Thermography Society Santiago, Chili, April 1984

Hobbins, W.B. Multimodality thermography's role in ultrasound breast. In Gautherie M, Albert E, Keith L et al., Thermal Assessment of Breast Health. Chapter 23. MTP Press, Ltd. Lancaster, England, pp 235-240, July 1984.

Hobbins, W.B., Abplanalp K, Barnes C, Miner S. Analysis of thermal class TH 5 examination in 37, 050 breast thermograms. In Gautherie M, Albert E, Keith L et al., Thermal Assessment of Breast Health. Chapter 25. MTP Press, Ltd. Lancaster, England, pp 249-255, July 1984.

Hobbin, W.B. Thermography + ultrasonography. In: Abernathy M, Uematsu S eds. Medical Thermology. Amer. Acad. of Thermology, Washington, D.C. 1986; pp. 246-249.

Hobbins, W.B., Abplanalp K, Barnes C, Miner S. Analysis of thermal class TH 5 examination in 37, 050 breast thermograms. In: Abernathy M, Uematsu S eds. Medical Thermology. Amer. Acad. of Thermology, Washington, D.C. 1986; pp. 250-255.

Presented: International Conference on Thermal Assessment of Breast Health Washington, D.C. July, 1983

American Academy of Thermology Johns Hopkins School of Medicine, October, 1983.

American academy of Thermology 14th Annual Meeting Crystal City VA May/June, 1985

514

Hobbins, W.B. Thermography and Ultrasonography. Medical Thermology, 1986

Presented: Third International Congress on the Ultrasonic Examination of the Bresat Tokyo, Japan, June 1983

International Conference on Thermal Assessment of Breast Health Washington, D.C. July 1983

Hobbins, W.B. Double Blind Study of Effectiveness Transcurtaneous Progesterone in Fibrocystic Breast Conditions Monitored by Thermography.

Presented: Breast Diseases IV International Congress of Senology Paris, France, September, 1986

Jiang LJ, Ng FY et al "A Perspective on Medical Infrared Imaging". J Med Technol 2005 Nov-Dec;29(6):257-67

Lawson RN. Implication of surface temperatures in the diagnosis of breast cancer. Canadian Medical Association Journal 1956; 75-309. [#144].

Lawson RN. Thermography- a new tool in the investigation of breast lesions. (Reprinted in THERMOLOGY, 1(2): 115-119, 1985). Canadian Services Medical Journal 1957; 13:517-524. [#72].

Lawson RN, Chughtai MS. Breast cancer and body termperature. Can Med Assoc J 1963; 88:68-70. [#1437].

Lawson RN, et al. Breast cacner and heptaldehyde (preliminary report). Can Med Assoc J 1956; 75: 486. [#1440].

Spitalier, H., Giraud, D. et al. "Does Infrared Thermography Truly Have a Role in Present Day Breast Cancer Management?" Biomedical Thermology pp.269-278, 1982

Stark. A., Way, S. "The Screening of Well Women for the Early Detection of Breast Cancer Using Clinical Examination with Thermography and Mammography". Cancer 33: 1671-1679.

Y.R. Parisky, A. Sardi, R. Hamm, K. Hughes, L. Esserman, S. Rust, K.Callahan, "Efficacy of Computerized Infrared Imaging Analysis to Evaluate Mammographically Suspicious Lesions". AJR:180, January 2003

**Articles on breast thermography research:**

"Beyond Mammography - An Examination of Breast Thermography" by Len Saputo, M.D., Townsend Letter for Doctors and Patients, June 2004

"Efficacy of Computerized Infrared Imaging Analysis to Evaluate Mammographyically Suspicious Lesions" American Journal of Radiology, January 2003

"Infrared Imaging of the Breast" The Breast Journal, July/August 1998, Volume 4, Number 4

"What You Should Know About Breast Thermography" by Len Saputo, M.D.

"Factors likely to Effect the Efficacy of Mammography" Journal of the National Cancer Institute Volume 91, Number 10, May 19, 1999

"Breast Cancer Detection Demonstration Project" Cancer, 1982, Volume 32, Pages 194-225

"Breast Masses: Mammographic Evaluation" Radiology, 1989, Pages 173-303

"MRI of the Breast: state of the art" European Radiology, Volume 8, Number 5, June 1998

"Comparison of FDG-PET and dynamic contrast enhanced MRI" The Breast, Volume 12, Issue 1, February 2003, Pages 17-22

## 12. Breast Cancer Boot Camp

*Acupuncture: Review and Analysis of Reports on Controlled Clinical Trials.* Geneva: World Health Organization, 202. Print.

Anna L. Choi, Guifan Sun, et al. "Developmental Fluoride Neurotoxicity: A Systematic Review and Meta-Analysis." Environ Health Perspect. 2012 October; 120(10): 1362–1368.

<http://www.ncbi.nlm.nih.gov/pmc/articles/PMC3491930/.>

Atkins, Robert C. *Dr. Atkins New Diet Revolution.* New York: Harper, 2008.

Bernard, Alfred, Marc Nickmilder, Catherine Voisin, and Antonia Sardella. "Impact of Chlorinated Swimming Pool Attendance on the Respiratory Health of Adolescents." *Pediatrics.* 124.4 (2009): 110-1118. Print. <http://pediatrics.aappublications.org/content/124/4/1110.abstract>.

Carton, Robert. Interview by Andrew Saul. 2006. doctoryourself.com. Web. http://www.doctoryourself.com/carton.html.

"Flouride." *Sail Home.* N.p.. Web. <http://www.sailhome.org/Concerns/BodyBurden/Burdens/Fluoride.html>.

Garg, Vinod Kumar and Singh, Bhupinder. "Fluoride in Drinking Water and Fluorosis." Feb. 2007 <http://www.eco-web.com/edi/070207.html.>

Harvey, et al. "Cholesterol and health Uncovering the truth about America's demonized nutrient."*Biochemistry.* (2005): 235-238. Print.

HB 1416-Local – Final Version s 1723 http://www.gencourt.state.nh.us/legislation/2012/HB1416.html (25 April 2012)

Kuhnle, Gunter G. C., Caterina Dell'Aquila, Sue M. Aspinall, Shirley A. Runswick, Angela A. Mulligan, and Sheila A. Bingham. "Phytoestrogen Content of Foods of Animal Origin: Dairy Products, Eggs, Meat, Fish, and Seafood." *Journal of Agricultural and Food Chemistry*56, no. 21 (2008): 10099-0104. doi:10.1021/jf801344x.

"Lard Is the New Coconut Oil." Return to Now. May 14, 2018. Accessed September 26,2017. http://returntonow. net/2017/09/26/lard-new-coconut-oil/.

Lee, John, and Virginia Hopkins. *What your doctor may not tell you about menopause*. New York: Warner Books, Inc., 1996. Print.

Lee, John, and David Zava. *What your doctor may not tell you about breast cancer*. New York: Warner Books, Inc., 2002. Print.

Levy, SM, B Broffitt, et al. "Associations between fluorosis of permanent incisors and fluoride intake from infant formula, other dietary sources and dentifrice during early childhood." *Journal of the American Dental Association*. 141.10 (2010): 1190-1201. Print.

Lundell, Dwight. "Heart Surgeon Speaks Out On What Really Causes Heart Disease." *Sign of the Times*. Quantum Future Group, 01 Mar 2012. Web. <http://www.sott.net>.

Masterjohn, Chris. "Synthesis of Steroid Hormones From Cholesterol." *Cholesterol and Health*. N.p., 02 September 2005. Web. <http://www.cholesterol-and-health.com/Steroid-Hormones.html>.

"Milk Fat Built for Digestion." International Milk Genomics Consortium. Accessed September 03, 2017. http://milkgenomics.org/article/milk-fat-built-digestion/.

Moritz, Andreas. *Heal Yourself with Sunlight*. U.S.: Ener-chi Wellness Press, 2010.

Ober, Clinton, Stephen T. Sinatra, and Martin Zucker. *Earthing: The Most Important Health Discovery Ever?* Sydney, N.S.W.: Read How You Want, 2014.

"Omega-3 Fatty Acids: Fact Sheet." *WebMD.* N.p., 30 Mar 2011. Web. <http://www.webmd.com/healthy-aging/omega-3-fatty-acids-fact-sheet>.

"Top 11 compounds in US drinking water." *Newscientist.* Newscientist, 12 Jan 2009. Web. <http://www.newscientist.com/article/dn16397-top-11-compounds-in-us-drinking-water.html>.

San-Xiang Wang,[1] Zheng-Hui Wang, et al. "Arsenic and Fluoride Exposure in Drinking Water: Children's IQ and Growth in Shanyin County, Shanxi Province, China." Environ Health Perspect. 2007 April; 115(4): 643–647. <http://www.ncbi.nlm.nih.gov/pmc/articles/PMC1852689/>.

Sisson, Mark, and Mark Sisson. *The New Primal Blueprint: Reprogram Your Genes for Effortless Weight Loss, Vibrant Health, and Boundless Energy.* Oxnard, CA: Primal Blueprint Publishing, 2017.

Thompson, Lilian U., Beatrice A. Boucher, Zhen Liu, Michelle Cotterchio, and Nancy Kreiger. "Phytoestrogen Content of Foods Consumed in Canada, Including Isoflavones, Lignans, and Coumestan." *Nutrition and Cancer* 54, no. 2 (2006): 184-201. doi:10.1207/s15327914nc5402_5.

Vine, DF, JCL Mamo, et al. "Dietary oxysterols are incorporated in plasma triglyceriderich lipoproteins, increase their susceptibility to oxidation and increase aortic cholesterol concentration of rabbits." *Journal of Lipid Research.* 39. (1998): 1995-2004. Print.

Weber, Charles. "The Damaging Effects of Fluoride for Teeth on Thyroid and Brain, and a Cure." <http://charles_w.tripod.com/fluoride.html.>

"What Is Vitamin D? What Are The Benefits Of Vitamin D?." *Medical News Today.* Medical News Today, 29 Jan 2013. Web.

Ying Rong, Li Chen, et al. "Egg consumption and risk of coronary heart disease and stroke: dose-response meta-analysis of prospective cohort studies." BMJ 2013; 346e; 8539 (Published 7 January 2013) <http://www.bmj.com/content/346/bmj.e8539.>

Zava, David T., Charles M. Dollbaum, and Marilyn Blen. "Estrogen and Progestin Bioactivity of Foods, Herbs, and Spices." Hypertension (High Blood Pressure). Accessed September 03, 2018. http://www.cancersupportivecare.com/estrogenherb.html.